D1707074

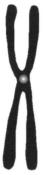

Oncogenes
Aneuploidy
and AIDS

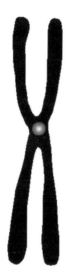

Oncogenes
Aneuploidy
and AIDS

A Scientific Life & Times of
Peter H. Duesberg

Harvey Bialy

Institute of Biotechnology
Autonomous National University of México
Cuernavaca, México

Published by
The Institute of Biotechnology of the Autonomous National University of México, Avenida Universidad, Colonia Chamilpa, Cuernavaca, 62210, Morelos, México

Distributed by
North Atlantic Books, P.O. Box 12327, Berkeley, California 94712

Cover design by Suzanne Albertson
Text design by Paula Morrison

Printed in the Unites States of America
Distributed to the book trade by Publishers Group West

Oncogenes, Aneuploidy, and AIDS: A Scientific Life and Times of Peter H. Duesberg is produced by the Society for the Study of Native Arts and Sciences, a nonprofit educational corporation whose goals are to develop an educational and crosscultural perspective linking various scientific, social, and artistic fields; to nurture a holistic view of arts, sciences, humanities, and healing; and to publish and distribute literature on the relationship of mind, body, and nature.

Library of Congress Cataloging-in-Publication Data

Bialy, Harvey.
    Oncogenes, aneuploidy, and AIDS : a scientific life and times of Peter H. Duesberg / by Harvey Bialy.
        p. ; cm.
    Includes bibliographical references and index.
    ISBN 1-55643-531-2 (pbk.)
    1. Duesberg, Peter. 2. Molecular biologists—United States—Biography.
3. AIDS (Disease)—Research—History. 4. Cancer—Genetic aspects—Research—History.
    [DNLM: 1. Duesberg, Peter. 2. Molecular Biology—Biography. 3. Acquired Immunodeficiency Syndrome—etiology. 4. History of Medicine, 20th Cent.
5. Neoplasms—etiology. 6. Oncogenes—Biography. WZ 100 D853b 2004] I. Title.
    QH506.D84B53 2004
    572.8'092—dc22
                                    2004008802

1 2 3 4 5 6 7 8 9 DATA 09 08 07 06 05 04

For my children: Tara, Ezra Thelonious, and Benjamin. And in loving memory of my father Louis, my mother Dorothy, and my friend Edward Dorn.

Acknowledgments

This book would not be except for the following people. I thank them equally and alphabetically: Margaret Akpan, Alejandro Alagon, Peter Duesberg, Daniel Fendel, Robert Leppo, Martin Pato, Zaida Penton, and Roberto Stock. I also wish to make it abundantly clear that the opinions expressed in these pages are solely my own and in no way reflect an official position of either the Institute of Biotechnology of Mexico's National University or its community.

Contents

1

"What's in a Name?"

When I ran into Peter in the fourth-floor library of U.C. Berkeley's Molecular Biology and Virus Laboratory in the fall of 1982, he was riding high, although I wasn't. I had just returned to the East Bay after a disastrous two years as a senior lecturer in microbiology at the University of Calabar in southeastern Nigeria. My stay climaxed in a student revolt that destroyed the vice chancellery, and perhaps due to my '60s Berkeley background, I was accused of encouraging. Actually, the advice I gave my students was that the proper response to the egregious but predictable behavior of the administration was to refuse the proffered diplomas at the upcoming graduation—not to trash their offices, as they were planning with war drums literally beating in the courtyard of the main student hostel. What the vice chancellor and his deputies did was have a large emergency electrical generator installed to provide power for themselves and not the science blocks and dormitories, both of which had been without electricity for months.

I came to the library to check the recent issues of *Nature* and *Science* for employment opportunities, my departure from Calabar hardly being well planned, and had not seen Peter for almost ten years. But as we were friendly in my graduate student days, he put down the stack of bound journals he was carrying, and with a characteristically ready smile, greeted me warmly.

"What and how was I doing, and what was I doing back at the MBVL?" I can't remember whether my narrative of the circumstances sketched above resembled the humorous version I tend to tell today or whether it was melodramatic and depressed. Probably the latter, considering the dire monetary straits I was in. But whichever version, Peter would have made light of it in a way that even his most embittered present-day critics still refer to as "infectious." I have often thought it is this particular inner quality, his adamantine and irrepressible sense of humor that more than any other allowed him to survive and continue to be scientifically productive throughout the tough times that were to come.

Eventually he let me get around to asking what he was up to.

At this very moment, he explained, gesturing at the piles of open journals and legal pads filled with notes that occupied one entire table of the not overly large departmental library, he was working on an invitation from another Peter. This one, Peter Newmark, was the deputy editor of *Nature,* and characteristically of *Nature* then, he was interested in having a critical appraisal of the already glamorous and well-funded field of 'oncogenes' from one of its leading lights. The following year Newmark would become a colleague of mine in the Macmillan publishing family, when I succeeded in finding more or less legitimate employment as the scientific editor of *Bio/Technology.*

Peter had obviously taken to the task with the same tenacity and furious intellect I remembered so well from Wednesday seminars where he would sometimes reduce otherwise-articulate visiting speakers to stammering inanities by gently insisting on answers to exactly the questions they didn't want to hear, a habit that continues to the present.[1] Unfortunately, he was hard at work on what would become the first of a series of scholarly critiques of "oncogene theory" at a most inopportune moment. The new gene cloning and sequencing technologies were poised to transform molecular biology from a rigorous discipline of proving that alterations in DNA sequence (mutations) have particular functional consequences to simply identifying individual mutations (because we could do that now with such relative ease) and inferring altered functions, almost at whim. He could not have picked a worse time to rethink more than a decade's work.

It is sadly true that the essential importance of constant questioning—especially the very ideas you helped shape and conclusions you helped establish—is not so highly esteemed as it once might have been, and every scientist who overtly challenges a weighty prevailing idea finds him- or herself in hot water. But Peter's almost continuous rethinking of the problem he has been working to solve now for thirty-five years—understanding the actual genetic basis of cancer—put him in a pot near boiling. How much heat he might have been able to avoid, and how much more readily his subsequent experimental work in cancer genetics might have been accomplished and received had only he kept his mouth shut about AIDS, we will never know. But for Peter, such silence was and is unthinkable.

Nonetheless, this library encounter was several years before publication of another invited review, in which he first set down the reasons for his profound misgivings with pronouncing a recently identified retrovirus the cause of AIDS. This review appeared in the journal *Cancer Research* in 1987 and sealed his scientific fate for a dozen years. When we spoke in 1982 he was diligently, and with a certain naiveté (indeed he "was even feeling a little sorry for those guys"), preparing the ground of his future demise for the pages of *Nature*—the most widely-read scientific journal in the world.

He began explaining to me the arguments and questions that were taking form while he dissected the ten years or so of scientific literature since his identification of the very first oncogene, and proceeded with logic and data to challenge almost every idea I had about the genes of cancer viruses. As he did so, I forgot my desperate finances and re-experienced the mind-rattling excitement I always thought was the special thrill that made otherwise-normal people become scientists.

So what are these oncogenes, and what did Peter point out in his 1983 *Nature* review that made, and continues to make, many powerful cancer molecular biologists more than a little uncomfortable?

Peter H. Duesberg had his scientific temperament forged in a molecular biology that was founded in—and which its practitioners adhered to almost religiously—the discipline of hypothesis formulation and testing. It was about as classical as science gets. In fact, all molecular biology was in the years before it became biotechnology was the formulating and testing of alternative hypotheses, mostly about the gene-protein relationships in the commonest of bacteria and the viruses that like to live with and on them. Such activity requires a precise language in order to clearly delineate the lines along which alternative hypotheses can be tested. In 1982, "oncogene" still had a very particular meaning: a gene that causes cancer—a definition much less diffuse than the collection of archetypes its linguistic roots signal in our collective brain, or the collection of functions (ranging from normal cellular controls to malignancy) under which the term now passes in the scientific literature. But it was far from proven then that normal cells harbored genes that could cause cancer, and what Peter did in the review that appeared in the Bastille Day 1983 issue of *Nature* was painstakingly point this out. It is still not proved that normal human cells contain particular genes which can cause them to become cancerous, and between then and now he has not stopped pointing.

In 1982 it was still generally accepted in the scientific community of cancer molecular biologists that the only really known cancer-causing genes were those belonging to a very rare kind of virus termed a transforming retrovirus. "Transformation" is another word that had, and still does have, a specialized meaning for cancer biologists; it denotes the conversion of a normal cell into a cancerous one. Such viruses had been one of the major objects of study of this elite group since the early 1970s, when Duesberg and his then-close friend and co-worker Peter Vogt succeeded in biochemically defining the first retroviral oncogene.[2] But in 1982 it was not yet a matter of general consensus, although very soon to become one, that cells possessed their own oncogenic simulacra waiting to bring on all sorts of cancers when "activated or inactivated" by a long list of possible mutations. Thus Peter could, without (he thought) raising any offense, provocatively title his *Nature* review with a question: *Retroviral transforming genes in normal cells?* It begins with what was an innocuous and universally acknowledged fact:

> *Animal retroviruses fall into two classes, the rare highly oncogenic class with transforming* (onc *or* onco) *genes and the almost ubiquitous class without* onc *genes.*[3]

Little did he imagine that while engrossed in attempting to sort out what was and was not legitimately known about the relationship between these very rare viral genes and their cellular relatives, another friend, Robert Gallo, was equally busy preparing the way to announce that one of the "almost ubiquitous" types of retroviruses was the cause of the millennium's final, and most fearsome, plague. This announcement would come fully U.S-government certified, but without much prior scientific scrutiny, less than one year after publication of the *Nature* review.

How such an ordinary virus became so special is told from Peter's unique perspective in his popular-language book *Inventing the AIDS Virus*[4] and is a subject of the middle chapters of this. For now, we return to seeing why publishing a highly technical, didactic critique could be such a big deal. It really did no more than insist cancer molecular geneticists remain attached to demonstrating the truths of inferences about the biological function of cellular genes that they have drawn from data showing only that such genes are related in form to their viral counterparts.

Tumor retrovirologists had always been confronted by an embarrassing contradiction between their objects of study and the objective of their studies. Namely, these extremely uncommon viruses had never caused a single outbreak, let alone epidemic of cancer in any animal, although in the laboratory they are the most efficient carcinogens known. Therefore, what could studying their genes—the objects of Peter and the other superior experimentalists working in this rarefied field—possibly have to do with human cancer?

The 'oncogene hypothesis,' formalized in 1969 by cancer biologists Robert Huebner and George Todaro,[5] sought to resolve this somewhat paradoxical situation by postulating that the transforming (*onc*) genes of retroviruses preexist in normal cells as latent cancer genes that can be transduced by retroviruses or activated by carcinogens.

At that time the only experimental systems in which transduction (the movement of a gene from its normal location into the genome of a virus) had been demonstrated were rather mundane ones involving a few common gut bacteria and certain of the viruses (called lysogenic bacteriophage) that share a special relationship with them. These viruses can incorporate their complete set of genes into the host DNA and essentially disappear for a long winter. But occasionally, when their hibernation concludes for one or another reason, they take a piece of the host's genetic package with them as they leave. These cozy bacteria-bacteriophage relationships, termed lysogeny, are the sole reason it was even conceivable a virus that caused cancer in the laboratory could have acquired its oncogenic ferocity from the same kind of cell it was now making malignant.

The early seventies were especially good years for the onco-gene idea. Howard Temin proved his twelve-year-old hypothesis that retroviruses behave exactly like lysogenic bacteriophage when he isolated an RNA-directed, DNA polymerase activity directly from a retrovirus,[6] thus making the analogy with bacterial systems concrete instead of inferential. The discovery of this very odd (at the time) enzyme also required a revision of the hitherto "sacred" central dogma of molecular *DNA makes RNA makes Protein*—to the much less elegant-sounding *DNA makes RNA (that sometimes also makes DNA) makes Protein*. The association of this enzyme with viruses that could cause cancer lent an additional panache to the idea that their transforming genes had derived from oncogenic, cellular precursors.

The other major support for Huebner and Todaro was provided by the molecular biology "wunderkids," Peter Duesberg (working at Berkeley's MBVL) and Peter Vogt (at USC). In a series of beautifully conceived and difficult-to-perform experiments, reported between 1970 and 1975, they succeeded in precisely defining a viral transforming gene.[2,7,8] This made it possible to test the oncogene hypothesis directly.

By 1982–83 the evidence was quite conclusive, from many studies that by then included sequencing a number of cloned cellular and viral genes: Exactly as the oncogene hypothesis required, the *onc* genes of retroviruses came from the chromosomes of their hosts.

So what was the problem?

Although it resolved one difficulty—how a highly infrequent virus-promoted natural cancer could be relevant to an extremely common human disease—the oncogene hypothesis raised another thorny problem, as Peter's *Nature* review points out.

It would appear paradoxical for normal cells to have evolved and maintain a battery of perhaps 16 known onco-

genes which, when carried by retroviruses, are the fastest acting and most inevitably carcinogenic agents known to date.[3]

In attempting to provide an adequate resolution to this paradox, Duesberg began to go in a direction that within a very few years would remove him from the "must-speak list" of every major cancer molecular biology symposium, while turning a fifteen-year, one-thousand-percent batting average in obtaining U.S. National Institutes of Health funding to zero.

Comparisons between the (real) *onc* genes of retroviruses and the (hypothetically oncogenic) proto-*onc* genes of cells had indeed proved the cellular origin of transforming viral sequences. But they proved neither the structural identity nor the functional equivalence of these genetic homologs, to use the present idiom. In fact, what these numerous studies showed was that the viral and cellular genes differed substantially from one another in their structures. And because retroviruses contain special signals (called promoters) that dictate how much of a gene's product a cell can make that are hundreds of times stronger than the cell's own, they are likely to differ greatly in the amounts of actual oncogenic proteins produced.

These differences seemed to Peter to be important. He devoted the remainder of the article's seven thousand words to addressing them, and in the best molecular biology tradition, did so by examining the experimental and epistemological status of alternative current hypotheses about the structure—function relationship between *onc* and proto-*onc* genes. He referred to these alternative views as the qualitative and quantitative models.

Both models held that viral *onc* genes arose from transduction of cellular genes. But the qualitative model required that the transduction event create an essentially new genetic entity, while the other viewed the transduced cellular proto-*onc* gene and the viral *onc* gene as basically the same, differing only in the quantity with which they, or their particular protein products, were present. In a normal cell the proto-*onc* gene was silent, or expressed to a very low level, and in the cancer cell this latent oncogene was expressed more actively, i.e., activated. Or so went the version at the time. Such distinctions were very shortly to be completely obliterated and all but disappear from the scientific discourse of cancer geneticists.

Gene cloning technology was enabling almost anybody to work with what just a few years earlier had been an unthinkably precious and almost impossible-to-obtain material: well-defined molecules of DNA. At the same time, these revolutionary methods for manipulating genes made it possible to separate forever the cellular proto-*onc* gene from its unsettling conceptual origins in virus-mediated transformation assays. Mutation and oncogene theories of cancer had not yet fully merged, but the time when they would was only months away.

Thus Duesberg's pedagogical approach was perceived by his peers as being more than a little retrograde. "Minor discrepancies" of the sort Peter was "carping on" were "going to be explained by future experiments which would tell us many things that we didn't know now." I was often to hear such sentiments from scientists whose frequently highly publicized work didn't survive the light of Peter's high-minded and intense scrutiny. In response, Peter remains fond of alluding to the biotechnology division of Dupont that sells to cancer researchers essentially healthy mice that have been engineered to carry an "activated oncogene" in every single cell of their warm, furry bodies with the advertising slogan, "Shorten the path to knowledge."

At the time, the qualitative model was known as the protovirus hypothesis, and its major proponent was the Nobel laureate Howard Temin, who remained, until his untimely death from cancer in 1994, friendly to Peter and (at least in this area) supportive of his efforts. Perhaps because the *Nature* review came down heavily in Temin's corner. Peter remembers: "Howard was the only one of the gang who called to say how much he liked it."

But as stated earlier, the evidence for the quantitative model wasn't too bad, and depending on which side of the Bay Bridge your laboratory was located, must even have looked pretty good. Sufficiently so, at least to the future Nobelist J. Michael Bishop, to have already endorsed the redesignation of proto-*onc* genes as "(*c*) oncogenes" and to refer to them as "enemies within" in the pages of *Cell* in 1981,[9] thus removing the last vestige of their evolutionary history as experimental objects. Genetic enemies within? A most peculiar choice of metaphors for a biologist, although maybe not from one whose father was an Anglican priest. But it seemed strange enough to Peter, who called attention to the phrase's odd logic by quoting it at a key juncture in his review. Rather than confront the paradox, it embraces it as axiomatic. Of course complex organisms would evolve and maintain an entire repertoire of potentially deadly genes. Why not? Instead of a handful of real *onc* genes that were epistemologically troublesome, and even with the polymerase chain reaction (PCR) just around the corner, difficult to isolate because it was, and is, no trivial task to work cleanly with retroviruses and their very unstable RNA genomes—just ask Robert Gallo, or Max Essex or Robin Weiss—cancer molecular biologists now had an almost limitless field in which to search for important, potentially deadly genes—a field ripening for harvest under the dawning, golden sun of biotechnology. In 1983 sixteen real *onc* genes were known; today there are close to a hundred oncogenes listed in the most important molecular biology graduate-level textbooks, and the one for the next cancer is just waiting to be published. Over the same time, as we shall see in subsequent chapters, the nature of biological scientific publishing was changing every bit as profoundly as the semantic bedrock of the biology it reported.

At first sight, the close sequence homologies between viral onc *genes and cellular prototypes suggested that normal cells contain retroviral* onc *genes, in accord with the oncogene hypothesis. That, in turn, led to the quantitative or dosage model in which enhanced dosage of a normal gene is postulated to be sufficient to cause cancer. Consistent with this view, cellular prototypes of viral* onc *genes were named cellular (c) oncogenes (38) and referred to as enemies from within the cell (39). The alternative view, consistent with the protovirus hypothesis, is the qualitative model in which vital differences exist between the structure and function of the viral* onc *genes and their cellular prototypes. These two models are not mutually exclusive, since many different mechanisms may lead to the same cancers. There is now ample sequence information to suggest differences between viral* onc *genes and proto-*onc *genes but still insufficient genetic and functional knowledge to determine whether cellular proto-*onc *genes are indeed cellular oncogenes; hence, the term proto-*onc *is used here rather than* c-onc *to emphasize this uncertainty. However, the following arguments suggest that most available data favour the qualitative model for the conversion of cellular sequences into oncogenic agents.*[10]

As is almost always true, especially in science, the devil is in the detail. In the review's next pages, Peter becomes the devil's advocate by examining in excruciating detail the hard evidence for and against the structural and functional equivalence of *onc* and proto-*onc* genes. Unfortunately, by the time these arguments were published, nobody really cared.

In molecular biology, structure and function go together like "love and marriage" in the song. And in the molecular biology in which Peter honed his scientific acumen—one without the option of material gratification—the only song anybody was singing was some version of "my brain's bigger than yours." This meant that no one would dare present as anything more than a working hypothesis a conclusion based on an incomplete demonstration that a particular mutation was responsible for a difference in function.

Ultimately this would mean having an x-ray crystallographic analysis of the protein (the gene in question's product) in both the normal and mutant forms in which the particular difference (attributable to the mutation in the gene) is not only evident in an altered three-dimensional structure, but in which the altered form can be directly related to differences in the functional properties of the protein. It's a tall order, and one that is rarely filled. It is (or was) known as a complete genetic analysis, and accomplishing it was the goal of every molecular biologist worthy of the name. Peter's and my friend Alvin John Clark, who began teaching me bacterial genetics in 1966, has had a marvelously productive life in science doing just that. He completed a single genetic analysis, beginning in 1965 with the isolation of a mutant bacteria unable to recombine its DNA properly, and finishing almost thirty years later with completely satisfying explanations, from the biological to the atomic levels, of why this is, how it happened, and what it means.

But Peter was by no means presenting such a steep challenge in the review article. Short of the proof that comes with crystals, there are many steps that can be taken to show that the products of two genes are likely to have similar functions based on analysis of only the gene parts of the gene-protein totality.

A virus, like everything else biological, has limits to its size. It cannot, obviously, be larger than its host, nor can it package unlimited amounts of genetic material into its protein coat, no matter how elastic. Retroviruses are extremely compact creatures. Basically they contain only three genes, thus they do not have very much leeway to either add new genetic information directly or exchange part of what they have for genetic material from the cell.

What Peter shows is a scientific literature replete with unimpeachable data, much of it from his own laboratory, demonstrating (and nobody has ever argued that it doesn't) that the structures of viral *onc* genes are not identical to their cellular progenitors, and on that basis alone no conclusions about the normal functions of their cell-derived parts can be legitimately drawn. In fact, some *onc* genes are composed of elements from the virus and two different cellular genes. Claiming that both cellular progenitors are oncogenes seems like a long stretch. Peter concludes his examination of the evidence bearing on the structural equivalence of *onc* and proto-*onc* genes as follows:

> *From this data, it would appear that viral* onc *genes and cellular proto-*onc *genes are not isogenic. Available structural evidence favours the hypothesis that either deletion and mutation of cellular sequences or the addition of virus-specific information, such as Δgag, or both are needed to confer transforming function on proto-*onc *sequences transduced by viruses. In some cases, elements from several cellular genes appear necessary to generate an oncogenic virus. That is to say, qualitative changes are the norm.*[3]

He then goes on to review the existing data concerning the functional equivalence of *onc* and proto-*onc* genes.

When biologists use the word "function," it is almost always accompanied by the word "assay." Assays are experimental systems for testing the properties of something, and their use is fundamental to the practice of science. In cancer biology, the best assay for whether a cell has been transformed is to inject its clonal descendants (in as small numbers as possible) into immunologically defective animals and see if the animals develop malignant tumors. This, like obtaining crystal structures, is not so often or so easily accomplished; therefore assays are used that are faster, less expensive, and serve as indicators of whether putting the cells into animals is likely to give the expected result. Morphological transformation is one such important assay, where the ability of a cell to escape from its normal growth controls and form a visible colony on a laboratory dish is the experimental endpoint.

In keeping with the times (and what was an unspoken but nonetheless real desire to free modern cancer molecular biology of its complicated origins in oncogenic retroviruses), a new type of transformation assay emerged in the early 1980s that used purified DNA instead of viruses as the vectors with which to deliver genes, whose oncogenic activity was being interrogated, into cells. The first results of these transfection assays, as they are known, heavily favored the qualitative model, insofar as no cloned proto-*onc* gene was able to transform primary cells, as each of their viral *onc* counterparts could do so reproducibly and efficiently. Not to be deterred in their efforts to establish, beyond the need to question, the existence of latent cellular oncogenes, cancer molecular biologists introduced a variation of the new, naked DNA assay in which they replaced cultured primary cells by a special cell line, developed by Green and Todaro in Boston and called NIH 3T3. This singular change in the functional assay for cancer genes is crucial to the final stages in the evolution of today's almost completely insubstantial oncogene (defined in the 1997 edition of the *Oxford Dictionary of Biochemistry and Molecular Biology* as "any gene associated with cancer"), and one of the key reasons that Peter's criticisms would be side-stepped by the scientists whose conclusions he was questioning.

Primary cell cultures are those obtained from freshly dissected adult or embryonic animal tissue. Such cells are presumably as genetically normal as it is possible to obtain and are the first choice for testing the effects of an introduced gene (or anything else). Very importantly they have exactly one complement of chromosomes, and it is almost unspeakably unfortunate that they cannot be maintained in this balanced genetic state indefinitely. After a relatively few divisions, most of the explanted cells give up the ghost and become disorganized, dissolving gels of biochemicals. However, once in a while, a mutant cell appears which has the useful, if not miraculous, property of being able to continue to divide until the last cow comes home. But. These types of cultures, known as cell lines, unlike primary cultures are not even close to genetically normal, possessing wildly aberrant numbers of chromosomes. In fact, Peter could refer to the mouse NIH 3T3 cell line as "preneoplastic" (cancerous) without editorial argument.

In one set of highly regarded experiments using these 3T3 cells, Ed Scolnick (later to become director of corporate research at Merck), working at the NIH, fused the cellular prototype of the Harvey (no relation) sarcoma virus transforming gene, *ras,* to a promoter from the virus, and thus created in the test tube something close to an artificial transforming retrovirus.[11] When this was transfected into 3T3 (and only into 3T3) cells, colonies of cells tumorigenic for mice could be obtained—although this did not occur nearly as frequently as with the virus, where even when primary cells are used, every single infection leads to a cancerous transformation. Whether Scolnick's result supports the quantitative or qualitative model was a matter of scholarly debate at the time, and now is of little import. What is important is that it and a few similar "landmark" publications involving proto-*ras* and 3T3 cells were the only experimental bases upon which the functional oncogene was being built. All other proto-*onc* genes failed to transform even 3T3 cells.

How persuasive conclusions based on such foundations will be is very much a matter of who's trying to convince whom. This is something biotech entrepreneurs knew from the beginning, when they made certain their boards of directors contained biologists with names of high repute who could be counted on to explain to potential investment bankers and the media the "company's science," as it would horribly come to be called in the popular press and among unbelievably young editors at prestigious scientific journals.

The *Nature* review's last section is entitled "Proto-*onc* genes as potential cancer genes," and it is as accurate and relevant now (twenty-plus years later) as it was then.

> *Clearly, the identification of* onc *genes has moved viral carcinogenesis from the romantic into an academic age. The same cannot be said for the suspected role of proto-*onc *genes in cancer. As yet there is no functional and no consistent circumstantial evidence that proto-*onc *genes directly initiate and maintain cancer like the* onc *genes of retroviruses. There is also no such evidence that proto-*onc *genes encode one of the multiple initiation and promotion events that create virus-negative cancers (81, 96, 117, 118).*
>
> *... So far retroviral* onc *genes are the only proof that altered proto-*onc *genes can be cancer genes. There is as yet no conclusive example that an unaltered proto-*onc *gene can function as a cancer gene simply through enhanced transcription or gene amplification. Complete genetic definition and assays for the biological function of normal and mutated proto-*onc *genes are now necessary to understand their possible role in carcinogenesis.*[12]

While Peter's article was being prepared for publication, two papers appeared, one in *Nature* and the other in *Science,* which seemed to forcefully address the challenge in the final sentence. These first results of an enterprise that is now denoted by the expensive term "functional genomics" are the underlying reason most molecular biologists would feel intellectually comfortable with the newly emerging oncogene, even though proto-*onc* and *onc* genes are clearly not the same genetic units. The papers showed that the Simian sarcoma virus *onc* gene, *sis*, derives from a gene that had been very recently cloned (in the days when cloning a working mammalian gene was still an impressive display of laboratory skills, not simply the start of a graduate thesis) and shown to function as a "growth factor."[13,14] Since "everyone knows" that cancer is a disturbance of a cell's normal growth controls, what could be more natural than attributing true oncogene status to the *c-sis* proto-*onc* gene (aka platelet-derived growth factor, or PDGF)?

All the pieces were now in place to guarantee that the once-clear differences between quantitative and qualitative interpretations of what an oncogene represented would be forever obscured. It only remained for the word "activate" to acquire a new meaning, without losing its old one. How "turned on" also came to mean "turned into" is a subject of the next chapter, in which mutations marry with oncogenes and Peter becomes the lone voice in a forest that is no longer anything other than its rapidly multiplying trees.

Chapter 1 Notes

1. On November 18, 1999, Frank McCormick, Director of the University of California San Francisco Comprehensive Cancer Center and Cancer Research Institute, and founder of Onyx Pharmaceuticals, gave a SRO seminar in the old MBVL ground-floor auditorium. I asked Peter if any of the luminaries present spoke to him. "Oh, the usual nods, and as usual I was allowed one question. Frank had been talking all the time about 'the guardian of the genome,' protecting DNA from damage.— *[The gene and protein that go by this epithet, p53, is among the more studied of the 35,000 or so genes that make up the human genome, and we will become reasonably well acquainted with it in due course. But for now, simply its ponderous designation will serve.]*—So I asked him: Couldn't he be a little more specific about what damage it was guarding against? I thought we had concepts of mutation, deletion, rearrange-

ment, etc., all these things we know about so well thanks to molecular genetics, and here we are talking like Boveri a hundred years ago about 'damage to DNA.' Is it point mutation? I ask. No, it's not point mutation. Ok. So it's overlooking point mutations. What *is* it guarding against? Then he came with single-stranded DNA. So I said it would be very busy preventing all cells from dividing since double-stranded DNA is made from single-stranded pieces. Oh, no, he meant 'abnormal' single-stranded DNA. Now even some students began to laugh. Botchan *[the seminar chairman]* then declares the discussion absurd and asks for the next question."

2. Duesberg, P. H., and Vogt, P. K. 1970. Differences between the ribonucleic acids of transforming and nontransforming avian tumor viruses. *Proc. Natl. Acad. Sci. USA* 67:1673–1680.

3. Duesberg, P. H. 1983. Retroviral transforming genes in normal cells? *Nature* 304:219–225.

4. Duesberg, P. H. 1996. *Inventing the Aids Virus.* Regnery Publishing, Inc., Washington, D.C.

5. Huebner, R. J., and Todaro, G. 1969. Oncogenes of RNA tumors viruses as determinants of cancer. *Proc. Natl. Acad. Sci. USA* 64:1087–1094.

6. Mizutani, S., Boettiger, D., Temin, H. M. 1970. An RNA-dependent DNA polymerase and a DNA endonuclease in virions of Rous sarcoma virus. *Nature* 228:424–427.

7. Duesberg, P. H., Vogt, P. K., Beemon, K., and Lai, M. 1974. Avian RNA tumor viruses: mechanism of recombination and complexity of the genome. *Cold Spring Harbor Symp. Quant. Biol.* 39:847–857.

8. Wang, L. H., Duesberg, P. H., Beemon, K., and Vogt, P. K. 1975. Mapping RNase T-1-resistant oligonucleotides of avian tumor virus RNAs: sarcoma-specific oligonucleotides are near the poly(A) end and oligonucleotides common to sarcoma and transformation-defective viruses are at the poly(A) end. *J. Virol.* 16:1051–1070.

9. Bishop, J. M. 1981. Enemies within, the genesis of retrovirus oncogenes. *Cell* 23:5–6.

10. Duesberg, P. H. 1983. Retroviral transforming genes in normal cells? *Nature* 304:219–225. [The convention used throughout this book for references within quotations is they will be presented in the order in which they occur in the text of the quotation, and in the format of the journal in which the article appeared.]

38. Coffin, J. M. et al. *J. Virol.* 40:953–957 (1981).

39. Bishop, J. M. *Cell* 23:5–6 (1981).

11. Chang, E. H., Furth, M. E., Scolnick, E. M., Lowy, D. R. 1982. Tumorigenic transformation of mammalian cells induced by a normal human gene homologous to the oncogene of Harvey murine sarcoma virus. *Nature* 297:479–483.

12. Duesberg, P. H. 1983. Retroviral transforming genes in normal cells? *Nature* 304:219–225.

81. Logan, J. & Cairns, J. *Nature* 300, 103–105 (1982).

96. Cairns, J. *Nature* 289, 353–347 (1981).

117. Knudson, A. G. *Cancer* Vol. I (ed. Becker, F.) 73–88 (Plenum, NY, 1981).

118. Berenblum, I. *Cancer* Vol. I (ed. Becker, F.) 451–484 (Plenum, NY, 1981).

13. Doolittle, R. F., Hunkapiller, M. W., Hood, L. E., Devare, S. G., Robbins, K. C., Aaronson, S. A., Antoniades, H. N. 1983. Simian sarcoma virus onc gene, v-sis, is derived from the gene (or genes) encoding a platelet-derived growth factor. *Science* 221:275–277.

14. Waterfield, M. D., Scrace, G. T., Whittle, N., Stroobant, P., Johnsson, A., Wasteson, A., Westermark, B., Heldin, C. H., Huang, J. S., Deuel, T. F. 1983. Platelet-derived growth factor is structurally related to the putative transforming protein p28sis of simian sarcoma virus. *Nature* 304:35–39.

2

Hoof-beats on the Road to the Prize

In the winter of 1984, I had been the scientific editor of *Bio/Technology* (or *Bioslash* as we affectionately and quickly called it), the brand-new, Manhattan-based publishing venture of London's Macmillan Journals for only a few months when I attended my first professional meeting at which everyone wore a suit. The symposium, organized by Stan Crooke and George Poste, president and vice president, respectively, for corporate research at SmithKline & French, was held in a downtown hotel of SK&F's Philadelphia headquarters. Its subject—receptor biochemistry, biotechnology, and drug development—was chosen for two reasons. The company's bread-and-butter anti-ulcer prescription, Tagamet, was one of the very few drugs at the time that could be considered a rational therapeutic, and the biochemical basis for its activity involved very specific interactions with a particular "receptor" protein on the surface of the cells lining the stomach.

The second reason for the meeting and the one that made it so timely and exciting was the recent spate of discoveries from molecular cloning laboratories that certain cellular growth-promoting proteins were related to viral oncogenes. Since growth factors function by becoming intimate with unique, complementary-shaped protein partners called receptors that are on the surface of cells—thereby initiating a chain of connected biochemical reactions that climaxes with the cell duplicating its chromosomes in preparation for division—the promise of at last being able to develop anti-cancer drugs that were truly specific, and thus free of the agonies of chemotherapy, seemed very real indeed.

In trying to understand how otherwise skeptical scientists could so wholeheartedly embrace the flawed reasoning that the structural similarity between viral *onc* genes and certain cellular genes implies that they are functional equivalents, I keep coming back to this statistically unimpressive coincidence: Some viral oncogenes derive from cellular genes whose normal functions appear to concern proliferation. "If you hear hoof-beats, think horses," as J. Michael Bishop put it, giving his imprimatur to the nouveau oncogene with this memorable (if not logically rigorous) phrase in an article for *Annual Reviews of Biochemistry*[1] that was contemporaneous with Peter's *Nature* review but considerably more popular.

It was equally obvious that these cellular genes could, by a variety of easily imagined genetic mechanisms such as mutation, have their normal functions subverted to the oncogenic ones of the extremely rare, transforming retroviruses to which they were related. And the modifier now applied to these multiple, postulated but completely unproved mechanisms was "activated." It was on everyone's lips at the cocktail and reception the first night of the meeting. Activated oncogenes were the answers to cancers. There were, however, a few considerations that might have dampened all this enthusiasm, at least a little. For one—as many of these same people were to show ten or so years later, when they developed the powerful set of technologies that has enabled deciphering the genomes of a large number of complex organisms (including the human variety)—the number of genes involved in mitosis (cell division) represents a significant fraction of the entire genetic repertoire. Thus picking up a piece of a "growth control gene or its receptor" and making an oncogene out of it may be rare not because the cellular proto-*onc* is a special bird but because assembling and maintaining an oncogenic virus involves a series of highly unlikely biochemical events. Although this precise argument was not really available in early 1984, it could have been made on the grounds that mitosis is probably the most complicated and certainly one of the more important things a cell does. Therefore, it should not be surprising that a large fraction of the gene pool is devoted to it. Another implication—that it is very unlikely any single one of this large number of genes would be enough to cause a cancer—goes directly to the heart of cellular oncogene theory.

A second reason for taking these discoveries with a few grains of salt is more biological, and that everyone at the meeting either did know or should have known. Cancer is not really a disease of uncontrolled growth. A cancer cell may divide faster or slower than its normal parent. Its malignant properties (as we will examine in later chapters) derive from the almost total disruption of a differentiated metabolism. That is to say, a pancreatic cancer cell is cancerous because it no longer remembers either the form or function of the normal pancreas cell from which it devolved, and not because it replicates its chromosomes at odd times. Exactly this view was put forward by the noted cancer biologist Henry Harris in the pages of *Nature,* as recently as January 2004, when he wrote: "But however complex the ultimate phenotype of a malignant cell might be, it would reduce confusion if it could be agreed that cancer, in the first instance, is not a disease of cell multiplication, but a disease of differentiation."[2]

Nobody in the ballroom that night appeared to have any interest in such considerations, however, as it is almost impossible to avoid the elation that comes with the first glimpse of a previous *terra incognita*. Gene cloning technologies, and new computer algorithms with which to compare long genetic sequences, were providing just those first glimpses of a hitherto impenetrable biochemical-genetic landscape. Simultaneously, giant pharmaceutical companies were on the verge of going for biotech big time.[3]

This is not to imply that the symposium itself was unduly influenced by commercial or economic considerations. And neither, emphatically, were its speakers, whom Stan and George had invited to discuss cutting-edge receptor biology for three days with their company researchers. Quite the contrary, in today's celebrity scientist journalistic parlance, they were all "world class," and the level of presentations was impressive to the extreme. There was even much critical discussion and lively questioning about particular experimental details and individual conclusions, if not overarching theory. One such detail, involving NIH 3T3, gave the initial impetus to a warm and longstanding relationship with George Poste, whom I would later invite to chair *Bio/Technology*'s board of scientific advisors.

In the few years since its introduction to the experimental palette of cancer molecular biologists, the NIH 3T3 cell line had become the favorite system for testing the effects of suspected human cancer genes, although it was unclear whether it detected primary cancer genes (those that actually initiated or maintained a malignant transformation) or secondary genes that were involved in "tumor progression." And it was a question very much on Poste's agenda, although I had no idea of that at the time. The following year he would publish an important (but largely unappreciated) paper in the *Proceedings of the National Academy of Sciences*[4] in which he showed "that 'normal' untransfected NIH/3T3 cultures contain sub-populations of cells that express malignant properties, and that transfection of NIH/3T3 cells with activated c-Ha-ras-1 accelerates formation of metastases." This provided definitive experimental evidence that assays using this cell line at best detected secondary events.

So when I asked George during our first conversation the opening night of the symposium whether he had read Duesberg's

Nature review and did he think it related to the interpretations that everyone was giving to the growth factor and growth factor receptor results, I was not as prepared as I might have been for his almost effusive reply. Indeed he had read the review. As usual, Peter's arguments were compelling, and he raised a number of important issues many would prefer he hadn't. High on the list was the use of 3T3 assays to probe oncogenic function. Nonetheless, Poste did think it was meaningful that retroviral oncogenes derived from cellular genes involved in growth control, and it was now a matter of elucidating the precise mechanisms that converted them into direct agents of cancer. As to whether simple point mutation was a sufficient mechanism, and whether using 3T3 cells was the correct way to address the question, he was pretty sure the answer to both of those questions was no.

My reason for asking about point mutations was because of some findings that were generally considered to be persuasive evidence that normal cellular genes could be turned into oncogenes (activated) by changing one genetic letter (nucleotide) for another.

In 1982, Robert Weinberg and his colleagues at MIT and the NIH published a paper in *Nature* entitled "Mechanism of activation of a human oncogene"[5]—the first use of "activation" to mean a qualitative change in the hypothetical proto-oncogene, rather than a quantitative change in the amount of its product. The paper so impressed the editors they invited a special editorial from John Cairns to comment on how the "secrets of cancer" were now beginning to be revealed.[6] In this article, Weinberg, Scolnick, and others showed that the genetic sequence of the proto-*ras* DNA from a bladder cancer cell line differs from the *ras* DNA of normal human cells by only one letter in the approximately six hundred letters that together spell proto-*ras*. This particular alteration in genetic spelling (mutation) has the effect of changing one of the two hundred or so amino acids that compose the protein molecule specified by the proto-*ras* gene—designated "p21," in which the "p" stands for protein and the "21" for the molecular mass of the "p," in this case 21 thousand Daltons. In the normal cell, the amino acid glycine is located at a particular position in the protein, and in the proto-*ras* encoded p21 from the bladder cancer cell line, the very closely related amino acid valine is present. Because the 3T3 experiments purported to show that this mutation was specifically responsible for the transforming ability of proto-*ras* DNA from the cancer cell line, Weinberg (and almost everyone else) was content to conclude that it was also the cause of the bladder cancer from which the cell line derived. Needless to say, Peter was not. His reasons for rejecting it, and similar conclusions, are detailed in the review he titled "Activated Proto-*onc* Genes: Sufficient or Necessary for Cancer?" and that appeared in the May 10, 1985, issue of *Science*.[7]

Unlike the *Nature* article, which was commissioned by its deputy editor, the impetus for this second look at oncogene theory came from Duesberg himself. Prior to Newmark's invitation, he had as he puts it, "been a good foot soldier in Huebner's *Wehrmacht*," doing his experiments, enjoying his success, and "not really thinking too much about the bigger picture." But given Peter's pit bull temperament, once he did, there was no letting go. The questions about the relevance of single genes to common human cancer he began to consider then would become more and more refined over the following decade until, in the best tradition of science, they would lead, as we will see, to a reformulation of cancer genetics in terms that not only make biological sense, but are rigorously quantitative and powerfully predictive. Over the same period of time, these persistent questions would in another (though not particularly noble) scientific tradition earn him close to total vilification by his former peers whose elaborately decorated cathedrals were under siege. But in the middle of 1984, the cement was still a little wet and the cathedrals were not quite completed, let alone decorated and fortified (even though reification of the "genetic enemies within" idea of cancer had proceeded essentially uninterrupted), and Peter still had enough clout with editors of major journals to convince Eleanor Butts at *Science* to give him the chance to reexamine developments in the field since the emergence of the cloned oncogene.

The review begins in a considerably more combative style than the analysis of a few years previous, perhaps because he was a little annoyed at the minimal impact of the more high-toned *Nature* article, and perhaps, as Peter contends, since there was little other than rhetorical illusion supporting the 1985 version of the oncogene, the situation called for a more forceful prose. In either case, its opening sentences are nothing if not direct: *"A primary objective of cancer investigators is the identification of cancer genes. Despite their efforts, this objective has not met with much success."*[7]

While acknowledging in the article's title that the word "activation" no longer meant what it did just a few years previous, Peter then set out to examine the available evidence for each of two then-current hypotheses that sought to explain human cancer in terms of these "activated oncogenes." And he posed his investigation in the form of what was, this time, a purely rhetorical question, as he would go on to show that neither of the favored models could muster anything more than rather tenuous, circumstantial evidence that "activated oncogenes" (alone or in combination) were sufficient or even necessary for the development of the tumors with which they were sometimes associated.

*The roles of proto-*onc *genes as accidental progenitors of retroviral* onc *genes have made them the focus of the search for cellular cancer genes. The postulated role of cellular proto-*onc *as cancer genes was initially tested by many investigators in view of a "one gene-one cancer" hypothesis and*

. . . .

more recently in view of a "multigene-one cancer" hypoth-
esis. The one gene-one cancer hypothesis postulates that
activation of one inactive cellular oncogene is sufficient to
cause cancer. [7]

In framing the hypotheses in this way, Peter is recalling the
"one-gene, one-enzyme" hypothesis of Beadle and Tatum in the
1940s, the essential proof of which, at least for micro-organisms,
was among the earliest triumphs of molecular biology and contributed in a major way to forming the intellectual bias of the
cancer molecular biologists they fathered. Peter continues:

It is based on the oncogene hypothesis of Huebner and
Todaro (60). Some investigators have postulated that acti-
vation is the result of increased dosage of a given proto-onc
gene product. . . . Others have suggested that proto-onc
genes are activated by mutations or rearrangements in the
primary DNA sequence. The multigene-one cancer hypoth-
esis postulates that an activated proto-onc gene is neces-
sary but, unlike the corresponding viral gene, not sufficient
to cause cancer. A quantitatively or qualitatively activated
proto-onc gene is postulated to function either as initiation
or as maintenance gene together with another gene, in a
multistep process (54, 55, 68–74).[8]

Thus, by 1985, quantitative and qualitative models of cancer
gene conversion had seamlessly joined. Cellular genes were now
considered to be turned into cancer genes by a change in their
structure through mutations and by changes in the frequencies
with which their protein products were produced. In almost imper-
ceptible increments, the new molecular oncology had put itself in
bed with the extremely popular view that mutagens are carcinogens. But until then, this view had no specific genes on which to
blame the carcinogenic effects of certain chemicals and ionizing

radiations, although Bruce Ames in the biochemistry department of UC Berkeley had made a career in the 1970s with his slogan "carcinogens are mutagens." On its basis, Ames developed what is now the most widely used chemical mutagen screen in the world (and which bears his name). The marriage would turn out, at least for the two groups of scientists involved, to be a match made in heaven. But in terms of the logical imperatives that are supposed to govern scientific thinking, it was close to a complete disaster. What had been, until that moment, a still unproved, rigorously testable hypothesis—that the structural progenitors of viral *onc* genes in cells could become their functional equivalents in the absence of the virus—was now a series of potentially endless hypotheses about how many of these genes it took to create a cancer, and what were the genetic and biochemical mechanisms involved in their various "activations." It was clearly a major advance for cancer molecular biologists and biotechnologists, if not yet for cancer patients, who have been patiently waiting for the U.S. government to win the "War on Cancer" since Richard Nixon declared it when it was obvious that the war in Vietnam was not going as planned.

In what would turn out to be a futile attempt to get this sterile marriage annulled, Peter used more than seven full pages, prominently positioned in an extremely powerful scientific journal, to unimpeachably demonstrate that there was no convincing functional evidence on which to believe that either of the *only* two "oncogenes" for which there was any functional evidence at all was causally involved in the cancers for which it was held responsible. That this article made as little impact as it did is a testimony to the almost instantaneous rapidity with which the "activated cellular oncogene" attained the epistemological status of a real theory, like Darwinian evolution or quantum mechanics.

Peter gave (and continues to give) little weight to the "how likely is it to find fish in a milk glass" arguments of proponents of the *onc* gene growth-factor coincidences (this particularly choice vignette is from the pen of Harold Varmus,[9] who was clearly inspired by his co-Nobelist-to-be J. Michael Bishop's prescient hoof-beats). He briefly refers to these findings in an early paragraph as follows: *"The normal functions of proto-*onc *genes are poorly understood. On the basis of* in vitro *assays, one of them appears to be a growth factor, another a growth factor receptor, and two others resemble genes of the yeast cell cycle."*[7] and does not return to this argument again. Instead he focuses his dissecting microscope on the experimental bases supporting the fundamental tenet of oncogene theory—that specific, normal cellular genes can go crazy and cause cancer. Because, in the absence of such proof, all the high-tech molecular biology and biochemistry in the world is only so much "pouring from the empty into the void"[10] as far as offering meaningful insight into the genetic abnormalities of the cancer cell.

But granting existential reality to the oncogene most definitely was good for cancer molecular biologists. Among whom, the more prominent could each lay claim to his or her own "onco-" and, as we shall see, possibly their favorite "anti-onco-"gene as well, with which to shorten simultaneously "the paths to knowledge" and the advancement of their own careers. Yet Peter has remained firm (to the point of frequently driving his scientific adversaries to Nixon-like "expletives deleted") in maintaining that unless and until a cloned cellular gene (or genes) can be shown to perform in an equivalent experimental system in the same way that viral *onc*-genes do (i.e., turn normal cells cancerous), it is folly to pretend they are the same.

At the time Peter composed this review for *Science,* the cancer-is-caused-by-activated-oncogenes hypothesis essentially rested on the results of a few key experiments with two oncogenes. One of them, *ras,* we have already met. The other, code-named *myc* (pronounced as in Jagger), was initially described by Duesberg,

Bister, and Vogt in 1977 and derives from MC29, a miniscule, transforming chicken retrovirus.[11] Two years later, Bishop succeeded in finding its cellular version[12] proto-*myc*, which would become celebrated, in part, for leading to the designation of the first oncogene that did not have a retroviral counterpart from which to infer its malignant properties. This Botticelli-like, full-sprung-from-a-seashell, cancer gene,[13] called *Blym* (for B-cell lymphoma), as we will soon see, was identified completely by the use of the new molecular cloning technologies and 3T3 cells. There are many who regard this as a praiseworthy accomplishment.

The idea that proto-*myc* activation played a causative role in B-cell lymphomas of animals and humans came initially from observations that the amount of the gene's primary molecular output (transcript), the aptly called messenger RNA (mRNA) that serves as the template on which the ultimate protein product of the gene is fashioned, is frequently enhanced in retroviral lymphomas of chickens.[14] On the basis of this, Bishop and Varmus postulated that transcriptional activation of proto-*myc* is the cause of the cancers, which appear in a small percentage of animals infected by one of the avian leucosis viruses.[15] Unlike true oncogenic retroviruses, these so-called "chronic transforming" viruses do not have *onc* genes, and the cancers they are said to cause appear after latent periods of more than six months, compared to the few weeks required for those induced by their "acutely" transforming but much less common relatives. (Peter would have much to say about these viruses in the 1987 review article for *Cancer Research* that we examine in the next chapter.) The hypothesis of Bishop and Varmus (and others, such as George Klein) was termed "downstream promotion," and it is a somewhat tortured attempt to make cellular proto-*onc* genes relevant to cancer in the absence of transforming retroviruses.

The term "downstream promotion" derives as follows. Recall that retroviruses contain signals (promoters), which determine how many mRNA molecules will be made (transcribed) from their genes that are one hundred to one thousand times more powerful than the promoters of their hosts. Since the words of the genetic dictionary are read in a particular direction, we can refer to sequences as being upstream or downstream of the beginning and end of a given gene. The downstream-promotion hypothesis postulates that the proto-*myc* gene is activated by the promoter of a retrovirus integrated into the cell's DNA upstream of its start, so that it now behaves functionally like the transforming gene of MC29. In accord with the hypothesis, hybrid mRNAs made of viral sequences at their beginning and cellular sequences in their more downstream parts were found in some tumors.[14] But subsequently, examples were reported in which the retrovirus was integrated downstream of proto-*myc*[15] or upstream but in the opposite transcriptional direction.[15] In these cases, of course, no hybrid RNAs are found, but to maintain the hypothesis proponents argue, almost *ad hoc,* that here the virus functions like a direction-independent promoter, called an "enhancer," even though it does not bear any striking similarity to known enhancer elements.

The hypothesis also runs into trouble, as Peter takes great pains to illustrate, because the chicken proto-*myc* differs considerably in its structure from the virus-cell, hybrid *myc* gene of MC29; thus even if it were activated, there is no compelling reason to think that proto-*myc*'s product would function biochemically in the same way as the viral gene. Peter also points out that the cancers induced by MC29 and the lymphomas attributed to the leucosis viruses are not the same diseases. Furthermore, downstream promotion does not explain the origin of about 20% of viral lymphomas in which proto-*myc* is not activated.[15]

Even more problematic is the fact that the exact places into which the leucosis viruses integrate themselves in the chromosomes of the chicken cells are not, as it is termed, site-specific, but the tumors they are said to induce are clonal. This means that the cancer is the product of a single malignantly transformed cell, because in all the cells of the cancer the leucosis virus is in precisely the same spot. It is inexplicable, therefore, how out of millions of cells infected by the virus, only one becomes cancerous, and that one is not defined by one (or a few) integration sites in every chicken lymphoma. Cancers induced by MC29, on the other hand, are polyclonal and arise quickly, as would be expected from a dominant, position-independent, viral carcinogen.

Explaining avian cancer, however, was not really the objective of oncogene theorists. Basically ignoring all the above problems but hearing a hoof-beat or two, they extended the activated-*myc* idea to the retrovirus-negative, human Burkitt's lymphoma. In this case, chromosome translocation was proposed as a mechanism of activating proto-*myc* function.[16-19] The main reason for this proposal is that proto-*myc* is located in chromosome 8 and a part of this chromosome, which includes proto-*myc*, is reciprocally translocated to the middle of an immunoglobulin gene of chromosome 2 in most, but not all, Burkitt's lymphoma cell lines that have been examined. But at best, only 50% of primary lymphomas show a chromosome 8 to 2 translocation, and in some cases it does not involve the *myc* gene directly, so it is difficult to see how proto-*myc* could be activated by being rearranged or placed in the environment of new transcription signals (promoters, enhancers), as the hypothesis would have it. Worse, the activation-by-translocation notion cannot offer even an *ad hoc* explanation for those Burkitt's lymphomas in which proto-*myc* remains in its original location while a region downstream of the gene is exchanged with chromosome 2.[20-23]

Having made these points, and a number of others too technical to be accurately conveyed here in a relatively unspecialized vocabulary, Peter goes on to consider the heart of the proto-*myc* activation hypotheses as they concern a real human cancer:

*There appears to be no consensus as to whether proto-myc
expression is enhanced in Burkitt's lymphoma cells, as compared to normal control cells. Some investigators report
elevated expression compared to normal B lymphoblasts
or lines (88), while others report essentially normal levels of
proto-myc mRNA (71, 86, 87, 89, 90–93). Enhanced proto-
myc transcription is not specific for B-cell lymphomas since
high levels of proto-myc expression are seen in non-Burkitt's
lymphomas (92), in other tumors (74), and in chemically
transformed fibroblast cell lines in which proto-myc is not
translocated or rearranged (41).*[24]

His conclusion from this portion of the evidence is unambiguous:

*Thus, there is no translocation, rearrangement, elevated
expression, or characteristic mutations of proto-myc common to all Burkitt's lymphomas investigated. This casts
doubt on the concept that any of the known proto-myc alterations are a sufficient cause (or even necessary) for Burkitt's
lymphoma.*[7]

After he has presented the case outlined above Peter turns to
the most crucial experimental question concerning proto-*myc*
and cancer. Does proto-*myc* DNA from tumor cells have transforming activity even partially as effective as the MC29 version?
When this question was asked by the Cambridge, Mass., molecular
onco-geneticists—using of course the 3T3 cell transformation
assay, with DNA from chicken or human B-cell lymphomas—the
answer was clear.

*No myc-related DNA was detected even though its pre-
sumed functional equivalent, the Δgag-myc gene of MC29,
is capable of transforming 3T3 cells (100, 101) and other
rodent cell lines (102).*[25]

However, the experiment appeared to produce one of those almost mythical "chance favors the prepared mind" moments of scientific serendipity because:

> *Instead, another DNA sequence termed* Blym *was identified by the assay (69, 103). On the basis of these results, the role of proto-*myc *in lymphomas has been interpreted in terms of a two-gene hypothesis. It has been suggested that activated proto-*myc *is necessary but not sufficient to cause the lymphomas (69, 74). It is postulated to have a transitory function that generates a lymphoma maintenance gene,* Blym, *which appears to be the DNA that transforms 3T3 cells and is thought to maintain the B-cell tumor. There is no proof for this postulated role of proto-*myc *as a lymphoma initiation gene, because the 3T3 cell transformation assay does not measure proto-*myc *initiation function and because there is no evidence that the two genes jointly (or alone) transform B-cells. Furthermore, it is also not known whether* Blym *is altered in primary Burkitt's lymphomas, since all of the transfection experiments were done with DNA from cell lines.*[26]

Exactly one year after this question appeared on page 627 of *Science*, James Devine, a member of the Harvard team that first reported the identification of the *Blym* oncogene only a few years before, wrote as follows in a paper published in the May 11, 1986, issue of *Nature*, titled "Mechanism of activation of HuBlym-1 gene unresolved."[27]

> I report here that there are no differences between the sequences of three recombinant DNA clones from Burkitt's lymphoma cell lines that cross-hybridize to (normal, human) HuBlym-1 but do not induce foci when transfected into NIH 3T3 cells, and the reported sequence of Burkitt's lymphoma

Blym. Also there is no obvious or consistent increase in the transcription of the *HuBlym-1* gene in Burkitt's lymphoma cell lines of the type that might otherwise have accounted for its transforming activity even in the absence of a mutation. How the *HuBlym-1* gene is activated therefore remains a mystery.[27]

Notice that the last sentence of Devine's abstract begins with "how"—consistent with the waffling language characteristic of weak hypotheses—and not as it more properly should, with "whether." But this semantic escape clause was not good enough to keep *Blym* from going blam, even among those who had been making a pretty good living from it. According to a Pub. Med. search, in the three years between its triumphal birth and Devine's 1986 paper, the *Blym* oncogene was the subject of sixteen publications in *Nature, Science,* and other high-toned journals, including a review in *Advances in Cancer Research.* Since the 1986 (let's call a spade a spade) retraction above, there have been an additional nine. Of these, the two most recent—one in 1994 and the other in 1993—by noted cancer molecular biologists J. D. Zhu and N. Ishigura, have the inspiring titles "Proto-oncogene expression in a human chondrosarcoma cell line: HCS-2/8" and "Specific expression of cellular oncogenes c-*myc* and c-*myb* in T-cell lines established from three types of bovine lymphosarcomas," and appeared in the *Japanese Journal for Cancer Research* and the *American Journal of Veterinary Research.*

Although it did not itself survive the rigors of the "cancer gene today, gone tomorrow" linguistic mutational process, the spawn of *Blym* nonetheless live on enshrined in the major graduate-level textbooks, and shaping the thinking of the next generation of cancer geneticists in the form of various versions of multiple, cooperating-oncogenes explanations of cancer that have provided a continuous parade of candidates and combinations—none of which has yet succeeded in doing what the tiniest virus imaginable, MC29, with only half a cellular proto-*myc* in its arsenal, can do so well. As we will see in subsequent chapters, cancer is indeed the result of an imbalance in multiple genes and their products, but these genes are neither reproducibly denumerable, nor can they legitimately be said to be cooperating.

Having dealt with one pillar of the experimental support for the idea that activated, specific genes are the causes of human cancers, Peter turned his attention to the other important "human oncogene" of the time, *ras*. Referred to as a "dominant-acting oncogene by Weinberg in a still well-cited 1981 *Nature* paper,[28] by Bishop in the *Annual Reviews of Biochemistry* in 1983,[1] and only one year later by Varmus in the *Annual Reviews of Genetics*,[9] Peter summarizes the status of the evidence concerning *ras* in a characteristically direct style.

The proto-Ha-ras gene from the bladder carcinoma cell line differs from normal proto-Ha-ras in a point mutation which alters the 12th p21 codon in exon 1 from normal Gly to Val (67,110). This mutation does not cause overproduction of the ras gene product (p21) in the 3T3 cell line (67) and does not change known biochemical properties of p21 (111). The single base change is thought to activate the gene to a functional equivalent of Ha-MuSV and to be the cause of the carcinoma because it is the apparent cause for 3T3 cell-transforming function (67, 112). However, this mutation has not been found in a survey of more than 60 primary human carcinomas, including 10 bladder, 9 colon, and 10 lung carcinomas (113), in 8 other lung carcinomas (114), and 14 additional bladder and 9 kidney carcinomas (115). Further, the mutated human proto-Ha-ras, which transforms 3T3 cells, does not transform primary rat embryo cells (54, 70) and, more significantly, does not transform human embryo

*cells (116). Transformation of primary cells would be
expected from a gene that causes tumors in animals. Thus
the mutated proto-ras gene does not correspond to the viral
model which transforms primary mouse, rat (117, 118), and
human cells (119–123).*[29]

From this catalog of experimental challenges, the only ones
that seem to have mattered are those concerning functional assays.
The technical but extremely important point for cellular oncogene theory about the role of particular mutations in "activating" even the 3T3 transforming function of proto-*ras* would
become an ongoing debate between Peter and Weinberg. Sadly,
what began as a spirited scientific battle in the finest tradition
of dueling hypotheses would degenerate on Weinberg's part as
we will shortly see, to name-calling when he referred to Peter as
"intellectually dishonest" at a major cancer symposium near the
end of 1985.

Peter's other challenge—providing an experimental system,
free of artifacts, in which one or more defined genes would reproducibly transform a normal, diploid human cell—is even more
important because it goes to the absolute center of oncogene theory. And it also remains unmet, though not, as we will now and in
subsequent chapters see, from lack of effort.

To explain why mutated proto-Ha-*ras* transforms preneoplastic 3T3 cells, but not rat or human embryo cells, Weinberg
(and others) proposed—somewhat boldly, since it was without
very much experimental or conceptual precedent—that mutated
proto-Ha-*ras* is only one of at least two activated genes that are
necessary to induce cancer.[30-32] This "two-gene, one-cancer"
hypothesis was tested when primary rat cells were transfected
with a mixture of the mutated human proto-Ha-*ras* and either
the DNA form of MC29 or "activated" proto-*myc* from a mouse
cancer[30] as helper genes. None of these genes was able to transform

rat embryo cells alone (MC29, remember, is a chicken virus and will not by itself do anything to a normal rat cell), but some cells were transformed by the artificially mixed genes. Why this particular combination, you ask? The rationale given by the MIT geneticists was that *myc* would function in a manner similar to the way it did when cooperating with *Blym*, i.e., as a transient initiator that could immortalize the cells. The irony, in the light of subsequent findings, is that they were quite right in the first part of their supposition, although obviously not exactly in the way they imagined. But even if *myc* in fact had such an "immortalization" function, the ability to divide indefinitely in tissue culture is not an essential property of cancers, since cells from many primary tumors cannot be so maintained. Perhaps with more truth, the answer to the question of "why *myc* and *ras*?" is contained in the well-known maxim, "If one's only tool is a hammer, every problem looks like a nail" (or in this case, two nails). Duesberg comments on these results as follows:

> *The study with* myc-*related helper genes did not show that the transformants contained and expressed the added DNAs; not tested in this study was the question of whether unaltered forms of proto-*ras *or proto-*myc, *together with an altered helper gene, are sufficient to register in this assay.*[7]

Peter would go on to spend a fair number of the NIH's taxpayer-provided dollars (when he was still receiving them) to answer this last question, and in so doing demonstrate convincingly that these highly-touted results are no more than experimental artifacts generated by the DNA transfection protocols used and dependent upon the helper gene to provide a viral promoter. Exactly like the experiments of Scolnick a few years earlier, these newer demonstrations had done nothing more than create an artificial transforming retrovirus. However, despite the unchallenged papers by Duesberg in the *Proceedings of the National Academy of Sciences (USA)* in 1988 and 1991,[33,34] Baltimore, Lewin, and Watson have not seen the need to correct or even question their prominent textbook endorsements of these mixes of *myc* and *ras* where they receive the same historical importance, for example, as Al Hershey and Martha Chase's truly landmark piece of molecular biology in which they proved, a half century ago, that DNA was the molecule of the gene, and began, although they had no idea, the biotechnology revolution.

Some of Peter's sparest scientific prose is reserved for the article's "Conclusions" section where, as in the *Nature* review, he makes a series of points, which although unheeded are not because of that, any less pertinent or true.

The preponderance of 3T3 cell-transformation negatives among the above-described tumors suggests that either no genes have caused the negative tumors or that the assay failed to detect them. That only ras-*related proto-*onc *genes have been detected in human tumors indicates another limitation of the 3T3 assay. Since the proto-*ras *mutations detected by the 3T3 assay do not transform primary cells, it is possible that they are not relevant for tumor formation.... As yet, viral* onc *genes are the only "activated" proto-*onc *genes that are sufficient to cause tumors and that act as autonomous, dominant cancer genes in susceptible cells.*

*... The proposals that altered proto-*onc *genes are necessary but not sufficient for tumor formation are a significant departure from the original view that they were equivalents of viral* onc *genes. They do not address the question why these genes are assumed to have oncogenic functions different from those of the viral models. Ironically, these proposals suggest that activated proto-*onc *genes are functional subsets of viral* onc *genes, whereas viral* onc *genes*

*are structural subsets of proto-*onc *genes. Functional proof
for multiple, synergistic transforming genes and consistent
correlations between altered proto-*onc *genes and specific
tumors are needed to support the view that proto-*onc *genes
are necessary for multigene carcinogenesis.*[7]

As Peter was marshaling these arguments, I attended my second scientific gathering at which the dress code was 180 degrees
from the Cold Spring Harbor meetings that until my job with
Bio/Technology had been the only kind I knew. But while the
SK&F meeting was recognizably a scientific symposium, and a
very good one, this *Nature*-organized event was closer to a
celebrity showcase.

The early eighties were good for both the burgeoning biotechnology industries and the scientific journals read by its practitioners. In 1982, *Nature* turned a profit for the first time in its
hundred-year-plus history. This was mostly due to a phenome-
nally increased display advertising revenue that itself was largely
a result of increased spending by the companies that manufac-
tured the reagents and equipment that were much more in demand
than just a few years previously. The ensuing windfall profit was
the reason the bosses in London were receptive to starting a U.S.
monthly devoted to biotechnology when Bob Ubell (brother of
the late TV science journalist, Earl) first approached them with
the idea.

I don't remember who originally had the idea that holding a
meeting at a posh hotel in Boston in 1984, inviting a carefully
selected group of "internationally renowned" cancer biologists
to speak for forty minutes each, and charging a hefty admission
could be a cash cow (although I do remember being drafted by
Diana Berger, the first ever conference coordinator in the NY
offices, to write some advertising copy for the event). But who-
ever it was midwifed an entire service industry in biotechnology

conferences. Four hundred people actually paid money (though mostly, then and now, it was company and taxpayer dollars) to hear (in no particular order) John Cairns, Ray White, Robert Weinberg, Philip Leder, Robert Gallo, and a few others hold forth on "The Molecular Biology of Cancer." Who in the MBVL or Harvard Biology Labs in 1968 would have thought this possible? The event was so successful that I was asked by our publisher, Gary Rekstad, to organize a for-profit *Bio/Technology* conference *muy pronto,* which I did, choosing New Orleans over Boston as a venue.

Much more important to the course of subsequent events than a superstar science show, however, was that by sponsoring this meeting, *Nature,* with all its history and prestige, was giving a fulsome, very public endorsement to the unproved oncogene. Peter's arguments didn't have the chance of the proverbial snowball in summer after that.

At the speakers' dinner the night before the scientific sessions began, I met John Maddox, *Nature*'s famous editor (with whom Peter and I were to have a series of fascinating exchanges concerning recently discovered deadly viruses until he retired—with a knighthood—in 1995), and Peter Newmark, *Nature*'s deputy editor,—the generally-acknowledged molecular biology brain of the journal who told me later in the evening that he frequently had to rework Mr. Maddox's editorials because of silly mistakes that came from John not having any formal education in advanced biology. So of course I asked Dr. Newmark, *"Vhere vus Herr Doktor Professor Duesberg?"* "Oh, did I know Peter?" *"Indeed, we had been friends since 1966 in Bezerkeley."* Sensing an ally, Newmark admitted that of course he had wanted Duesberg to be there, but that Maddox, acting on the advice of others (something he would do a lot of in the future when it came to Peter), had vetoed the idea. "Since Duesberg didn't 'believe in' oncogenes, what was the point in having him speak?"

In my naiveté, I assumed that one would want to have a seriously considered dissenting voice; especially one to which *Nature* had so boldly given a large number of dissenting words only months before. But as I must have made clear by now, this was a different sort of scientific meeting, although prototypical. It set, among other unfortunate precedents, placing a higher premium on consensus than reasoned discourse.

But before I appear too cynical, let me say that at the time I was much more sanguine about the new biotechnologies, and being somewhat younger, not completely immune to all the sudden glamor. My most pleasant memory of the event now is seeing John Cairns again. I had gotten to know John when he was the director of the Cold Spring Harbor Laboratory, and I attended the annual phage meetings in the late 1960s. I had not seen him since.

In his 1978 book, *Cancer, Science and Society,* he had written insightfully about mutation theories of cancer as follows: "One of the problems is that most mutations lead to loss of functions, rather than the creation of new function."[35] Although he would never become an outspoken supporter of Peter's oncogene critique, Cairns was as close to a moderating voice as the 1984 *Nature* symposium would have.

My contemporaneous summary of the meeting appeared shortly after the fact in *Bio/Technology,* although rendered almost unintelligible by the "front of the book" editor of the time, who was pressed for space and didn't know very much molecular biology. Nonetheless, the following bits survived, and in light of what was to come, are not without interest.

Robert Gallo of the NIH presented his work on the relationships between human T cell lymphotropic viruses. He proposed a "complementarity" between HTLV-I, a chronic transforming virus, and HTLV-III, a genetically related virus that appears to have quite opposite effects. In an extended discussion, which went well beyond the results presented in his recent paper in *Science,* Gallo raised the possibility (as did Samuel Broder presenting the clinician's view) that these viruses may be involved in a much wider range of lymphoid neoplasias than is currently believed.[36]

But the big hit of the three-day event was provided by Phil Leder from MIT, who gave the paying customers their money's worth by revealing, while it was still in the press at *Cell* [37] (the third, along with *Nature* and *Science,* of the important competing journals of modern molecular biology), the world's first transgenic "onco-mouse." This was about as new as it could get, and the collective gasp of the lap-dog science journalists from the major dailies was audible. Leder's presentation afforded me the opportunity to ask my one question. It concerned a control experiment that he did not mention in his talk.

Control experiments are designed to make certain that the variables to which one assigns meaning are in fact the important ones. Conclusions from imperfectly controlled experiments aren't worth too much. My question concerned whether Leder had made transgenic mice that carried the same synthetic proto-*myc* genes as the onco-mice but contained internal deletions (i.e., they were missing a piece from their middles) in order to control for nonspecific positional activation of other proto-*onc* genes that might occur because of the large number of "black box" genetic events in their breeding. Leder acknowledged that this was a good question, and they were in the process of doing exactly those controls. I don't know whether they have been done since, but they did not appear as a *note added in proof* in the *Cell* paper. I do know, however, the number of paths to knowledge that the "Onco-Mouse," has shortened between then and now is smaller than the bank statements whose digits it has lengthened.

Exactly like the 1983 *Nature* review, the 1985 *Science* article was, with absolute certainty, widely and even carefully read, and subsequently, with no further ado, completely ignored. Except, with near certainty, it provoked both Bishop and Weinberg to their own review articles that quickly followed the Duesberg frontal assault on the oncogene. Peter's *Science* review has been cited 147 times thru 1998. J. Michael Bishop's, which appeared in *Trends in Genetics*[38] four months later, a bush-league journal when its citation index is compared to that of *Science,* received half as many in the same period. And Robert Weinberg's response, which was published in *Science*[39] in November, was referenced more than 700 times. Between them, Bishop and Weinberg manage to cite Peter once.

Bishop's review, already titled "Trends in Oncogenes," is a poor-man's version of his 1983 *Annual Reviews* treatment of essentially the same material, an article that has been cited a whopping 1,512 times. But while short on scholarship, it does contain splendid metaphors like "the first outlines of a biological 'roadmap' to cancer" in which "oncogenes impinge on the chain of command that directs the response to polypeptide growth factors"; exaggerations such as "DNA taken from a variety of tumor cells can transform select cells in culture, as if it contained an active oncogene of the sort we were once accustomed to finding only in viruses"; somewhat contradictory equivocations, as exemplified by, "but there is no direct evidence that this is the means by which these genes function in normal cells or induce neoplastic growth"; freshman biochemistry mistakes like using the terms "activity" and "function" interchangeably when referring to enzymes;, and of course several stampedes of hoof-beats. The one that follows this spirited defense of 3T3 cell assays is typical:

> The use of gene-transfer (or 'transfection') to identify oncogenes has been criticized because the mouse 3T3 cell commonly used in the assays is itself abnormal. But the 3T3 cell

should be viewed in this setting as nothing more than a sensitive indicator that can be used to ferret out genetic lesions. The mounting abundance of these lesions, their restriction to neo-plastic cells, their reproducible occurrence in diverse experimental tumors, their phenotypic effects on both established and primary cultures of cells, and the evidence of biological selection for specific mutations all conjoin to make a powerful argument: it seems likely that mutant oncogenes are more than innocent bystanders or mere pawns in the tumors where they are found.[38]

And in keeping with the paper's trendy title, Bishop treats us to the words of internationally renowned cancer authority Norman Mailer—who "has reminded us that the genesis of cancer is not a simple matter"—to explain multigene carcinogenesis: "None of the doctors have a feel for cancer.... The way I see the matter, it's a circuit of illness with two switches. Two terrible things have to happen before the crud can get its start. The first cocks the trigger. The other fires it."[38]

Oh yes, the single reference to Duesberg, P. H., *Science* 228: 669–677 (1985) follows a few sentences later: "Some observers quarrel with these findings, faulting the fabric before it is fully woven." Extending this science by metaphor to its logical inference, one might counter that indeed, a fabric woven from a misplaced spindle is fatally flawed from inception. But Bishop saved, as many skilled debaters do, his most powerful argument for last: "Where there is smoke, there is usually fire."

Weinberg's counter was of a different sort. Receiving equal space as Peter, he avoids referring, even in passing, to his colleague's six-month-old predecessor by changing the ground from a discussion of experimental proof of function to "The Action of Oncogenes in the Cytoplasm and Nucleus." He essentially dismissed Peter's entire critique by declaring in the opening paragraphs:

Oncogene research has changed substantially over the past several years. Initial emphasis concerned the identification of oncogenes present in tumor virus genomes and in the genomes of a number of different types of tumor cells. Together, various experimental routes have led to the characterization of at least 30 different oncogenes originating from the cellular genome and 10 or more found in the genomes of DNA tumor viruses. Having catalogued these genes and their structures, workers are now moving into a new phase in which mechanistic problems are confronted: how do oncogenes and their encoded proteins convert normal cellular metabolism to that of a tumor cell? What regulatory pathways are perturbed by onco-genes, and how can their various modes of action be interrelated?

This review attempts to synthesize much of the currently available data on these issues. It is written with the belief that much of the information about oncogenes will eventually be understandable in terms of a small number of mechanisms and that the outlines of some of these are gradually becoming apparent.[39]

Even for those who have raised equivocal language to new standards, the escape clause in this last sentence is truly extraordinary. With promises like these, it is not surprising that twenty years later, we are still waiting for the first biochemical pathway whose disruption by a point or otherwise mutated oncogene or genes is necessary, let alone sufficient, *"for the crud to get its start."*

But Weinberg's lack of appreciation for the finer points of academic debate would go well beyond neglecting to acknowledge the existence of a prominent critic or his critique. In an auditorium at the dedication symposium for the $60 million Eli Lilly Biomedical Research Building at the end of 1985, he would cross the line between argument and outrageous attack.

By now I was accustomed to jacket and tie meetings. I was not, however, accustomed to seeing Peter at them, especially as his name did not appear on the program that arrived a few weeks before, along with an invitation to be one of the few journalists in attendance.

When we ran into each other at the reception he was quite cheerful, having just convinced David Baltimore, one of the session chairs, to allow him fifteen minutes the next morning in which to present some experimental results that directly addressed the mechanism of activation of proto-*ras*. I had not seen David for a long time and was looking forward to renewing an old relationship that twenty-four years earlier had set me irrevocably on my own career path. As a graduate student at the Rockefeller Institute in 1962, he and a few others organized a special summer course for prospective biology students on their way to college. I was lucky enough to be one of those chosen the first year the course was offered, and I immediately felt affection for this bearded, sandaled, Pall Mall chain-smoking, beatnik oddball among the otherwise very conservative-appearing cadre of Rock Tech students. Peyton Rous, with whom we ate lunch in the same magnificent dining hall every day for six weeks, never failed to look askance at his attire.

I will always remember the first question David challenged us to answer by the next day. Sitting on the desk, he held up a Petri dish with a lawn of bacteria that had been infected with virus. And calling our attention to the dark spots on the plate, he said that all the important conclusions of molecular genetics depended on the fact that each of the spots resulted from the infection of one bacteria by a single virus. As the infected culture grew, he explained, the virus would multiply and after a short time have spread sufficiently to produce a crater of dead cells, or plaques. Therefore, by counting easily visible plaques, one could accurately count invisible virus particles. The challenge was to provide an experimental proof this was so. The next morning all of us had arrived at the correct answer. Dilute, in series, a solution containing bacteria-eating virus, add known amounts of several dilutions to growing cultures of bacteria, and count the number of resulting plaques. If one virus was sufficient to produce a plaque, then a ten-fold dilution would produce ten-fold fewer plaques. But if two particles, for example, were required, then a ten-fold dilution would produce a hundred times fewer and so forth. This simple experiment left a lasting impression, and I used it to begin every course I ever taught in molecular biology. Viruses are single-hit pathogens.

When I asked Peter how he came to be in Indianapolis at all, he explained that Irving Johnson had personally requested his presence. Irving was the head of research at Eli Lilly, and a member of *Bio/Technology*'s board of scientific advisors, which explained my invitation. He is also the first pharmaceutical executive to see the potential for recombinant DNA technologies to revolutionize the industry.[40] Irving had read Peter's *Science* review with some interest, and he was looking forward, as was I, to a lively exchange the next day. Little did we imagine what was to come. In his graciously-allowed fifteen minutes at the end of Baltimore's session, Peter presented primary data from his laboratory that showed:

> *Molecularly cloned Harvey proviral vectors carrying viral* ras, *normal rat proto-*ras *and recombinant* ras *genes in which the virus-specific* ras *codons 12 and 59 were replaced by proto-*ras *equivalents each transformed aneuploid mouse 3T3 cells after latent periods that ranged from 4 to 10 days.... Thus specific* ras *codons are not necessary for transforming function.*[41]

In an effort, both desperate and successful, to stop Peter in his tracks at a moment when there was a real sense that prominent scientists, including David, were listening with attention Weinberg attacked this conclusion by impugning its experimental foundation in the crudest, and cruelest, possible way. Even Irving's carefully edited phrasing that appears in the proceedings of the symposium is chilling:

> Dr. Weinberg said that a graduate student in his laboratory had made exactly analogous constructions to those described by Dr. Duesberg and had got exactly opposite results.[42]

As Weinberg was unwilling or unable to provide any specific data to back up his insinuation of experimental ineptitude, the ensuing exchange between the two distinguished professors was naturally a bit heated, causing David to quickly declare it a personal matter best reserved for the coffee break. Peter was to publish the same data he presented that fateful morning a few months later in the *Proceedings of the National Academy*[43] where neither Weinberg nor anyone else has sought to challenge it. Neither, of course, have they ever cited it, nor has the contradictory data yet to appear in any MIT Ph.D. thesis, fortunately for the anonymous graduate student, and the reputations of his thesis committee. If Peter was a lonesome cowboy before this travesty, "leper at a beauty pageant" describes his subsequent treatment, although he was to enact some measure of revenge. Not too long after, he soundly defeated Weinberg in fair debate at a prestigious cancer symposium of the Weizmann Institute held in Eilat, Israel. After this event Weinberg complained to another scientist, Josh Fidler, about the "level of hostility he felt towards himself and the oncogene concept."[44]

In 1986 Peter received a Fogarty fellowship to spend a year at the NIH probing the roots and branches of cancer genes; was awarded a five-year, highly competitive National Institutes of Health Outstanding Investigator Grant; and was inducted into the U.S. National Academy of Sciences at the still-young age of fifty. As we will see in the following chapters, none of this was to do him much good.

Chapter 2 Notes

1. Bishop, J. M. 1983. Cellular oncogenes and retroviruses. *Ann. Rev. Biochem.* 52:301–354. This article has received well over 1500 citations in the scientific literature. Peter's contemporaneous *Nature* review has been cited approximately 100 times.

2. Harris, H. 2004. Tumor suppression: Putting on the brakes. *Nature* 427:201.

3. Fujimura, J. H. 1996. *Crafting Science: A Sociohistory of the Quest for the Genetics of Cancer.* (Cambridge, MA: Harvard University Press).

4. Greig, R. G., Koestler, T. P., Trainer, D. L., Corwin, S. P., Miles, L., Kline, T., Sweet, R., Yokoyama, S., Poste, G. 1985. Tumorigenic and metastatic properties of "normal" and ras-transfected NIH/3T3 cells. *Proc. Natl. Acad. Sci. USA* 82:3698–3701.

5. Tabin, C. J., Bradley, S. M., Bargmann, C. I., Weinberg, R. A., Papageorge, A. G., Scolnick, E. M., Dhar, R., Lowy, D. R., Chang, E. H. 1982. Mechanism of activation of a human oncogene. *Nature* 300:143–149.

6. Logan, J., and Cairns, J. 1982. The secrets of cancer. *Nature* 300:104–105.

7. Duesberg, P. H. 1985. Activated proto-onc genes: Sufficient or necessary for cancer? *Science* 228:669–677.

8. *Ibid.* References therein:

   60. R. J. Huebner and G. J. Todaro, *Proc. Natl. Acad. Sci. USA* 64, 1087 (1969).

   54. H. Land, L. F. Parada, R. A. Weinberg, ibid., 304, 596 (1983).

   55. H. Land, L. F. Parada, R. A. Weinberg, *Science* 222, 771 (1983).

   68. G. M. Cooper and P. E. Neiman, ibid., 292, 857 (1981).

   69. G. M. Diamond, J. Cooper, M. A. Ritz, Lane, ibid., 305, 112 (1983).

   70. H. E. Ruley, ibid. 304, 602 (1983).

   71. P. Leder, J. Battev, G. Lenoir, C. Mouldine et al., *Science* 222, 76(1983).

72. I. M. Adams, S. Gerondakis, E. Webb, L. M. Carcoran, S. Gory, *Proc. Natl. Acad. Sci. U.S.A.* 80, 1982 (1981).

73. G. Klein and E. Klein, *Carcinogenesis* 5, 429 (1984).

74. D. J. Slamon, J. B. deKemion, I. M. Verma, M. J. Cline, *Science* 224, 256 (1984).

9. Varmus, H. E. 1984. The molecular genetics of cellular oncogenes. *Ann. Rev. Genet.* 18:553–612.

10. A favorite phrase of G. Gurdjieff, used frequently in *All and Every-thing: Beelzebub's Tales to His Grandson* (New York: E. P. Dutton & Co., 1964).

11. Duesberg, P. H., Bister, K., and Vogt, P. K. 1977. The RNA of avian acute leukemia virus MC29. *Proc. Natl. Acad. Sci. USA.* 74:4320–4324.

12. Sheiness, D., and Bishop, J. M. 1979. DNA and RNA from unin-fected vertebrate cells contain nucleotide sequences related to the puta-tive transforming gene of avian myelocytomatosis virus. *J. Virol.* 31:514–521.

13. Goubin, G., Goldman, D. S., Luce, J., Neiman, P. E., Cooper, G. M. 1983. Molecular cloning and nucleotide sequence of a transforming gene detected by transfection of chicken B-cell lymphoma DNA. *Nature* 302:114–119.

14. Hayward, W. S., Neel, B. G., and Astrin, S. M. 1981. Activation of a cellular onc gene by promoter insertion in ALV-induced lymphoid leukosis. *Nature* 290:475–480.

15. Payne, G. S., Bishop, J. M., Varmus, H. E. 1982. Multiple arrange-ments of viral DNA and an activated host oncogene in bursal lymphomas. *Nature* 295:209–214.

16. Leder, P., Battey, J., Lenoir, G., Moulding, C., Murphy, W., Potter, H., Stewart, T., Taub, R. 1983.Translocations among antibody genes in human cancer. *Science* 222:765–771.

17. Adams, J. M., Gerondakis, S., Webb, E., Corcoran, L. M., Cory, S. 1983. Cellular myc oncogene is altered by chromosome translocation to an immunoglobulin locus in murine plasmacytomas and is rearranged similarly in human Burkitt lymphomas. *Proc. Natl. Acad. Sci. USA* 80:1982–1986.

18. Klein, G. 1983. Specific chromosomal translocations and the gen-esis of B-cell-derived tumors in mice and men. *Cell* 32:311–315.

19. Rowley, J. D. 1983. Human oncogene locations and chromosome aberrations. *Nature* 301:290–291.

20. Gelmann, E. P., Psallidopoulos, M. C., Papas, T. S., Dalla-Favera,

R. 1984. Identification of reciprocal translocation sites within the c-myc oncogene and immunoglobulin mu locus in a Burkitt lymphoma. *Nature* 306:799–803.

21. Croce, C. M., Thierfelder, W., Erikson, J., Nishikura, K., Finan, J., Lenoir, GM., Nowell, P. C. 1983. Transcriptional activation of an unrearranged and untranslocated c-myc oncogene by translocation of a C lambda locus in Burkitt. *Proc. Natl. Acad. Sci. USA* 80:6922–6926.

22. Erikson, J., ar-Rushdi, A., Drwinga, H. L., Nowell, P. C., Croce, C. M. 1983. Transcriptional activation of the translocated c-myc oncogene in Burkitt lymphoma. *Proc. Natl. Acad. Sci. USA* 80:820–824.

23. Hollis, G. F., Mitchell, K. F., Battey, J., Potter, H., Taub, R., Lenoir, G. M., Leder, P. 1984. A variant translocation places the lambda immunoglobulin genes 3' to the c-myc oncogene in Burkitt's lymphoma. *Nature* 307:752–755.

24. Duesberg, P. H. 1985. Activated proto-onc genes: Sufficient or necessary for cancer? *Science* 228:669–677.

88. J. Erikson et al., *Proc. Natl. Acad. Sci. USA* 80, 7581 (1983).

71. P. Leder, J. Battev, G. Lenoir, C. Mouldine, W. Murphy, H. Potter, T. Stewart, R. Tate, *Science* 222, 765 (1983).

86. Hollis et al., *Nature* (London), 307, 752 (1984).

87. M. Davis, S. Malcolm, T. H. Rabbitts, *Nature*(London), 308, 286 (1984).

89. J. Battey et al., *Cell* 34, 779 (1983).

90. E. H. Westin et al., *Proc. Natl. Acad. Sci. USA* 79, 2490 (1982).

91. R. T. Maguirq, T. S. Robins, S. S. Thorgersson, C. A. Hedman, ibid. 80, 1947 (1983).

92. P. H. Hamlyn and T. H. Rabbitts, *Nature* (London), 304, 135 (1983).

93. R. Taub et al., *Cell* 36, 339 (1984).

74. D. J. Slamon, J. B. deKemion, I. M. Verma, M. J. Cline, *Science* 224, 256 (1984).

41. J. Campis, H. E. Gray, A. B. Pardee, M. Dean, E. Sonenshein, *Cell* 36, 241 (1984).

25. *Ibid.* References therein:

100. N. G. Copeland and G. M. Cooper, *J. Virol.* 33, 1199 (1980).

101. J. A. Lautenberger, R. A. Schulz, C. F. Garon, P. H. Tsichlis, T. S. Papas, *Proc. Natl. Acad. Sci. USA* 78, 1518 (1981).

102. K. Quade, *Virology* 98, 461 (1979).

26. *Ibid.* References therein:

69. Diamond, G. M. Cooper, J. Ritz, M. A. Lane, *Nature* 305, 112 (1983).

103. G. Goubin, D. S. Goldman, J. Lute, P. E. Neiman, G. M. Cooper, *Nature,* 302, 114 (1983).

74. D. J. Slamon, J. B. deKemion, I. M. Verma, M. J. Cline, *Science* 224, 256 (1984).

27. Devine, J. M. 1986. Mechanism of activation of HuBlym-1 gene unresolved. *Nature* 321:437–439.

28. Shilo, B. Z., Weinberg, R. A. 1981. Unique transforming gene in carcinogen-transformed mouse cells. *Nature* 289:607–609.

29. Duesberg, P. H. 1985. Activated proto-onc genes: Sufficient or necessary for cancer? *Science* 228:669–677.

67. C. J. Tabin et al., *Nature* (London) 300, 143 (1982).

110. D. J. Capon, E. Y. Chen, A. D. Levinson, P. H. Seeburg, D. V. Goeddel, *Nature* 302, 33 (1983).

111. T. Finkel, J. D. Channing, G. M. Cooper, *Cell* 37, 151 (1984).

112. E. P. Reddy, R. K. Reynolds, E. Santos. M. Barbacid, *Nature* 300, 149 (1982).

113. A. P. Feinberg, B. Vogelstein, M. J. Droller, S. B. Baylin, B. D. Nelkin, *Science* 220, 1175 (1983).

114. E. Santos et al., ibid. 223, 661 (1984).

115. R. Muschel and G. Khoury, personal communication.

54. H. Land, L. F. Parada, R. A. Weinberg, *Nature* (London) 304, 596 (1983).

70. H. E. Ruley, *Nature* (London) 304, 602 (1983).

116. R. Sager, K. Tanaka, C. C. Lau, Y. Ebina, A. Anisowicz, *Proc. Natl. Acad. Sci. USA* 80, 7601 (1983).

117. J. J. Harvey and J. East, *Int. Rev. Exp. Pathol.* 10, 265 (1971).

118. J. A. Levy, *J. Natl. Cancer Inst.* 46, 1001 (1971).

119. S. A. Aaronson and G. I. Todaro, *Nature* (London) 225, 458 (1970).

120. S. A. Aaronson and C. A. Weaver, *J. Gen. Virol.* 13, 245 (1971).

121. V. Klement, M. Friedman, R. McAllister, W. Nelson-Rees, R. J. Huebner, *J. Natl. Cancer Inst.* 47, 65 (1971).

122. L. M. Pfeffer and L. Kopelvich, *Cell* 10, 313 (1977).

123. J. A. Levy, *Nature* (London) 253, 140 (1975).

30. Land, H., Parada, L. F., and Weinberg, R. A. 1983. Tumorigenic conversion of primary embryo fibroblasts requires at least two cooperating oncogenes. *Nature* 304:596–602.

31. Land, H., Parada, L. F., and Weinberg, R. A. 1983. Cellular onco-genes and multistep carcinogenesis. *Science* 222:771–778.

32. Ruley, H. E. 1983. Adenovirus early region 1A enables viral and cellular transforming genes to transform primary cells in culture. *Nature* 304:602–606.

33. Zhou, R.-P., and Duesberg, P. H. 1988. *myc* protooncogene linked to retroviral promoter, but not to enhancer, transforms embryo cells. *Proc. Natl. Acad. Sci. USA* 85:2924–2928.

34. Chakraborty, A. K., Cichutek, K., and Duesberg, P. H. 1991. Trans-forming function of proto-*ras* genes depends on heterologous promot-ers and is enhanced by specific point mutations. *Proc. Natl. Acad. Sci. USA* 88:2217–2221.

35. Cairns, J. 1978. *Cancer, Science and Society* (New York: W. H. Freeman and Co.).

36. Bialy, H. 1984. The molecular biology of cancer. *Bio/Technology* 2:848.

37. Stewart, T. A., Pattengale, P. K., and Leder, P. 1984. Spontaneous mammary adenocarcinomas in transgenic mice that carry and express MTV/*myc* fusion genes. *Cell* 38:627–637.

38. Bishop, J. M. 1985. Trends in Oncogenes. *Trends in Genetics* 2:245–249.

39. Weinberg, R. A. 1985. The action of oncogenes in the cytoplasm and nucleus. *Science* 230:770–776.

40. Hall, S. S. 1987. *Invisible Frontiers: The Race to Synthesize a Human Gene (New York: Atlantic Monthly Press)*.

41. Duesberg, P. H., and Cichutek, K. 1987, pp. 75-88. Ras genes trans-form without mutant codons and are possibly activated by truncation of a newly defined *ras* exon. A Perspective on Biology and Medicine in the 21st Century: Proceedings of a Dedicatory Symposium sponsored by Eli Lilly & Co., held in Indianapolis on 27–30 October, 1985, *International Congress and Symposium Series* 121, ed. Irving S. Johnson (London: Royal Society of Medicine Services).

42. Johnson, I. 1987. p. 88. Discussion of the Duesberg paper above. *In:* A Perspective on Biology and Medicine in the 21st Century: Proceed-ings of a Dedicatory Symposium sponsored by Eli Lilly & Co., held in Indianapolis on 27–30 October, 1985, *International Congress and Sym-posium Series* 121 (London: Royal Society of Medicine Services).

43. Duesberg, P. H., and Cichutek, K. 1986. Harvey ras genes trans-form without mutant codons, apparently activated by truncation of a

. . . .

5' exon (exon-1). *Proc. Natl. Acad. Sci. USA* 83:2340–2344.

44. Letter from George Poste to Peter Duesberg, September 21, 1987, preserved in the *Peter H. Duesberg Archive* of the Bancroft Library of the Univ. of California, Berkeley.

3

··

One for the Gipper

In the early fall of 1986 the Waxsman Institute of Rutgers University opened its biotechnology research center and David Praemer, Waxsman's director, graciously asked me to help him organize a one-day mini-symposium to commemorate the event. I took the opportunity to invite Barry Bloom from the Albert Einstein College of Medicine to speak about his work on leprosy, which was beginning to receive the attention it deserved. This was, in part, because one of the initial promises of the new biotechnologies was that recombinant DNA manipulations would allow effective vaccines against previously intractable diseases that affected, almost entirely, the world's poor. Unfortunately this promise has been all but forgotten, so that nobly ambitious and completely attainable projects—like the creation of a vaccine against malaria, which demonstrably kills more than one million children a year in the Third World—no longer appear prominently in the prospectuses of pharmaceutical companies or multinational world health organizations.

My other invitee was Peter, who was spending the year at the NIH in Bethesda, Maryland, on a Fogarty Fellowship. The telephone reports of what he was up to prompted me to ask him to speak about human leukemia viruses, another area of biotechnological interest since new tests with which to detect these viruses could be devised and patented. As opposed to proto-oncogenes and the concomitant intricacies of even an infantile cancer molecular biology, microbial disease agents were familiar concepts; and as the arguments Peter had outlined to me over the past few months were straightforward and provocative, I thought the audience at Rutgers would also enjoy hearing them. And they did. Driving back to NYC with Barry after the symposium, we spoke about Peter's engaging, humorous, and scientifically persuasive presentation of the case that human leukemia viruses were agents of leukemia in name only. We also agreed that his remarks at the end of the talk were probably a disservice to the previous forty minutes. In the closing moments, Peter said that many of the same arguments just presented with regard to HTLV-I (a so-called human leukemia virus) were also applicable to HTLV-III, one of the original three names for the virus now known as HIV—or, as it is designated in the *de rigueur* style manuals of newspapers like *The New York Times,* "HIV, the virus that causes AIDS," in case we might forget.

I remember saying to Peter after his talk that although I could find no fault with any of his remarks concerning retroviral cancers, I was not at all persuaded by these same arguments when applied to a retroviral pathogen, which, as HTLV-III was said to do, killed cells instead of making them grow abnormally. As he was hurrying to catch a plane, Peter's reply was brief, and in light of what was to come, unforgettable: "In a few months I will send you a manuscript that will answer your objections." The manuscript, "Retroviruses as carcinogens and pathogens: Expectations and reality," which appeared in the March 1987 issue of the journal *Cancer Research,*[1] is perhaps the defining article of Peter's life in science. Once committed to the standard of proof he demanded then, it was impossible for him to settle for anything less. And because AIDS quickly became the world's most fearsome disease, this commitment (some might say obsession) would consume his attention and result in disastrous professional consequences. It would also make it easy for his other scientific opponents to dismiss ongoing experimental tests and theoretical critiques of oncogene theory as the tired old horse of the guy who refuses to accept that HIV causes AIDS.

The circumstances under which the review was written bear an interesting symmetry to the 1983 *Nature* article that first opened the schism between Peter and his retrovirologist colleagues, who by 1986 had essentially all converted to the "genetic paradigm,"[2] as J. Michael Bishop would refer to the shift from the study of retroviral *onc* genes to the quest for transforming function in their cellular counterparts. Once the *Cancer Research* review was published, the rift, which had already widened significantly, would quickly become a chasm.

Peter was spending the year with Stuart Aaronson and Robert Huebner at the NIH's Tumor Virus Laboratory as the indirect result of a recent "site visit." Site visits are part of the due diligence process the NIH uses to make sure that the investigators who are spending American taxpayer dollars are doing so in a reasonable fashion. That Peter was still a designated "inspector general" speaks both to his unblemished reputation as a peerless experimentalist (despite Weinberg's aspersions at the Lilly Symposium) and the fact that the NIH was the last bastion of retroviral tumor biology, and so the home of his few remaining allies. During the course of the site visit, Peter had spoken at length to Aaronson about the ongoing controversy between himself and Weinberg concerning the need for specific mutations to "activate" the 3T3 transforming functions of proto-*ras*. Both Aaronson and Huebner agreed that this was an absolutely critical question, and they suggested to Peter that he spend a year in their lab doing a few more experiments to nail the point down. They were so enthusiastic about these experiments that they arranged a prestigious Fogarty Fellowship, which would give Peter the opportunity to complete this work in an unrestricted environment free of teaching and the other academic duties of Berkeley.

There was probably more to the invitation than purely the desire to midwife emergent truth. The rapid rise of the cellular oncogene concept was making it clear that "oncogenes" were very likely to be the subject of a Nobel Prize sometime soon, and which group of cancer geneticists would be its beneficiary was still an open question. Would it go to the first generation of onco-geneticists, who following in Peyton Rous' footsteps (who received his Prize in 1966, at the age of eighty-seven) had finally figured out what it was that made the Rous sarcoma virus tumorigenic? Or would the prize go to the relative newcomers who had all but eliminated the virus from the cancer causation equation? Peter's incorrigible efforts to preserve the scientific premise of proving functionality before assigning the prefix "onco" to any but viral genes was seen by Huebner, Aaronson, Gallo, and others at the NIH as being definitely beneficial to their cause. In line with these expectations, Peter's stay did provide the final elements of the demonstration of what it took to convert a normal cellular proto-*ras* gene into an oncogenic variant by showing that the addition of a Harvey sarcoma virus promoter to an unaltered (or native) proto-*ras* gene was the critical variable in conferring transforming function.[3] The rest of his time, however, was spent in a way that made at least one of his Fogarty supporters, Robert Gallo, wish he had never heard of Peter H. Duesberg.

This came about because another NIH senior scientist, Peter Mage, was then editor of *Cancer Research,* and in much the same spirit as Peter Newmark a few years earlier, he invited his namesake to look at the evidence that retroviruses without *onc* genes play any significant role in cancer. Gallo was the prime mover in floating the idea that a retrovirus he had isolated and named HTLV-I was the cause of adult T-cell leukemia, and he was also the most prominent proponent of the idea that another human retrovirus—which he had obtained from Luc Montagnier at the Institut Pasteur and claimed to have independently isolated[4-7]—was the cause of AIDS. The analysis by Duesberg that appeared in 1987 would demolish the former idea. If that was not enough to end their collegial relationship, the fact that Peter would go on in the same article to seriously undermine the logical and scientific bases (if not yet the popularity) of the latter hypothesis, certainly was.

When I asked Peter why he was not content with restricting the 1987 critique to the relevance of retroviruses to human cancer, and leaving AIDS alone, his answer was immediate.

It was largely a personal matter. I could not refrain from looking hard at any hypothesis Bob [Gallo] was behind. It's exactly as Gunther [Stent] said to me when we talked about this very point years ago: "If Crick publishes it, you read it thinking it right. With Gallo, it's the opposite." In addition, there was the complete improbability of the virus-AIDS hypothesis on first principle, and I just couldn't ignore it.

The first principle Peter was referring is that the defining characteristic of retroviruses is an absolute dependence on continued division of their host in order to complete their own life cycles. Thus retroviruses do not typically kill cells. The fact that they sometimes did the opposite, i.e., caused cells to grow uncontrollably, was the reason the entire NIH Tumor Virus Laboratory even existed.

To summarize the situation as it was when Duesberg accepted Mage's invitation: Despite its overall lack of success in winning the war on cancer,[8-10] the NIH had garnered three apparent victories by focusing essentially all of its resources for fifteen years on retroviruses. First, the identification of retroviral *onc* genes by Duesberg and Vogt led directly to the elaboration of the cellular oncogene concept. Secondly, after years of fruitless effort, a virus was identified that could be epidemiologically associated (albeit as we shall see rather unimpressively) with an almost numerically insignificant human leukemia. And lastly, the same drastic laboratory manipulations had been adopted to identify a human retrovirus unlike any the world had ever known. This latter achievement prompted U.S. Secretary of Health and Human Services Margaret Heckler in her 1984 press conference announcing the identification by a "U.S. government scientist of the probable cause of AIDS" to proudly claim justified all the time, money, and effort that had been put into the virus-cancer program of the NIH.[11] Peter had already made it clear what he thought of the first victory. In "Retroviruses as Carcinogens and Pathogens: Expectations and Reality" he would be just as emphatic regarding the remaining two.

Like the previous reviews, the one in *Cancer Research,* which ran under the journal's section heading as a "Perspective," is exhaustive. In this case, consuming twenty-two full pages and containing 278 literature references. As anyone who knows Peter, or has ever debated him, will attest, this encyclopedic knowledge of a vast scientific literature, in several languages, is quite real. With such a comprehensive overview (compiled, years before Pub. Med., "the old-fashioned way, one paper at a time"), charges of selective citation in order to bolster only one's own position are not really credible. And similarly to its predecessors, the *Cancer Research* review is written with the authority of someone who had spent by then almost twenty years working with these notoriously tricky viruses so impeccably that not a single experimental flaw was present in 120 peer-reviewed scientific papers he authored and of which they were the subject.[12] The same, unfortunately, cannot be said of his soon-to-be implacable, and powerful, scientific adversaries, Robert Gallo and Myron Essex, whose problems with keeping a clean laboratory are near legendary among molecular biologists.

The first part of the "Perspective" deals with retroviruses as agents of cancer. Then, as now, most of the data available for analysis came from animal retroviruses and their associated tumors; the relevance to human cancer remains completely restricted to the opening paragraphs justifying grant applications. I will not attempt therefore to reconstruct Peter's elegantly interwoven continuity of various, sometimes quite complicated, arguments, that even his most ferocious opponents acknowledge is masterful. But with regard to HTLV-I, the best candidate for a clinically relevant human cancer virus, he makes the following points.

*HTLV-I or ATLV (adult T-cell leukemia virus) was originally isolated from a human cell line derived from a patient with T-cell leukemia (71). It replicates in T-cells (27) and also in endothelial cells (76) or fibroblasts (77). The virus was subsequently shown, using antiviral antibody for detection, to be endemic as latent, asymptomatic infections in Japan and the Caribbean (27). Since virus expression is undetectably low not only in healthy but also in leukemic virus carriers, infections must be diagnosed indirectly by antiviral antibody or biochemically by searching for latent proviral DNA. Due to the complete and consistent latency, the virus can be isolated from infected cells only after acti-*vation in vitro *when it is no longer controlled by the host's antiviral immunity and suppressors. Therefore the virus is not naturally transmitted as a cell-free agent like other pathogenic viruses, but only congenitally, sexually, or by blood transfusion, that is, by contacts that involve exchange of infected cells (13, 27).*

It is often pointed out that functional evidence for the virus-cancer hypothesis is difficult to obtain in humans because experimental infection is not possible. However, this argument does not apply here since naturally and chronically infected, asymptomatic human carriers are abundant. Yet most infections never lead to leukemias and none have ever been observed to cause viremias (the presence in blood or other tissue of significant numbers of infectious virus particles). Moreover, not a single adult T-cell leukemia was observed in recipients of blood transfusions from virus-positive donors (13, 78, 79), although recipients developed antiviral antibody (81).

The incidence of adult T-cell leukemia among Japanese with antiviral immunity is estimated to be only 0.06% based on 339 cases of T-cell leukemia among 600,000 antibody-positive subjects (78). Other studies have detected antiviral antibody in healthy Swedish donors (268) and in 3.4% of 1.2 x 10^6 healthy Japanese blood donors (79). Further, it was reported that 0.9% of the people of Taiwan are antibody-positive, but the incidence of the leukemia was not mentioned (80).

In conclusion, the tumor risk of the statistically most relevant group of retrovirus infections, namely the latent natural infections with antiviral immunity, is very low. It averages less than 0.1% in different species, as it is less than 1% in domestic chickens, undetectably low in wild mice, 0.04% in cattle, and 0.06% in humans.[13]

Of course, it could be argued that a low incidence is exactly what is seen in most viral and other microbial diseases in which not everyone infected succumbs. The reason for this, however, is that in such cases the incidence of disease represents the proportion of the infections that have managed to avoid the host's immunologic and other defenses. It does not reflect a spectrum of pathogenic potential across the invading microbe. But this otherwise valid argument is not applicable to ATL and HTLV-I, since the virus is totally immunologically suppressed in both healthy and leukemic carriers, as Peter emphasizes in the passage quoted above.

Yet even if one were to make the *ad hoc* hypothesis that in one in a thousand human carriers of HTLV-I the virus does something (after all, science is full of surprises) to induce a leukemia, such a hypothesis could still not explain the single most problematic fact for cancer virologists of all persuasions. Cancer is a monoclonal disease. Each T-cell leukemia is derived from a single, initially transformed cell. Thus, even if only one percent of a person's susceptible T-cells were infected, this would still mean that one cell in one million becomes cancerous, and then only after the 10–100 generations corresponding to the ten- to twenty-year interval between infection and disease. The arithmetic is straightforward. The probability of a cell infected with HTLV-I turning malignant is one in a million (the number of infected cells) multiplied by 10–100, or one in 10–100 million.

But biologists, even of the molecular variety, are not noted for being overly enamored with these kinds of arguments, preferring empiricism to calculation. And as we have emphasized numerous times, functional demonstration is the ultimate requirement for all theories of causation. So if HTLV-I is an agent of transformation, even with extremely low efficiency, it should be possible to show this using primary human T-lymphocytes growing in culture, where enough cells could be infected for enough time to observe even a very rare cancerous conversion. If accomplished, such a demonstration would be the first example of a retrovirus without an *onc* gene capable of a malignant transformation, and almost certainly earned Gallo the Nobel he has coveted for as long as anyone has known him.

However, the best that he, his close friend and sometime collaborator Flossie Wong-Staal, and others from their laboratory could produce was a report of experiments in which they were able to occasionally generate an immortal T-cell line after infection with HTLV-I.[14] As noted before, continuous growth in culture is not at all equivalent to malignant transformation, and is not a general property of cancerous cells biopsied from human patients. Nonetheless, even this "partial success" is not without serious problems. Peter comments on them as follows:

> *The assay infects about 5 x 10^6 primary human lymphocytes with HTLV-I. However, less than one of these cells survives the incubation period of 30 to 60 days, termed "crisis" because the resulting immortal cells are monoclonal with regard to the proviral integration site, and because only 4 of 23 such experiments generate immortal cells (115). Since no virus expression is observed during the critical selection period of the immortal cell and since some immortalized cells contain only defective proviruses (115), immortalization is not a viral gene function. Further it is unlikely that the integration site of the provirus is relevant to the process of immortalization, since different lines have different integration sites (115). Indeed, spontaneous immortalization of primary human lymphocytes has been reported applying this assay to simian viruses (113).... Finally, immortalized cell lines with defective viruses (115) or no viruses (113) indicate that immortalization is a virus-independent, spontaneous event.[15]*

To a first approximation, this constellation of arguments would seem to have had as little effect as those mustered against cellular oncogenes in the pages of *Nature* and *Science*. HTLV-I remains in the major textbooks as the cause of ATL, and the U.S. Red Cross spends about $10 on every unit of donated blood to test for antibodies to this virus, even though no instance of transfusion-related ATL has ever been recorded. But this is a relatively small price to pay for the propaganda value of being able to say "the

American blood supply is free of leukemia viruses."

A closer look, however, reveals a slightly different picture. Real-world indicators of the popularity (importance) of a scientific hypothesis are how much money is spent on it; which and how many laboratories work on the problem; and how many and in which journals their findings are published. By any of these measures, retroviral leukemias (and lymphomas) are the last subject any professor working today on cancer would advise her students to study. The almost total scientific obscurity into which the entire field of human cancer retrovirology has fallen is exemplified by a review article, "Human retroviruses: their role in cancer,"[16] which appeared at the very end of 1999. Its author, William Blattner, a long-time colleague of Gallo from the NIH, moved with his friend to the University of Maryland when Gallo was given his own Institute of Human Virology in 1995, despite being an unindicted co-conspirator in several criminal investigations involving HIV.[4,6,17,18]

Significantly, the article was published in the *Proceedings of the Association of American Physicians,* a journal of such minor importance that the Institute for Scientific Information—which invented the currently used and all-important rating system for scientific journals, called the "impact factor"—places it at number 73 out of the 100 publications in its category of General Medicine. That the review appears in such a journal is not accidental. As Blattner admits in the paper's abstract: "After a long latent period, adult T-cell leukemia/lymphoma (ATL) occurs in 1 per 1000 carriers per year, resulting in 2500–3000 cases per year worldwide."[16] Hard to get too excited about these kinds of numbers.

Further, it is only in a journal read (if at all) by physicians that Blattner could claim the following: "For human T-cell leukemia virus 1 (HTLV-I), the viral regulatory *tax* gene product is responsible for enhanced transcription of viral and cellular genes that promote cell growth by stimulating various growth factors and through dysregulation of cellular regulatory suppressor genes, such as *p53*."[16] This somewhat bold, although characteristically vague, attribution of a tumorigenic activity to a gene of HTLV-I is close to nonsensical. Since the putative activating protein of HTLV-I is essential for replication, all cells in which the virus replicates should be transformed. This is clearly not the case. Further, this gene cannot be relevant for transformation since human HTLV-I-infected leukemic cells do not even produce viral RNAs or proteins.

A similar reassignment to the scientific backwaters, however, was not to befall Gallo's other human lymphotropic virus, HTLV-III, which is the subject of more than 130,000 papers, a large number of which are published in the most prominent journals, and has consumed upwards of $50 billion since its identification in 1984.

The second part of Peter's *Cancer Research* "Perspective" concerns the pathogenic potential of this remarkably close genetic relative of HTLV-I that now travels with a universally accepted passport stamped "HIV, the virus that causes AIDS."

It is probably fair to write that almost everyone reading this book would agree with the following: The virus known as HIV is said to cause AIDS, after unpredictable periods averaging more than ten years, by progressively destroying a key component of the human immunologic defense system called the T4-cell. As a result of this, the victim becomes abnormally susceptible to a large variety of other microbial pathogens, which themselves are the direct causes of the AIDS-defining diseases. It may therefore come as a surprise to learn, as Peter and I were to discover from a fax we received on March 2, 1995, that John Maddox does not.

Writing in regard to his decision to withdraw a previous offer in the pages of *Nature* earlier in the year in which we were challenged to reply to some recent papers he had published[19] that claimed to provide, after twelve years, a "new view of HIV," he rejected this presentation of the "old view" given above as follows: "On the contrary, the 'HIV-hypothesis' is much simpler: HIV causes AIDS, in some manner not understood; most of those infected will develop the disease."[20]

John can perhaps be excused for being a little giddy, as he was only months away from retirement and had just been knighted. Plus, the landmark papers of David Ho and his colleagues, as we will see by the end of this chapter, really did provide an entirely new view of HIV, and one that has quickly undone almost a century of hard work by prior generations of virologists. But Maddox's version notwithstanding, hypotheses of disease causation are usually more specific. Thus, in a style that will by now be familiar, Peter could examine the evidence that supported the "complicated" version of the HIV-AIDS hypothesis presented above without facing the accusation, contained in the same letter, of resorting to "the old Goebbels' technique, that of creating a straw man from a farrago of indefensible propositions and then knocking it down."[20]

Considering Peter's childhood in the outskirts of a war-ravaged Frankfurt, and the censorship and persecution of scientists in Nazi Germany, Maddox's remark is, at best, insensitive. In fact it caused Peter noticeable pain and anger, although by then he had been very publicly accused on numerous occasions of apparently much worse, and his professional life was in shambles.

But let's examine just where things did stand regarding the evidence that HIV is a pathogenic retrovirus that kills T4-cells and thereby causes AIDS, in March 1987 when the virus-AIDS hypothesis was not quite the statement of belief with which Mr. Maddox confuses it. In Peter's words:

The isolation in 1983 of a retrovirus from a human patient with lymphoadenopathy, a typical symptom of AIDS, led to the proposal that the virus, now termed lymphadenopathy-

....

associated virus, is the cause of AIDS (26). Related viruses, termed HTLV-III, ARV, or HIV (209), have since been isolated from about one-half of the AIDS patients that have been sampled (210–214). In the United States about 26,000 AIDS cases and 15,000 AIDS fatalities have been reported between 1981, when the disease was first identified (215), and October 1986 (216).... Antibody to the virus is found in about 90% of AIDS patients and correlates with chronic latent infection by the virus (217–221). Because of the nearly complete correlation between AIDS and immunity against the virus, the virus is generally assumed to be the cause of AIDS (13, 27). Accordingly, detection of antiviral antibody, rather than virus, is now most frequently used to diagnose AIDS and those at risk for AIDS (27, 217–224).[21]

And after spending several thousand words assessing the totality of the available scientific literature on the relationship between this retrovirus and AIDS, he concludes as follows:

At this time the hypothesis that the virus causes AIDS faces several direct challenges. (a) First it fails to explain why active antiviral immunity, which includes neutralizing antibody (225–227) and which effectively prevents virus spread and expression, would not prevent the virus from causing a fatal disease. This is particularly paradoxical since antiviral immunity or "vaccination" typically protects against viral pathogenicity. (b) The hypothesis is also challenged by direct evidence that the virus is not sufficient to cause AIDS. This includes (i) the low percentage of symptomatic infections, (ii) the fact that some infected groups are at a relatively high and others at no risk for AIDS, (iii) the long latent period of the disease (Section B), and (iv) the genetic evidence that the virus lacks a late AIDS function. Since all viral genes are essential for virus replication (28, 245), the virus should kill T-cells and hence cause AIDS at the time of infection rather than 5 years later. (c) The hypothesis also fails to resolve the contradiction that the AIDS virus, like all retroviruses, depends on mitosis for replication yet is postulated to be directly cytocidal (Section D). (d) The hypothesis offers no convincing explanation for the paradox that a fatal disease would be caused by a virus that is latent and biochemically inactive and that infects less than 1% and is expressed in less than 0.01% of susceptible lymphocytes (Section D). In addition the hypothesis cannot explain why the virus is not pathogenic in asymptomatic infections, since there is no evidence that the virus is more active or further spread in carriers with than in carriers without AIDS.[22]

We will look at some of the responses over the years to several of these challenges in the next chapter. For the remainder of this one, however, we will focus on the most serious of them: How could such an apparently biochemically inactive virus cause so much havoc? It was for finally providing what was advertised as a resolution of this "paradox" that David Ho found himself on the cover of *Time* magazine as "Man of the Year" in 1996.

In the months after the published version of the *Cancer Research* review appeared, I telephoned a number of friends and working acquaintances to elicit their opinions. Among them were Walter Gilbert, George Poste, and Anthony Fauci, all—to a greater or lesser degree—committed to the virus-AIDS hypothesis. Yet not one characterized Peter's argument as "a farrago of indefensible propositions" created solely for the purpose of demolishing it. In fact, the only significant difference in their replies centered on his use of the term "paradox." To those scientists inclined, for one or another reason, to view the virus-AIDS hypothesis sympathetically, Peter's catalog of oddities came under the heading of "mysteries to be explained by future research," as Jay Levy was to phrase it later in the pages of *Nature*.[23] Indeed, the most frequently used counter-argument to the critique above was some version of: AIDS is new; therefore its cause is new. And if HIV is a new retrovirus, why shouldn't it have new properties? It was, after all, as Paul Simon wrote in his haunting song *Boy in the Bubble*, "a time of miracles and wonders, and lasers in the jungle." Or as Howard Temin, the best living authority on "new" as it applied to both molecular biology and retrovirology, argued— joining his name to those of Blattner and Gallo in the pages of *Science* in 1988—since RNA had recently been shown to be able to function as an enzyme (a property previously reserved only for proteins), HIV could just as plausibly be the cause of AIDS.[24]

But to those inclined to be a little skeptical about the hypothesis, the same counter-argument assumed a very different form: Attributing hitherto unobserved and unorthodox properties to a recently described virus that had not been shown to be significantly genetically different from its well-known and essentially harmless relatives was quite a radical idea. Therefore it required substantial experimental evidence before it could, or should be, taken seriously.

In 2000, I asked Peter something I had asked before: Why didn't he write a hefty NIH grant, like most of his buddies, to study some abstruse retroviral phenomena for which he otherwise might not be able to find funding in the rapidly shrinking field of cancer retrovirology, by claiming they were or could be related to HIV and AIDS? His answer was the same each time. *"Believe me, if I could have come up with a single experiment that I might have done to disprove the hypothesis, I would have written a grant in a minute. But there was no way I could take a dollar to work on pretense."*

Since it is apparently true that one cannot prove a negative, Peter was left only to point out inconsistencies and lacunae in the virus-AIDS hypothesis. As noted above, the single most important inconsistency between traditional medical virology and a viral explanation for AIDS lay in the issue of how much virus actually is present in persons infected and either symptomatic or free of AIDS-defining diseases.

When I telephoned Anthony Fauci in the summer of 1987 that was mostly what we talked about. We began by agreeing it was a shame he was not able to attend Peter's Fogarty Lecture at the NIH, although he had of course read the article when it appeared in *Cancer Research*. Then he asked me which of the arguments did I think was strong enough to counter the already massive amount of accumulated consensus? My answer was that I could find no way to reconcile the miniscule amounts of viral gene expression in infected T-cells, and the corresponding extreme difficulty in isolating virus from AIDS patients with the hallmark of their AIDS diagnosis—namely the non-regenerable amputation of the T-cell arm of the immune system. He replied by agreeing that this was indeed the best point Peter had made, but that some very recent papers had already addressed it. The problems were mainly technical ones that had to do with assaying this particular retrovirus in standard ways, but there were now reliable new techniques showing significant viral activity that coincided with a drastic depletion of T-cells.

Some readers might discern a certain resonance with the NIH 3T3 cell and the lack of functional proof of cellular transforming activity associated with proto-oncogenes before its adventitious arrival. When standard assays fail to provide the required answers, new ones with which to keep a popular hypothesis afloat can always be devised. The references that Fauci provided a few days later prompted an editorial commentary for *Bio/Technology* entitled "Where is the Virus? And Where is the Press?"[25] in which I pointed out an obvious and fatal flaw in these first-generation new techniques[26-29] for measuring HIV by means of a surrogate biochemical marker, instead of the real biological parameter, infection.

In this case, the biochemical surrogate for infectious HIV is called "p24 antigenemia" and it was supposed to detect the number of HIV particles present in a patient's serum by measuring the amount of a particular virus protein with a molecular mass of 24 kiloDaltons that is at the core of HIV and every other infectious retrovirus. Today almost nobody, including AIDS physicians, even remembers the term, let alone uses the results of such assays in assessing the clinical status of their patients. Instead, they rely on the second-generation of assays that detect surrogate biochemical markers as the basis to administer potent, toxic "anti-viral" chemicals. These tests, made familiar by David Ho and *Nature* in 1995,[30] produce a number suggestively termed the "viral load," which has so clearly supplanted "p24 antigenemia" it outscored its predecessor by 2,250 to 82 in scientific publications in the scant five years between then and the end of the last century.

But first-generation surrogates first. The spate of papers Fauci sent claimed to have answered the central problem of so little virus and so much disease by demonstrating that in fact there was ample virus present in the blood of patients during the late stages of AIDS. But they made this claim based on an assay that detected a virus-specific protein, not the virus itself. Since viral protein is present in an infected person in different forms, e.g. in the blood, as part of an infectious virus or complexed with antibodies that effectively render it incapacitated, or inside phagocytic white blood cells where it is also non-infectious, the results of tests based on measuring virus protein might be difficult to interpret correctly. In fact, the problem turns out to be severe enough to render the tests worthless. The amounts of protein reported in these papers imply a quantity of infectious virus of more than 100,000 particles per milliliter of blood, because the authors claim to detect upwards of 50 picograms (pg) of p24 protein per milliliter. A picogram is one thousand billionth of a gram. Not much, but a retrovirus is one thousand times lighter, and only one half of its weight is p24. The appropriate long division shows that 50 pg correspond to 100,000 virus particles, an amount that if actually present would not require any special biochemical assay to detect. Such quantities of virus would be easily observed by electron microscopy or by standard biological assays. Yet none of the papers showed anything resembling such a real viremia, and one[26] reported that no virus at all could be found in thirty-one "antigenemic" patients, even after extensive *in vitro* cultivation of more than one million of their T-cells, accompanied by the harsh treatments necessary to wake a sleepy retrovirus like HIV.

The authors of the various studies I questioned in the *Bio/Technology* piece never answered these objections in print: perhaps because they "could not take time from their busy schedules to correct my simple-minded and erroneous calculation," as I was informed on a few occasions. Or maybe, because the basic error was not in the calculation but in the assay itself, they simply "could not." In either case, the test never became particularly popular, as the citation numbers above reflect. Even in its heyday between 1987 and 1995, "p24 antigenemia" was cited in only 144 publications. Nonetheless, viral antigenemia would become the basis for a remarkable exchange between Prof. Duesberg and one of his formidable scientific foes in Washington, DC, in the spring of 1988. The occasion was a panel discussion sponsored by the American Foundation for AIDS Research (AmFAR), Elizabeth Taylor's favorite charity.

The event, to which seventeen privileged journalists, of which I was one, were invited, was held on the campus of George Washington University and promoted by AmFAR as "A Scientific Forum on the Etiology of AIDS." It was, in the words of their fact sheet: "... convened to critically examine the evidence that human immunodeficiency virus (HIV) or other agents give rise to the disease complex known as AIDS. Data from laboratory, clinical, and epidemiological research will be presented and evaluated. The forum seeks no consensus, instead it is designed to permit discussion among experts on the conclusions the facts permit."

In contrast to these noble objectives, the actual purpose of the event was more accurately described after the fact by Michael Specter, a mainstream AIDS journalist for the *Washington Post,* who is no friend of Peter's, as follows: "Billed as a scientific forum on the cause of AIDS, it was really an attempt to put Duesberg's theories to rest."[31] A different and detailed account of the AmFAR forum by John Lauritsen, a Harvard-educated AIDS journalist who is Peter's friend, appeared in the *New York Native,*[32] a gay newspaper critical of much of mainstream AIDS reporting. The part of this account that pertains to antigenemia was riveting then and is even more so today. As it coincides perfectly with my own recollections, and has the dual advantages of being contemporaneous with the forum while withstanding the tests of publication and time as to its accuracy, I quote from it at length below. Lauritsen begins the relevant section by describing the demeanor of one of the high-ranking field officers in the new NIH war on AIDS.

> William Haseltine, Chief of the Laboratory of Biochemical Pharmacology at the Dana Farber Cancer Center of Harvard Medical School, appeared to be an angry man. His presentation was devoted largely to personal attacks on Duesberg, in a manner which two of my colleagues described as "brutal" and "vicious." Haseltine's anger can probably be attributed to Celia Farber's interview with Duesberg in *Spin* Magazine (January 1988), in which Duesberg stated: "William Haseltine and Max Essex, who are

two of the top five AIDS researchers in the country, have millions in stock in a company they founded that has developed and will sell AIDS kits that test for HIV. How could they be objective?"

When Celia Farber contacted Haseltine, he confirmed his and Essex's business arrangement with Cambridge Bio-Science, a company that sells HIV testing kits. Said Haseltine: "I deeply resent the implication that my business investments have affected my work." Haseltine accused Duesberg of "serious confusion and misrepresentation of fact." He said that when rational arguments don't hold up, Duesberg "has resorted to personal attack; he has impugned the motivations of individuals and institutions."

So much for background, now to the theatre itself:

The most dramatic moment in the forum came when Haseltine began showing his slides; it deserves a separate section:

In presenting his first slide, Haseltine said: "This gives us a summary of the virology. Dr. Duesberg asserts that during the later phases of the disease one does not see free virus in circulation. That is not generally reflected in the patients." Pointing to his projected graph he continued, "The black line represents either virus titer or viral antigens directly detectable in the circulation. It rises later in the disease. That rise is concomitant with the period when T-cells fall. So it is not the case, the central assertion he has made in his arguments, that one does not have viremia."

At this point Duesberg asked, "Why are there no units on that slide?" Haseltine's response was, "Don't interrupt me; I didn't interrupt you." Duesberg replied, "I merely asked why the slide has no units on it." Haseltine angrily refused to answer the question, and the chairman intervened, saying that questions would have to wait until the presentation was finished.

Perhaps Duesberg ought to have waited, but one can understand his impatience. Witnessing a fast-flowing stream of propaganda, he spotted something that was obviously wrong, and wanted to confront it before the moment was lost. That his suspicions were more than justified became clear later.

In the question period following Haseltine's presentation, Harry Rubin asked Haseltine if he could provide a reference for his statement that nude mice were capable of mounting a vigorous immune response [something he had casually asserted earlier, and which is completely untrue - HB]. Haseltine said that there was a large literature on nude mice: "If you haven't read it, how can I discuss it with you?" Rubin gently replied that perhaps he had read it, but that he had only asked for a reference.

Duesberg then requested that the slide be shown on the screen again, and asked if it were an accident that the slide had no units on it. Haseltine was unable to answer the question himself, and asked Dr. Robert Redfield of the Walter Reed Army Research Institute, sitting in the audience, to explain how the slide was prepared. Redfield said something to the effect that "different measurements were used," a grossly inadequate explanation. When Duesberg persisted, Haseltine became truculent, and said that Duesberg should read the literature, because there were different measures that could be used. With no satisfactory answer forthcoming, the chairman moved on.

The truth about the Slide Without Units came out in the evening, at a party at the home of Dr. Harris Coulter. In a relaxed and convivial mood, Redfield admitted, in the presence of Duesberg, Rubin, myself, and several other wit-

nesses that the graph had been prepared to illustrate a theoretical possibility. It had no units on it for the simple reason that it was not based on any data at all. In other words,
the slide was a fake.[32]

This pure invention of how HIV should behave if it were causing AIDS has, like other things untrue, found its way into textbooks and is the basis of official U.S. government explanations
of AIDS pathogenesis. Nonetheless, among most researchers the
problem of massive cell killing by miniscule amounts of virus
(David Ho's "new view" and the popular press notwithstanding)
remains the central unanswered question about the HIV=AIDS
equation, as a Pub. Med. search of the scientific literature using
"HIV and," pathogenesis, indirect cell killing, mechanisms of cell
killing, cytocidal effects, or similar terms will quickly verify.

Besides the telephone conversation with Fauci, I had another
encounter as a result of Peter's *Cancer Research* review that
involved me deeper in the growing AIDS controversy than I ever
intended, but which also nearly got me to the basement of the
White House. It was with George Poste in the autumn of 1987,
and the circumstances were similar to our very first meeting, only
this time I was the host, and the setting was a bit more exotic
than Philadelphia. I had been asked by Nam Hai Chua, the professor of plant molecular biology at Rockefeller University, to use
my offices at the journal to help organize another inaugural symposium. On this occasion the institution to be inaugurated was
an impressive state-of-the-art Institute of Molecular and Cell
Biology, and its location was Singapore, Nam's birthplace. It
turned out to be quite a grand event, with Sydney Brenner, the
senior scientific advisor to the center, giving the keynote address.
One of our other invitations went to George Poste. At breakfast the
morning before the meeting officially convened, I asked him to
intercede with *Bio/Technology*'s editor at the time, Douglas

McCormick, regarding a "Last Word" commentary I wanted to publish, and which Doug was having third or fourth thoughts about. George was the chairman of our board of scientific advisors, and the one person whose endorsement could assuage Doug's trepidation. The piece of course was from Peter, and it was entitled "A Challenge to the AIDS Establishment."[33]

With Doug present, I showed George the one-page commentary, which was essentially a restatement of the conclusions from the *Cancer Research* review quoted earlier. Since its publication just a few months earlier, I had probably twenty-five extended conversations with scientists in the biotechnology industries who had not read the article but had heard about it, and they agreed with me that Peter's ideas deserved a more visible stage among biotechnologists than *Cancer Research* provided.

To my delight, but not surprise in light of our previous discussions, George enthusiastically endorsed publishing the "challenge." He went on to say that he had given these arguments a great deal of thought since he first read them, and he believed he could respond to at least the crucial virological ones.

As did everyone else who honestly looked at the data, George agreed that there was much too little virus present to be destroying the entire T-cell arm of the immune system by direct infection. In fact, he pointed out, the virus which was used to provide antigens for the so-called "AIDS tests" was grown in culture in a cell line derived from the same T-cells it was said to be killing in the host, but that nonetheless continued to divide while producing thousands of virus particles per cell per day. This paradox, which Peter did not raise in the *Cancer Research* article, but which he would subsequently, suggested to George that the entire immune system was necessary for HIV to do any damage, and that it did its dirty work by provoking an autoimmune disease.

His reasoning went like this: The one apparently special feature of HIV that made Gallo's hypothesis plausible to most people was that the envelope protein, which coats the virus core, has a shape that makes it fit quite nicely with a particular receptor, called CD4, that defines the specialized type of T-cell HIV preferentially infects and is said to destroy. Wasn't it therefore possible that this same HIV protein might, over unpredictable times, provoke certain very inappropriate antibodies that would contact the CD4 receptor with disastrous consequences? This extremely ingenious idea, by assigning a kind of catalytic role based on a distinctive structural feature, neatly side-stepped two of the key objections to the virus-AIDS hypothesis. Only a little virus would be necessary, and additionally pathogenesis would require an intact immune system, thus explaining why even large amounts of virus did not kill T-cells when they were growing in culture, as would be expected if uncontrolled virus replication were the real culprit.

George's hypothesis had a number of other virtues, not the least of which was that it was testable, since it predicted the existence in symptomatic AIDS patients of particular autoantibodies. Such antibodies have never been found, and thus while a real scientific response to Peter's critique, catalytic autoimmunity did not turn out to be an adequate one. However, when some evidence supporting this view of indirect pathogenesis emerged a few years later, it was cause for John Maddox to write, for the first and only time, a few moderately kind words about Peter that he would almost immediately take back.[34, 35]

When George finished his explanation, I was inspired to ask if he might be willing to foot the bill for a one-day closed-door meeting of perhaps six prominent AIDS virologists and a few other scientists, including Peter, to discuss in a no-holds-barred, notebooks-and-references-in-hand manner, the critical issues surrounding HIV pathogenesis, and that I would undertake to edit for publication in *Bio/Technology*. He said yes.

Back in New York, I began telephoning possible participants.

Among those who agreed to take part, in addition to George and Peter, were David Ho (then an assistant professor at UCLA), Dani Bolognesi (an old compatriot of Peter's in the retrovirus cancer wars who had joined the HIV officer's club and was a professor at Duke University), and Walter Gilbert (who was dividing his time between Biogen and Harvard). I was never clear as to whether Gallo would attend or not, but I had numerous conversations with Howard Streicher, his second in command, concerning the possibility. Subsequent events, however, were to render this point so moot as to be inaudible.

During the ten years *Bio/Technology* was located at 64 Bleecker Street, an historic Louis Sullivan building in lower Manhattan, I received two phone messages that created a general buzz in the office. One was from Tina Turner, who called to say she had arranged tickets for my daughter and me to her concert that weekend; the other was from James Warner, who worked in the Reagan White House as a senior policy analyst (directly under Gary Bauer, Reagan's domestic policy advisor). While the call from Tina was a completely delightful reminder of my sixties Berkeley youth when I had gotten to know her slightly, the one from Warner recalled less pleasant memories of that time when Reagan was California's governor. Why would the White House possibly be calling me?

The answer involved Chuck Ortleb, the feisty editor of the *New York Native,* who apparently had tendrils stretching into the deepest corners of Washington. Through Chuck, Warner had learned of the upcoming meeting at SmithKline, and he was wondering if I might like to move the venue to the *uber*-boss' basement. You're kidding, right? Not at all. Gary and I only want to listen, along with one or two associates. We will not say anything or otherwise interfere, and we will not record anything, I promise.

The last promise was in reference to my tongue-in-cheek

remarks about some infamous White House recordings made by Reagan's southern California buddy when he occupied the Oval Office. Warner did not appear to be amused but assured me that yes, I could bring a technician to guarantee the conference was a private affair.

I posed another condition. I wanted to also bring along my doctor's diploma from Berkeley, which contained a facsimile of the Gipper's signature, and have the President sign it for real. When he agreed, this time clearly amused, I said I would contact the various people involved and get back to him.

Surprisingly, everyone thought this was a very interesting offer, and I was able to phone Warner pretty quickly with the good word. In this conversation, I suggested that the White House now contact Gallo and Fauci and invite them directly. I thought this would end the waffling from Gallo, and while Fauci was not on the original list, I imagined he would be available to take part in a meeting on his home turf, and that his presence would be desirable even though he was neither a virologist nor an otherwise particularly distinguished scientist.

The day of our 1987 Christmas office party I spoke with Jim Warner for the last time when he called to tell me that sadly the meeting was off. He had been advised that Anthony Fauci, far from reacting as I anticipated, threw a "small fit" when he was invited, and demanded to know why the White House was interfering in scientific matters that belonged to the NIH and the Office of Science and Technology Assessment.

I have never decided whether the cancellation of my autograph session with the Gipper was really a Christmas present in disguise, and as we will see in the next chapter, this was not the last time Fauci pre-empted a wider circulation of Peter's views. But I have always thought that the short-circuiting of the scientific meeting was a watershed moment in the battle over the etiology of AIDS. In any event, this entire episode made it vanilla plain, naïf that I am, that AIDS was as much, or more, a political condition as a medical one.

Because the possibility of the White House meeting had been leaked to the media, several stories about its cancellation appeared in the mainstream as well as gay underground press. According to Peter, the ensuing pressure was what led Fauci to contact Mathilde Krim (the head of AmFAR) and organize the debacle in DC a few months later. Meanwhile, the topic the meeting was intended to discuss—namely, possible mechanisms of HIV pathogenesis and their relevance to AIDS etiology—lost the second clause and became the subject of an ongoing, inconclusive series of prestigious Keystone Symposia (generally held to coincide with spring skiing in the Rockies), to which Peter never once received an invitation.

Scientifically, this remained the status of the debate over the role of HIV in AIDS until the end of 1994.

On January 19, 1995, a peculiar commentary appeared in the "News & Views" section of *Nature.* Referring to papers he had published the previous week—papers accompanied by press releases, news conferences, and the other assorted hoopla befitting the announcement of scientific breakthroughs—John Maddox wrote:

> The publication last week of two important articles on the dynamics of the infection of people by HIV is agreed to have been a important landmark in the process of understanding the disease called AIDS, but not everybody will be aware of that. Reporting of the event has been curiously selective. In particular, the British newspaper *The Sunday Times,* which as recently as a year ago was replete with accounts of how HIV can have little or nothing to do with the causation of AIDS, chose not even to mention the new developments in last Sunday's edition.

Is it planning a major account of how it came to be so misled, thus to mislead its readers? Or is it waiting for a sign from Professor Peter Duesberg, of Berkeley, California, who started the hare the newspaper followed eagerly for two years?

Despite this journal's severe line, some months ago, on Duesberg's right of reply to critics of his position, it is now in the general interest that his and his associates' views on the new developments should be made public. Duesberg was not available to take a single telephone call one day last week, nor able to return it, but one of his associates appeared to welcome the idea of a comment on the articles by Wei et al. and Ho et al. (*Nature 373*, 117–122 & 123–126; 1995). That will be eagerly awaited and will be published with the usual provisos—that it is not libelous or needlessly rude, that it pertains to the new results and that it should not be longer than it needs to be.[36]

John concluded his highly personalized and somewhat petulant editorial by introducing religion into the political-psychosexual-scientific stew AIDS had become, invoking charges of heresy against Peter and me, and sternly advising us: "Now may be the time to recant."

To many of *Nature's* readers this inelegant piece of writing from Maddox, replete with whining ire towards Rupert Murdoch's very local weekend tabloid, must have seemed a little out of place and otherwise odd. But the autocratic editor who expected people to be available whenever he called, and was filled with indignation when they were not, was so infuriated by Neville Hodgkinson's stories between 1992 and 1994, in which I was sometimes quoted,[37] that he attempted, unsuccessfully, to have the Managing Director of Macmillan present me with an ultimatum of either desisting in my public support of Peter, or be terminated as scientific editor of *Bio/Technology.*

When Peter and I did prepare our response to Maddox's gracious invitation, the "eagerly awaited" reply was rejected in the "Goebbels" fax referred to earlier, simultaneously with a decaying carrot in the form of "I will publish the essence of what you have to say, but only after I have gone over it with a fine-tooth comb with the intention of ridding it of various misrepresentations." The complete record of the exchange was eventually published as part of a supplement to *Genetica,* the world's oldest journal of genetics, at the end of 1995, under the title "Duesberg and the right of reply according to Maddox-*Nature,*" and it is reproduced in its entirety as an appendix to this chapter.

The papers that so impressed *Nature's* former editor purported to show that quite different from the generally accepted view that there was very little active HIV in AIDS patients, in reality the immune system was being hyper-stimulated by furious amounts of viral replication that went unnoticed because the virus-producing cells were being eliminated as quickly as they were being produced, at least for a while.

Ho and Wei arrived at their "new view" as a by-product of clinical studies they were doing in order to ascertain the effectiveness of a new class of anti-HIV drugs. These compounds, called protease inhibitors, act by blocking a key step in the reproduction cycle of HIV and all other retroviruses, and would become the first and basically only commercial success of a type of pharmaceutical biotechnology called combinatorial chemistry. In carrying out these studies, it was of course necessary to measure the amount of virus in their patient subjects. To do this Ho and Wei used a recently devised, ultra-sensitive biochemical assay based on the Nobel Prize-worthy invention of Kary Mullis, PCR, the polymerase chain reaction, which was also put to effective use by Michael Crichton in *Jurassic Park.* They called the number that their PCR assays gave either "viral load" or "plasma virion

RNA units," terms which imply the presence of biochemically active virus. But what is the relationship between a "viral load" and an infectious virus? One of the authors of the *Nature* papers provided an exact answer two years previously when he showed in the pages of *Science* that the PCR-based assay they used was 60,000 times more sensitive than traditional measures of infectivity.[38] A "viral load" of 100,000, the largest value reported in the *Nature* papers, divided by 60,000 is 1.7 infectious virus particles per milliliter of blood, exactly the same biologically insignificant levels of virus that had always been found.

For a while it looked as though Maddox might be right about the "importance" of his hail and farewell papers. Protease inhibitors have been credited with bringing about declining AIDS death rates, even though the rates began to fall in 1994, two years before the protease inhibitors were even in limited use.[39] And for his contribution, David Ho would enjoy an Andy Warhol fifteen minutes of fame that culminated in a *Time* magazine cover portrait. AIDS journalist Celia Farber captured this moment quite brilliantly when she wrote:

> It's telling, and perfectly symbolic that when AIDS researcher David Ho's face appeared on the cover of *Time* as Man of The Year, 1996, you couldn't see his eyes. Instead, a colorful swirl meant to represent HIV filled his glasses. George Orwell used precisely this image—a man whose eyes are gone, whose glasses have been filled with the refracting light of his ideology—to convey the triumph of politics over truth in his famous essay *Politics and The English Language*.[40]

But neither the mass media's support, nor Maddox's censoring of the point-by-point refutation of Ho and Wei's scientific contribution by Peter and me, could save the "new view" of HIV, which suffered from so many flaws that in the February 1998 issue of *Nature Medicine,* Mario Roederer, a noted HIV-AIDS researcher at Stanford, would write:

> There has been considerable debate about this simple hypothesis of Ho and Wei. Their 1995 *Nature* papers ignited a heated controversy that resulted in publication of several well-designed and informative studies, which raised serious doubts about this 'war'. In this issue of *Nature Medicine,* reports by Pakker et al. and Gorochov et al. provide the final nails in the coffin for Ho's and Wei's models of T-cell dynamics, an illusion of faulty assumptions and poor measurement techniques.[41]

Thus, after fifteen years spent burning tens of billions of research dollars, there was still no consensus among those working on the HIV-AIDS problem as to how exactly or even inexactly the "deadly virus" manages to be so deadly. In the words of Sir John Maddox, OBE, "HIV causes AIDS, in some manner not understood." As we will see by the end of Chapter 5, the ensuing years did not change this disastrous admission one iota.

Chapter 3 Notes

1. Duesberg, P. H. 1987. Retroviruses as carcinogens and pathogens: Expectations and reality.*Cancer Res.* 47:1199–1220.

2. Bishop, J. M. 1995. Cancer: the rise of the genetic paradigm. *Genes Dev.* 9:1309–1315.

3. Cichutek, K. and Duesberg, P. H. 1987. Conversion of *ras* genes to cancer genes. In: *Modern Trends in Human Leukemia VII: New Results in Clinical and Biological Research including Pediatric Oncology, Haematology and Blood Transfusion* 31:477–481. Eds.: Neth, Gallo, Greaves, and Kabisch (Berlin: Springer-Verlag).

4. Duesberg, P. H. 1996. *Inventing the Aids Virus* (Washington, DC: Regnery Publishing, Inc.).

5. Crewdson, J. "The Great AIDS Quest," *Chicago Tribune,* Nov. 19, 1989.

6. Lang, S. 1998. *Challenges* (New York: Springer).

7. Cohen, J. 1993. HHS: Gallo guilty of misconduct. *Science* 259:168–170.

8. Greenberg, D. S. "What Ever Happened to the War on Cancer?" *Discover,* March 1986, p. 55.

9. Epstein, S. S., et al. 1992. Losing the War Against Cancer: A Need for Public Policy Reforms. *International Journal of Health Services and Molecular Biology* 22:455–469.

10. Gunby, P. 1992. Battles Against Many Malignancies Lie Ahead as Federal War on Cancer Enters Third Decade. *Jour. Am. Med. Assoc.* 267:1891. A dozen years later, the war is still far from won, despite a certain amount of public perception to the contrary, as elegantly documented in the March 24, 2004 *Fortune* by the magazine's editor, Clifton Leaf, in an essay entitled: "Why We Are Losing the War on Cancer (and How to Win It)."

11. Altman, L. K. "Researchers Believe AIDS' Virus Is Found," *The New York Times,* April 24, 1984.

12. See Peter H. Duesberg's *Curriculum Vitae,* included at the end of this book.

13. Duesberg, P. H. 1987. Retroviruses as carcinogens and pathogens: Expectations and reality. *Cancer Research* 47:1199–1220. References cited therein:

> 71. Poiesz, B. J., Ruscetti, F. W., Gazdar, A. F., Bunn, P. A., Minna, J. D., and Gallo, R. C. Detection and isolation of type C retrovirus particles from fresh and cultured lymphocytes of a patient with cutaneous T-cell lymphoma. Proc. Natl. Acad. Sci. USA 77:7415–7419, 1980.

> 27. Wong-Staal, F., and Gallo, R. C. Human T-lymphotropic retroviruses. Nature (London) 317:395–403, 1985.

> 76. Hoxie, J. E., Matthews, D. M., and Ames, D. B. Infection of human endothelial cells by human T-cell virus. Proc. Natl. Acad. Sci. USA 81:7591–7595, 1984.

> 77. Yoshikura, H., Nishida, J., Yoshida, M., Kitamura, Y., Takaku, F., and Ikeda, S. Isolation of HTLV derived from Japanese adult T-cell leukemia patients in human diploid fibroblast strain IMR90 and the biological characters of the infected cells. Int. J. Cancer 33:745–749, 1984.

> 13. Weiss, R., Teich, N., Varmus, H., and Coffin, J. RNA Tumor Viruses. Ed. 2. Cold Spring Harbor, NY: Cold Spring Harbor Press, 1985.

78. Tajima, K., and Kuroishi, T. Estimation of rate of incidence of ATL among ATLV (HTLV-I) carriers in Kyushu, Japan. Jpn. J. Clin. Oncol. 15:423–430, 1985.

79. Maeda, Y., Furakawu, M., Takehara, Y., Yoshimura, Y., Miyumoto, K., Matsubara, T., Morishima, Y., Tajima, K., Okochi, K., and Hinuma, Y. Prevalence of possible adult T-cell leukemia virus-carriers among volunteer blood donors in Japan: a nation-wide study. Int. J. Cancer 33:717–730, 1984.

81. Okochi, K., Sato, H., and Hinuma, Y. A retrospective study on transmission of adult T-cell leukemia virus by blood transfusion: seroconversion of recipients. Vox Sang. 46:245–253, 1984.

268. Koprowski, H., DeFreitas, E., Harper, M. E., Sandberg-Wollheim, M., Sheremata, W., Robert-Guroff, M., Saxinger, C. W., Feinberg, M. B., Wong-Staal, F., and Gallo, R. C. Multiple sclerosis and human T-cell lymphoytropic retroviruses. Nature 318:154–160, 1985.

80. Pan, I.-H., Chung, C.-S., Komoda, H., Mai, J., and Hinuma, Y. Seroepidemiology of adult T-cell leukemia virus in Taiwan. Jpn. J. Cancer Res. 76:9–11, 1985.

14. DeRossi, A., Aldovini, A., Franchini, G., Mann, D., Gallo, R. C., and Wong-Staal, F. 1985. Clonal selection of T lymphocytes infected by cell-free human T-cell leukemia/lymphovirus type I: parameters of virus integration and expression. *Virology* 143:640–645.

15. Duesberg, P. H. 1987. Retroviruses as carcinogens and pathogens: Expectations and reality. *Cancer Research* 47:1199–1220. References therein:

115. DeRossi, A., Aldovini, A., Franchini, G., Mann, D., Gallo, R. C., and Wong-Staal, F. Clonal selection of T lymphocytes infected by cell-free human T-cell leukemia/lymphovirus type I: parameters of virus integration and expression. Virology 143:640–645, 1985.

113. Gallo, R. C., Wong-Staal, F., Markham, P. D., Ruscetti, F., Kalyanaraman, V. S., Ceccherini-Nelli, L., Dalla Favera, R., Josephs, S., Miller, N. R., and Reitz, M. S. Recent studies with infectious primate retroviruses: hybridization to primate DNA and some biological effects on fresh human blood leukocytes by simian sarcoma virus and gibbon ape leukemia virus. Cold Spring Harbor Conf. Cell Proliferation 7:753–773, 1980.

16. Blattner, W. A. 1999. Human retroviruses: their role in cancer. *Proc. Assoc. Am. Physicians* 111:563–572.

17. Crewdson, J. "In Gallo Case, Truth Termed A Casualty," *Chicago Tribune,* January 1, 1995.

18. Crewdson, J. "Defending the Indefensible Dr. Gallo," *Chicago Tribune,* January 6, 1995.

19. Maddox, J. 1995. Duesberg and the New View of HIV. "News and Views," *Nature* 373:189.

20. Letter from John Maddox to Peter Duesberg, preserved in the *Peter H. Duesberg Archive* of the Bancroft Library of the Univ. of California at Berkeley. See also *Appendix* to this Chapter

21. Duesberg, P. H. 1987. Retroviruses as carcinogens and pathogens: Expectations and reality. *Cancer Research* 47:1199–1220. References therein:

26 Barre-Sinoussi, F., Chermann, J. C., Rey, F., Nugeyre, M. T., Chamaret, S., Gruest, J., Danguet, C., Axler-Blin, C., Vezinet-Brun, F., Rouzioux, C., Rosenbaum, W., and Montagnier, L. Isolation of T-lymphotropic retrovirus from a patient at risk for acquired immune deficiency syndrome (AIDS). Science (Wash. DC) 220:868–870, 1983.

209. Marx, J. L. AIDS virus has new name—perhaps. Science (Wash. DC) 232:699–700, 1986.

210. Levy, J. A., Hoffman, A. D., Kramer, S. M., Landis, J. A., Shimabukuro, J. M., and Oshiro, L. S. Isolation of lympho-cytopathic retroviruses from San Francisco patients with AIDS. Science (Wash. DC) 225:840–842, 1984.

211. Gallo, R. C., Salahuddin, S. Z., Popovic, M., Shearer, G. M., Kaplan, M., Haynes, B. F., Palher, F. J., Redfield, R., Oleske, J., Safai, B., White, F., Foster, P., and Markham, P .D. Frequent detection and isolation of cytopathic retroviruses (HTLV III) from patients with AIDS and at risk for AIDS. Science (Wash. DC) 224:500–503, 1984.

212. Salahuddin, S. A., Markham, P. D., Popovic, M., Sarngadharan, M. G., Orndorff, S., Fladagar, A., Patel, A., Gold, J., and Gallo, R. C. Isolation of infectious T-cell leukemia/lymphoma virus type III (HTLV-III) from patients with acquired immuno-deficiency syndrome (AIDS) or AIDS-related complex (ARC) and from healthy carriers: a study of risk groups and tissue sources. Proc. Natl. Acad. Sci. USA 82:5530–5534, 1985.

213. Levy, J. A., Kaminsky, L. S., Morrow, M. J. W., Steiner, K., Luciw, P., Dina, D., Oshiro, L. Infection by the retrovirus associated with the acquired immunodeficiency syndrome. Ann. Intern. Med. 103:694–699, 1985.

214. Levy, J. A., and Shimabukuro, J. Recovery of AIDS-associated retroviruses from patients with AIDS or AIDS-related condi-

tions and from clinically healthy individuals. J. Infect. Dis. 152:734–738, 1985.

215. Gottlieb, M. S., Schroff, R., Schamber, H. M., Weisman, J. D., Fan, P. T., Wolf, R. A., and Saxon, A. Pneumocystis carinii pneumonia and mucosal candidiasis in previously healthy homosexual men: evidence of a new acquired cellular immuno-deficiency. N. Engl. J. Med. 305:1425–1431, 1981.

216. Centers for Disease Control. Weekly surveillance report, October 20, 1986.

217. Sarngadharan, M .G., Popovic, M., Brach, L., Schupbach, J., and Gallo, R. C. Antibodies reactive with human T-lymphotropic retroviruses (HTLV-III) in the serum of patients with AIDS. Science (Wash. DC) 224:506–508, 1984.

218. Blattner, W. A., Biggar, R. J., Weiss, S. H., Melbye, M., and Goedert, J. J. Epidemiology of human T-lymphotropic virus type III and the risk of the acquired immunodeficiency syndrome. Ann. Intern. Med. 103:665–670, 1985.

219. Kaminsky, L. S., McHugh, T., Stites, D., Volberding, P., Henle, G., Henle, W., and Levy, J. A. High prevalence of antibodies to acquired immune deficiency syndrome (AIDS)-associated retrovirus (ARV) in AIDS and related conditions but not in other disease states. Proc. Natl. Acad. Sci. USA 82:5535–5539, 1985.

220. Peterman, T. A., Jaffe, H. W., Feorino, P. M., Haverkos, H. W., Stoweburner, R. L., and Curran, J. W. Transfusion-associated acquired immunodeficiency syndrome in the United States. JAMA 254:2913–2917, 1985.

221. Clumeck, N., Robert-Guroff, M., Van De Perre, P., Jennings, A., Sibomana, J., Demol, P., Cran, S., and Gallo, R. C. Sero-epidemiological studies of HTLV-III antibody prevalence among selected groups of heterosexual Africans. JAMA 254:2599–2602, 1985.

222. Gottlieb, M. S., Wolfe, P. R., Fahey, J. L., Knight, S., Hardy, D., Eppolito, L., Ashida, E., Patel, A., Beall, G. N., and Sun, N. The syndrome of persistent generalized lymphodenopathy: experience with 101 patients. Adv. Exp. Med. Biol. 187:85–91, 1985.

13. Weiss, R., Teich, N., Varmus, H., and Coffin, J. RNA Tumor Viruses. Ed. 2. Cold Spring Harbor, NY: Cold Spring Harbor Press, 1985.

27. Wong-Staal, F., and Gallo, R. C. Human T-lymphotropic retro-

viruses. Nature (London), 317:395–403, 1985.

223. Curran, J. W., Morgan, M. W., Hardy, A. M., Jaffe, H. W., Darrow, W. W., and Dowdle, W. R. The epidemiology of AIDS: current status and future prospects. Science (Wash. DC) 229:1352–1357, 1985.

224. Sivak, S. L., and Wormser, G. P. How common is HTLV-III infection in the United States? N. Engl. J. Med. 313:1352, 1985.

22. Duesberg, P. H. *Ibid.* References therein:

225. McDougal, J. S., Cort, S. P., Kennedy, M. S., Cabridilla, C. D., Feorino, P. M., Francis, D. P., Hicks, D., Kalyanaraman, V. S., and Martin, L. S. Immunoassay for the detection and quantitation of infectious human retrovirus, lymphadenopathy-associated virus (LAV). J. Immunol. Methods 76:171–183, 1985.

226. Robert-Guroff, M., Brown, M., and Gallo, R. C. HTLV-III neutralizing antibodies in patients with AIDS and ARC. Nature (London) 316:72–74, 1985.

227. Weiss, R. A., Clapham, P. R., Cheingsong-Popov, R., Dalgleish, A. G., Carne, C. A., Weller, I. V. D., and Tedder, R. S. Neutralization of human T-lymphotropic virus type III by sera of AIDS and AIDS-risk patients. Nature (London) 316:69–72, 1985.

28. Sodroski, J., Goh, W. C., Rosen, C., Dayton, H., Terwilliger, E., and Haseltine, W. A second post-transcriptional trans-activator gene required for HTLV-III replication. Nature (London) 321:412–417, 1986.

245. Dayton, A. I., Sodroski, J. G., Rosen, G. A., Goh, W. C., and Haseltine, W. A. The trans-activator gene of the human T cell lymphotropic virus type III is required for replication. Cell 44:941–947, 1986.

23. Levy, J. A. 1988. Mysteries of HIV: challenges for therapy and prevention. *Nature* 333:519–522.

24. Blattner, W., Gallo, R. C., and Temin, H. M. 1988. HIV is the Cause of AIDS. *Science* 241:515–517.

25. Bialy, H. 1988. Where is the Virus? And where is the Press? *Bio/Technology (Nature Biotechnology)* 6:121.

26. Paul, D. A., Falk, L. A., Kessler, H. A., Chase, R. M., Blaauw, B., Chudwin, D. S., Landay, A. L. 1987. Correlation of serum HIV antigen and antibody with clinical status in HIV-infected patients. *J. Med. Virol.* 22:357–363.

27. de Wolf, F., Goudsmit, J., Paul, D. A., Lange, J. M., Hooijkaas, C., Schellekens, P., Coutinho, R. A., and van der Noordaa. J. 1987. Risk of

AIDS-related complex and AIDS in homosexual men with persistent HIV antigenaemia. *Br. Med. J. (Clin Res Ed)* 295:569–572.

28. Pedersen, C., Nielsen, C. M., Vestergaard, B. F., Gerstoft, J., Krogsgaard, K., and Nielsen, J. O. 1987. Temporal relation of antigenaemia and loss of antibodies to core antigens to development of clinical disease in HIV infection. *Br. Med. J. (Clin Res Ed)* 295:567–569.

29. Goudsmit, J., Lange, J. M., Paul, D. A., and Dawson, G. J. 1987. Antigenemia and antibody titers to core and envelope antigens in AIDS, AIDS-related complex, and subclinical human immunodeficiency virus infection. *J. Infect. Dis.* 155:558–560.

30. Ho, D. D., Neumann, A. U., Perelson, A. S., Chen, W., Leonard, J. M., and Markowitz, M. 1995. Rapid Turnover of Plasma Virions and CD4 Lymphocytes in HIV-1 Infection. *Nature* 373:123–126.

31. Specter, M. "Panel Rebuts Biologist's Claims on Cause of AIDS," *Washington Post,* April 10, 1988.

32. Lauritsen, J. "Kangaroo court etiology," *New York Native,* May 9, 1988. Reprinted in *Poison by Prescription: The AZT story.* Asklepios Press, NY, 1990.

33. Duesberg, P. H. 1987. A challenge to the AIDS establishment. *Bio/Technology (Nature Biotechnology)* 5:1244.

34. Maddox, J. 1991. AIDS research turned upside down. *Nature* 353:297.

35. Maddox, J. 1991. Basketball, AIDS and education. *Nature* 354:103.

36. Maddox, J. 1995. Duesberg and the New View of HIV. *Nature* 373:189.

37. Hodgkinson, N. 1992. Experts mount startling challenge to AIDS orthodoxy. *The Sunday Times (Focus),* April 26.

38. Piatak, M., Saag, M. S., Yang, L. C., Clark, S. J., Kappes, J. C., Luk, K. C., Hahn, B. H., Shaw, G. M., and Lifson, J. D. 1993. High levels of HIV-1 in plasma during all stages of infection determined by competitive PCR. *Science* 259:1749–1754.

39. Duesberg, P. H., Koehnlein, C., and Rasnick, D. 2003. The chemical bases of the various AIDS epidemics: recreational drugs, anti-viral chemotherapy and malnutrition. *J. Biosci.* 28:383–412.

40. Farber, C. "Science Fiction," *Gear Magazine,* March 2000.

41. Roederer, M. 1998. Getting to the HAART of T cell dynamics. *Nat. Med.* 4:145–146.

Appendix
Duesberg and the Right of Reply According to Maddox-*Nature*

Peter H. Duesberg and Harvey Bialy*

Department of Molecular and Cellular Biology, University of California, Berkeley, California 94720, USA. *Bio/Technology, 64 Bleecker Street, New York, New York 10012, USA

Genetica Monograph "AIDS: Virus- or Drug-Induced?" 1995. Kluwer Academic Publishers, Dordrecht, The Netherlands. Reprinted with Permission.

In 1993 John Maddox, the editor of *Nature,* commissioned a commentary refuting the hypothesis that drugs cause AIDS (Ascher et al., 1993). The piece described 215 patients each of which had used drugs (Duesberg, 1993a; Duesberg, 1993b; Duesberg, 1993c). In view of this Duesberg sent a letter to *Nature* arguing that the perfect correlation between drug use and AIDS confirmed, rather than refuted, the drug hypothesis. Maddox censored the letter and wrote an editorial "Has Duesberg a Right of Reply?" (Maddox, 1993). The editorial pointed out that the world's oldest science journal could not afford an open scientific debate on the cause of AIDS because of the perceived dangers of infectious AIDS.

In an editorial on January 19, 1995, Maddox promised to lift the censorship to give "Duesberg and his associates an opportunity to comment" on two *Nature* studies that in his opinion prove the HIV-AIDS hypothesis.

In the following we document how Maddox-*Nature* honors its commitments. Our documentation includes:

(i) A photocopy of Maddox' "News and Views" article of January 19, 1995;

(ii) A summary of a phone conversation between Maddox and Bialy;

(iii) Our letter to Maddox answering his invitation;

(iv) Our commentary on the two new *Nature* studies;

(v) Maddox' response to our commentary;

(vi) Our response to Maddox;

(vii) What *Nature* published from and about Duesberg and Bialy on May 18, 1995;

(viii) *Nature*'s final letter.

References:

Ascher, M. S., H. W. Sheppard, W. Winkelstein Jr., and E. Vittinghoff, 1993. Does drug use cause AIDS? *Nature (London)* 362:103–104.

Duesberg, P., 1993a. Aetiology of AIDS. *Lancet* 341:1544.

Duesberg, P., 1993b. HIV and the aetiology of AIDS. *Lancet* 341:957–958.

Duesberg, P. H., 1993c. Can epidemiology determine whether drugs or HIV cause AIDS? *AIDS-Forschung* 12: 627–635.

Maddox, J., 1993. Has Duesberg a right of reply? *Nature (London)* 363:109.

Duesberg and the New View of HIV

John Maddox, "News and Views," *Nature* 373:189, January 19, 1995

This journal has offered Dr. Peter Duesberg and his associates an opportunity to comment on last week's publications suggesting that the immune system reacts hyperactively to HIV infection.

The publication last week of two important articles on the dynamics of the infection of people by HIV is agreed to have been an important landmark in the process of understanding the disease called AIDS, but not everybody will be aware of that. Reporting of the event has been curiously selective. In particular, the British newspaper *The Sunday Times,* which as recently as a year ago was replete with accounts of how HIV can have little or nothing to do with the causation of AIDS, chose not even to mention the new developments in last Sunday's edition.

Is it planning a major account of how it came to be so misled, thus to mislead its readers? Or is it waiting for a sign from Professor Peter Duesberg, of Berkeley, California, who started the hare the newspaper followed eagerly for two years?

The reasons why the new developments are (or should be) an embarrassment for Duesberg are simply put. Almost from the outset of AIDS as a recognized disease in the early 1980s, the objective index of an infected person's state of health has been the concentration in the blood of T lymphocytes carrying the CD4 antigen. The more advanced the infection, the smaller the concentration of CD4+ cells.

But Duesberg was quick to point to a paradox in the observations: although the concentration of CD4+ cells might decline with the persistence of infection, there was no dramatic increase of the frequency of infected T cells as infection gave way to overt disease. Cell death by inter-cellular infection could hardly be consistent with that state of affairs.

In essence, the new developments resolve the paradox by showing that the T cells in an infected person's blood are likely to have been created only in the few days previously. There will not have been time enough for more than a small proportion of them to have become infected, while those that harbour virus will be killed off very soon. So the scarcity of T cells from which virus can be recovered in test-tube experiments is consistent with the assertion that the immune system is in overdrive from the onset of infection by HIV.

On this (new) view, the progressive decline of the CD4+ concentration with the duration of infection is rather a symptom of the underlying infection than the crux of its mechanism. What seems to matter is that there should be cells (including T cells) somewhere in the body (the lymph nodes are likely candidates) from which virus particles continue to leak into the blood plasma. In other words, Duesberg is right to have argued all along that the usually slow decline of CD4+ cells is not consistent with what one would expect from a specific cytotoxic viral mechanism. The explanation is that the CD4+ population in the blood at any time has been freshly created.

Despite this journal's severe line, some months ago, on Duesberg's right of reply to critics of his position, it is now in the general interest that his and his associates' views on the new developments should be made public. Duesberg was not available to take a single telephone call one day last week, nor able to return it, but one of his associates appeared to welcome the idea of a comment on the articles by Wei *et al.* and Ho *et al.* (*Nature* 373, 117–122 & 123–126; 1995). That will be eagerly awaited and will be published with the usual provisos—that it is not libelous or needlessly rude, that it pertains to the new results and that it should not be longer than it needs to be.

Meanwhile, one important question stands out like a sore thumb: why, after more than a decade of research, has it only now emerged that the response of the immune system to infection by HIV is hyperactivity rather than the opposite? Simon Wain-Hobson, writing in News and Views last week (*Nature* 373, 102; 1995), remarked that the investigators were able to reach their startling conclusions "by teaming up with mathematicians."

Intuitively, the sharp recovery of CD4+ cells in the first few days after the administration of antiviral drugs pointed to their rapid production by the immune system. But in retrospect the good fortune of the investigators is clear. Only with the advent of highly specific drugs directed against HIV was it possible to cut off viral production so abruptly that the decline in plasma viremia could form the basis for a model of viral production. New techniques for assaying the low levels of virus involved were also necessary; had the drugs been available only a few years earlier, these studies would have been impossible on that account.

In retrospect, the dynamics of the immune system would seem to be central to any consideration of the body's response to infection, by measles virus as well as HIV. And modelling of such processes as the production of lymphocytes (B as well as T cells) in the immune response should be a relatively easy task (compared with, say, the appearance of endless molecular species in the evolution of a molecular cloud).

To be sure, immunologists are no strangers to quantitation in this spirit. And the involvement of mathematicians is simply explained by the authors' desire to be sure that even experts in this area approved of their data analysis. But the rarity of such studies says something depressing about the state of biology, for all its modernity. Despite the explosion in molecular knowledge (including molecular knowledge of viruses), the information to perform this kind of quantitative modelling is almost never available. In this case, the relevant data have emerged only after a decade of intensive research, fuelled by intense public interest in a most unpleasant pathogen. But virology is not the only field in which biology would benefit from more quantitative methods.

What more is to come? Now that the basis for the low CD4+ T-cell count in AIDS patients is clear, further studies of the viral dynamics will be eagerly awaited. How much virus is produced by each productively infected cell? How fast is the virus produced by the lymph nodes? And what is responsible for killing the CD4+ T cells? If these last are indeed being destroyed by the CD8+ cells of the immune system, as Wain-Hobson suggests (and this remains to be seen), it will undoubtedly lend further support to the idea that individuals who are repeatedly exposed to HIV while remaining unaffected are protected by their cytotoxic T lymphocytes (Rowland-Jones *et al.*, *Nature Medicine* 1, 59–64; 1995).

The search for effective antiviral therapy will also benefit. Already Wei *et al.* have followed the emergence of mutants resistant to one drug, and studies of others, alone and in combination, will surely follow. Here too, improved quantitation of the size of viral pools in different tissues, and their respective replication rates, will be vital.

What does this mean for basic research on AIDS, the cause eloquently advocated a year ago by Dr. Bernie Fields (*Nature* 369, 95; 1994)? Wei *et al.* and Ho *et al.* have provided the basis for a much more pointed programme of investigation from which, no doubt, a complete picture of the dynamics of this hitherto perplexing disease will emerge. A return to basics seems already to have happened. The prospects of therapy are much more difficult to tell, but has a fuller understanding ever failed to deliver improvements of technique? The danger for the Duesbergs of this world is that they will be left high and dry, championing a cause that will have ever fewer adherents as time passes. Now may be the time for them to recant.

Summary of Phone Conversation between John Maddox and Harvey Bialy

On the afternoon of January 12, [1995] the day the *Nature* issue containing the Ho and Wei *et al.* papers appeared, and one day after the press conference announcing these landmark publications, I received a rare telephone call from my colleague, the newly knighted Sir John Maddox, editor of *Nature*. The essence of the ensuing conversation is summarized below.

After congratulating John on his recently acquired honorific, I asked to what did I owe the pleasure of his call. He then asked me what I thought of the "HIV-1 dynamics" papers. I replied by thanking him for publishing them, as they were so transparently bad, they would convince any reasonable scientist who had the endurance to read them that the HIV-AIDS hypothesis was absolutely intellectually bankrupt. I also chided him by saying that even Wain-Hobson didn't know what to make of them, judging by his incoherent "News & Views" piece that accompanied their publication.

To my surprise, his response to these remarks was remarkably devoid of any outrage. We discussed in a cursory manner some of the more obvious criticisms of the papers, such as their lack of controls, and the methodological and biological problems with their estimates of free infectious virus. I also mentioned that I thought it ironic that after years of denying that T cells turned over at the rate of 5% in two days, the HIV-AIDS protagonists were now at last admitting this well known fact. He responded by asking how did I explain the "dramatic increase in T cells after treatment with the protease inhibitor." I replied that this transient, hardly dramatic, increase was also a well known phenomenon called lymphocyte trafficking, which occurs in response to many chemical insults.

The conversation then changed direction and John said that he had, without success, been trying to reach Peter (Duesberg) to inform him that he was, in this instance, willing to rescind his previous "refusal of the right of reply" and would welcome a correspondence from Peter (and me) addressing what we perceived as the shortcomings of Ho and Wei *et al.* He promised me that if the piece was relevant, succinct and not personally rude; he would publish it "unslagged." When I asked him what this meant, he said that it would be published as received, without prior review and without a response appearing in the same issue. I said, "Do you mean it will be allowed to generate its own replies?" and he said, "Yes." I congratulated him on his willingness to open a proper scientific debate, and said I would communicate our conversation to Peter.

I was a bit surprised to see his editorial in the following week's *Nature* in which he went much further than our talk in offering the pages of *Nature* to uncensored debate. I was, however, not surprised to discover, some weeks later, that the invited response which appears unedited in this issue of *Genetica* was deemed "too long by half and too unfocussed" to warrant publication in his own "highly esteemed" (as in the BBC's *Goon Show*) journal.

Letter to John Maddox
from Peter Duesberg and Harvey Bialy

February 7, 1995

Sir John Maddox
Nature, Macmillan Publishing
4 Little Essex St.
London, WC2R 3LF England

Dear John,

As per your invitation, published in *News and Views,* "Duesberg and the new view of HIV," and your invitation to Harvey Bialy over the phone, "to comment on last week's publications" by Wei *et al.* and Ho *et al.,* we submit "Responding to 'Duesberg and the new view of HIV'" by Duesberg & Bialy. We are delighted that after years of editorials, News & Views, and letters and censored letters we have been invited at last to make our case in our own words.

As you can see, our report meets your criteria of "not libellous or needlessly rude, that it pertains to the new results and that it should not be longer than it needs to be." The length of our commentary is compatible with the results presented in the two papers covering 10 pages, and the challenges delivered by the two accompanying News & Views from you and Wain-Hobson.

We both respect your courage and integrity to undertake an uncensored debate on the HIV-AIDS hypothesis.

Best regards
Peter Duesberg
Harvey Bialy

P.S. A hard copy is in the mail. We can send a disc if that helps.

Responding to
"Duesberg and the New View of HIV"

Peter H. Duesberg and Harvey Bialy*

The editor of *Nature,* John Maddox, has issued a published invitation to "Peter Duesberg and his associates ... to comment" on two new studies by Wei *et al.*[1] and Ho *et al.*[2] that he feels lend strong support to the hypothesis that HIV causes AIDS.[3] Maddox credits us for having identified two paradoxes of this hypothesis, (i) "Duesberg was quick to point to a paradox ... [that] there was no dramatic increase of the frequency of infected T cells as infection gave way to overt disease," and that (ii) "Duesberg is right to have argued all along that the usually slow decline of CD4+ cells [T cells] is not consistent with ... a specific cytotoxic viral mechanism."[3]

According to Maddox, "the new developments are (or should be) an embarrassment for Duesberg," because they "resolve the paradox." But we do not see any reason why a scientist should be embarrassed for having pointed out paradoxes in the past, whichever way these paradoxes are subsequently solved. We also object to rhetoric personalizing a scientific debate. However, it is embarrassing that in the name of science clinical, public health, journalistic, and political decisions have been made in the past, based on a hypothesis that—we all agree now—was unproven at that time.

Since the HIV-AIDS hypothesis makes many assumptions that are bewildering to pre-HIV virologists, and since the new studies do not clearly define the HIV hypothesis, we shall first state the hypothesis and then explain why, in light of these "new" studies, it remains paradoxical.

In 1984 it was proposed that the retrovirus HIV can cause such diametrically different diseases as Kaposi's sarcoma, pneumonia, dementia, diarrhea, and weight loss.[4,5] All of these diseases and

over two dozen more are now collectively called acquired immunodeficiency syndrome (AIDS)[6] if antibody to HIV is present. But
many of these diseases, including Kaposi's sarcoma, lymphoma,
dementia, and weight loss, are neither consequences of, nor consistently associated with immunodeficiency.[7,8] For example
Kaposi's sarcoma and dementia have been diagnosed in male
homosexuals whose immune systems were normal.[9-13] As a cause
of these diseases HIV was proposed to follow an entirely unprecedented course of action:

1) HIV was proposed to cause immunodeficiency by killing T-
cells. But retroviruses do not kill cells.[14,15]

2) Within weeks after infection, HIV would reach moderate to
high titers of $10–10^4$ infectious units per ml blood,[16] sufficient to
induce antiviral immunity and antibodies (a positive "AIDS-
test"). According to Shaw, Ho and their collaborators, HIV activity is "rapidly and effectively limited" by this antiviral activity.[17,18]
Prior to antiviral immunity, HIV would neither kill T-cells nor
cause AIDS.[16,19] But all other viruses are primarily pathogenic
prior to immunity; the reason vaccination protects against disease. Not one virus exists that causes diseases only after it is neutralized by antiviral immunity.[20,21]

3) On average 10 years after HIV is neutralized, the virus is
postulated to cause AIDS diseases.[5,22] But all other viruses typically cause disease within days or weeks after infection, because
they replicate exponentially with generation times of 8 to 48
hours.[20,23,24]

4) As a consequence of antiviral immunity, the virus titer is
typically undetectably low prior to and even during AIDS.[25-29]
Only in rare cases HIV titers are as high as in the asymptomatic,
primary infection.[16,30] But in all other viral diseases the virus titer
is maximally high when viruses cause disease.[20,21]

5) Antiviral immunity would typically restrict HIV-infected
lymphocytes to less than 1 in 500—prior to and even during

AIDS.[14,26,27,30-32] But all other viruses infect more cells than the host can spare or regenerate when they cause disease.[20,21]

6) The hypothesis fails to shed any light on the causation of non-immunodeficiency AIDS diseases, like Kaposi's sarcoma, dementia, lymphoma, and weight loss, which make up 39% of all American AIDS cases.[8,33]

Today this HIV-AIDS hypothesis stands unproven and has failed to produce any public health benefits.[34-36]

The new studies are claimed by two *News and Views* articles from Maddox[3] and Wain-Hobson[43] to resolve the paradoxa, (1) how HIV kills T-cells, (2) how HIV causes AIDS, and (3) why HIV needs 10 years to cause AIDS. But we argue that the new studies have failed to resolve any of these paradoxa, in fact they have added new ones:

(1) *How HIV kills T-cells.* Until HIV appeared on the scene, retroviruses did not kill their host cells. This is the reason they were considered possible tumor viruses. Since retroviruses integrate their genes into the chromosome of the host, they can only replicate as long as the host survives integration and remains able to express integrated viral genes. Therefore a cytocidal retrovirus would be suicidal. Indeed, HIV proved to be non-cytocidal. It is mass-produced for the "AIDS-test" in immortal T-cells in culture at titers of 10^6 infectious units per ml.[37,38] Luc Montagnier and others have confirmed that HIV does not kill T-cells.[39-42] Hence the claim that HIV causes AIDS by killing T-cells is paradoxical.

The new papers have indeed resolved this paradox by shifting the paradigm: According to Maddox, T-cells "that harbour virus will be killed off very soon"—but not by HIV—by the immune system. Also consistent with a non-cytocidal virus, Wei *et al.* report that "the average half-life of infected PBMCs [peripheral blood mononuclear cells] is very long and of the same order of magnitude as the half-life of uninfected PBMCs." But, paradoxically, the same investigators also report that "the life span of virus-producing cells is remarkably short ($t_{1/2} = 2 \pm 0.9$ days)," although these cells are in the same system as their long-lived HIV-infected peers.[1] Ho *et al.* state that "there is virus- and immune-mediated killing of CD4 lymphocytes."[2] According to the *News and Views* article by Simon Wain-Hobson, "an intrinsic cytopathic effect of the virus is no longer credible."[43]

It is consistent with this "new view of HIV" that there is no correlation between virus titers and T-cell counts in the patients that Wei *et al.* and Ho *et al.* have studied. In some of Ho *et al.*'s patients, i.e. #303 and #403, a 100-fold variation in virus titers corresponds to no changes in T-cell counts. In Wei *et al.*'s patients, 100-fold variations in virus titers correspond to only 0.25 and 3-fold variations in T-cell counts—hardly a correlation to prove that HIV kills T-cells.

Since HIV is no longer viewed as a T-cell killer, the above paradox is solved. However, if T-cell killing via antiviral immunity were the cause of AIDS, we would have a bigger HIV-AIDS paradox than before. Since only 1 in 500 T-cells are ever infected, and most of these cells contain latent HIV not making viral proteins,[25,26,30,44] only less than 1 in 500 T-cells could ever be killed by antiviral immunity.

(2) *How HIV causes AIDS.* Until HIV appeared on the scene, the pathogenicity of a virus was a direct function of the number of virus-infected cells: the more infectious virus there was, the more cells were infected, and the more pathogenic an infection was.

But in typical AIDS patients HIV is so rare, that even leading AIDS retrovirologists from the US, like Robert Gallo, and the UK, like Robin Weiss, failed for years to isolate HIV from AIDS patients.[45,46] Likewise, virus-infected cells are so rare that they could not be found by George Shaw, the senior investigator of the new study by Wei *et al.*, nor by Gallo and their collaborators, in most AIDS patients[27]until the rare proviral DNA could be amplified with the polymerase chain reaction (PCR).[31,44,47]

Although the new studies never mention the percentage of infected T-cells, Maddox confirms the status quo: "the scarcity of T-cells from which virus can be recovered in test-tube experiments is consistent with the assertion that the immune system is in overdrive from the onset of infection by HIV." But the new studies claim on average 10^5 units of "free virus"[1] or "plasma virion" per ml blood[2] in AIDS patients. That should be enough virus to eliminate all remaining T-cells of these patients, 105 per ml, within the two days HIV needs to replicate[48]—unless, as Maddox suggests, the "new techniques for assaying the low levels of virus involved were also necessary"[3] (amplifying viral RNA with the polymerase chain reaction), possibly because no infectious HIV could be detected by conventional infectivity tests.

Indeed, Wei *et al.* acknowledge "substantial proportions of defective or otherwise non-infectious virus." "To determine whether the viral genomes represented in total viral nucleic acid correspond to infectious virus ..." they had to resort to the same techniques that the "old HIV hands," as Wain-Hobson calls them,[43] had used to isolate HIV from rare infected lymphocytes of AIDS patients: "We cocultivated PBMCs ... with normal donor lymphoblasts in order to establish primary virus isolates." Shaw together with some of the investigators of Wei *et al.* had shown in 1993 how to convert "plasma viral RNA" to infectious virus. They concluded that the "quantitative competitive PCR" is "as much as 60,000 times more sensitive"[49] than infectious virus.[16,19] Divide 10^5 "plasma viral RNA" units by 60,000 and you have 1.6 infectious units per ml, a number that is consistent with numerous previous reports (see above). Ho and a different group of collaborators just published a paper in which they show that over 10,000 "plasma virions," detected by the "branched DNA signal-amplification assay" used in their *Nature* paper correspond to less than one (!) infectious virus.[50] Thus Wei *et al.* and Ho *et al.*

both reported titers of 10^5 biochemical virus-units that really correspond to one or even less than one infectious virus. However, infectivity is the only clinically relevant criterion of a virus.

In other words, there is no evidence for infectious virus in Wei and Ho *et al.*'s patients. Wei and Ho *et al.* had apparently detected non-infectious virus that had been neutralized by "the immune system [that] reacts hyperactively to HIV infection"—just as Maddox suggests. Infectious virus was only obtained by activating latent HIV from a few infected cells out of millions of mostly uninfected cells from a given AIDS patient. Such virus activation is only achieved by growing cells in culture away from the hyperactive immune system of the host, just as the "old HIV hands" used to do it, when they tried to isolate HIV from AIDS patients.[45,46] Thus the paradox of too few viruses to cause immunodeficiency remains unresolved.

In view of the evidence that there are no more than 1.6 infectious HIVs per ml blood in Wei's and Ho's patients, one wonders whether the 10^5 viral RNAs per ml are real or are an artifact reflecting inherent difficulties in quantifying the input number of "plasma viral RNA" molecules after many rounds of amplification by the PCR. The problem with the quantification of input RNAs—after 30 to 50 rounds of amplification by the PCR[51]—is like calculating the number of the original settlers in America, from the current number of Americans and their current growth rates. But even if the 10^5 "plasma viral RNAs" per ml were real, it is hard to guess where they came from in view of "the scarcity of T-cells from which virus can be recovered ..." acknowledged by Maddox.[3]

However, the apparent lack of infectivity of the "free virus" or "virions"[2] resolves the paradox of the coexistence of 10^5 T-cells with 10^5 plasma viral RNAs per ml blood in Ho *et al.*'s and Wei *et al.*'s AIDS patients.[1] Even HIV cannot kill T-cells that it does not infect. The fact that over 99% of T-cells in persons with AIDS are not infected by HIV,[14, 26, 27, 31, 32, 44] is definitive evidence that there is no infectious HIV in typical AIDS patients. Clearly, in AIDS patients with 1.6 infectious HIV units per ml something other than HIV must cause AIDS.

In earlier efforts to resolve the paradox, that there is too little HIV in AIDS patients to cause AIDS, both groups have observed huge discrepancies between virus titers and AIDS symptoms. In 1993, George Shaw and colleagues have described otherwise identical AIDS patients of which 5 contained 0 infectious HIV per ml, and 22 contained between 5 and 10^5.[16,19] In 1989, David Ho *et al.* have also described 40 AIDS patients with virus titers ranging from less than 1 to 10^5 infectious units per ml.[30] In 1993, Ho *et al.* even reported 12 AIDS patients, including 8 who had AIDS "risk factors," who were totally HIV-free: "Specific antibody assays, viral cultures, and polymerase chain reaction (PCR) techniques" for HIV were all negative. Their T-cell counts ranged from 3 to 308 per μl.[52]

There is only one consistent hypothesis to reconcile the bewildering ranges of HIV titers in Ho's and Shaw's patients with the role of the virus in AIDS: HIV is a passenger virus, rather than the cause of AIDS. Indeed, non-correlation between the titers of a virus and disease, and between the very presence of a virus and disease, is one of the hallmarks of a passenger virus. Both Ho *et al.* and Shaw *et al.* have failed to understand that rare correlations between a virus-at-high-titer and a disease are the hallmark of a passenger virus, and that consistent correlations between a virus-at-high-titer and a disease are the hallmark of causative virus.[8,53,54] Therefore they have, contrary to their claims, established HIV as a passenger virus of AIDS patients.

(3) *Why HIV needs 10 years to cause AIDS.* Until HIV appeared on the scene, the latent period from infection to disease was a function of the generation time of a virus. A virus that replicates in 2 days and produces 100 viruses per generation would cause disease in about two weeks—provided there is no antiviral immu-

nity. This is because 100 viruses infect 100 cells producing 100 x 100 or 10,000 viruses 2 days later. Within 14 days of such exponential growth 10^{14} cells—the equivalent of a human body—would be infected. Therefore the latent periods of pathogenic retroviruses, like Rous sarcoma virus, and non-retroviruses like flu, measles, mumps, herpes, hepatitis, mononucleosis, chicken pox are all 7 to 14 days.[23.] Since HIV replicates in 2 days, like all other retroviruses,[48] and since according to Ho an infected cell produces over 1000 viruses per 2 days,[32] HIV should cause AIDS— if it could cause AIDS—just as fast as other viruses.

Yet, as Maddox points out, the failure of HIV to cause AIDS within weeks after infection presents another paradox for the HIV-AIDS hypothesis, "... the usually slow decline of CD4+ cells is not consistent with what one would expect from a specific cytotoxic viral mechanism." Indeed, both studies confirm the paradox. Since the AIDS patients contain 10^5 "free viruses/virions" and 10^5 T-cells per ml plasma, the plasma of these patients should be T-cell free within 2 days, the generation time of HIV. But Ho *et al.* report that the T-cells of AIDS patients are either steady or even increasing over 1 month, and Wei *et al.* report that the T-cells of their patients remain either steady or decline slowly over 5 to 8 months.[1,2]

Even if there are 50 times more T-cells in hidden reservoirs— as Ho *et al.* Report—they, too, should be infected within two weeks, because according to Wei *et al.*, the "plasma viral RNA" titer can rise two orders of magnitude within two weeks. In fact, the ability of HIV to increase from 10^3 "plasma viral RNA" units to 10^5 units per ml described by Wei *et al.* should only be a fraction of the real "dynamics of the infection of people by HIV,"[3] since it occurred despite the presence of two DNA chain terminators, AZT and ddI, used as anti-HIV drugs in addition to a new coded antiviral drug.

Therefore it remains paradoxical that—dated from the time

of HIV infection—AIDS occurs at entirely unpredictable times, currently estimated to average 10 years.[5] To determine whether the currently unpredictable time from HIV infection to AIDS can be reconciled with a viral mechanism at all, one needs to know whether HIV kills T-cells, how much *infectious* virus there is, and the *percentage of infected cells* at a given time. Since the new studies by Wei *et al.* and Ho *et al.* provide none of these data, all new calculations "on the dynamics of the infection of people by HIV … in the process of understanding the disease called AIDS" are worthless.

However, the hypothesis that HIV is a passenger virus provides a consistent explanation for the unpredictable time intervals between HIV infection and AIDS. It is one hallmark of a passenger virus, that the time of infection is unrelated to, and independent of the time when a disease occurs—just as with HIV and AIDS. Another hallmark of a passenger virus is that its titer and even its presence are not correlated with disease—just as was shown above for HIV and AIDS.

The simplest interpretation of the slow decline of T-cells in Ho's and Wei's AIDS patients is a non-viral cause, e.g. long-term intoxication.[7] Take for example the slow decline of liver cells in long-term alcoholics or of lung cells in long-term smokers.

Maddox seems concerned that "reporting of the new event has been curiously selective." Perhaps even science reporters begin to wonder how much further the virus-AIDS hypothesis can be stretched to explain its most obvious failures and inconsistencies: Why is there no vaccine? Why does American/European AIDS stay in the classical risk groups, male homosexuals, intravenous drug users and transfusion recipients? Why do AZT-treated HIV-positives get AIDS?[55,56] Why do 918 HIV-positive male homosexuals who had "avoided experimental medications on offer" and chose to abstain or significantly reduce their use of recreational drugs …" remain AIDS-free, long-term survivors?[57] Why did the

T-cells of 29% of 1,020 HIV-positive male homosexuals and former intravenous drug users from the placebo arm of a clinical AZT trial increase up to 22% over two years—despite the presence of HIV?[58] Why did the T-cells of 14 out of 31 HIV-positive hemophiliacs treated with highly purified factor VIII increase up to 25% over three years—despite the presence of HIV?[59] Why is there not a single study showing that HIV-positive 20- to 50-year-old men or women who are not drug users or recipients of transfusions ever get AIDS?[60]

Why did neither Ho et al. nor Wei et al. identify the risk groups their patients came from or indicate whether they had Kaposi's sarcoma, dementia, or diarrhea or lymphoma? Can they exclude that recreational drugs used by AIDS risk groups, like nitrite inhalants, amphetamines, and cocaine, are immunotoxic or carcinogenic?[61] Why is it that among 10 long-term (10 to 15 years) survivors of HIV recently described by Ho et al.[50] "none had received antiretroviral therapy ..."? Can Wei et al. and Ho et al. exclude that the DNA chain terminators, AZT and ddI, that their patients received in addition to the new experimental drugs do not play any role in the "slow decline of CD4+ cells"? Are they aware that the manufacturer of AZT says in the *Physician's Desk Reference* that "it was often difficult to distinguish adverse events possibly associated with zidovudine [AZT] administration from underlying signs of HIV diseases ..."?[62] Are they aware that the DNA chain terminators were developed 30 years ago to kill growing human cells for chemotherapy, not as anti-HIV drugs?

It seems to us that the "new developments" of Wei et al. and Ho et al. are a Mayday of AIDS virologists—rather than a "virological mayhem."[43]

Acknowledgments

We thank Serge Lang (Yale University), Siggi Sachs (UC Berkeley), and Russel Schoch (UC Berkeley) for critical comments. Supported by the Council for Tobacco Research, USA, and private donations.

References

1. Wei, X., *et al. Nature* 373, 117–122 (1995).

2. Ho, D. D., *et al. Nature* 373, 123–126 (1995).

3. Maddox, J. *Nature* 373, 189 (1995).

4. Gallo, R. C., *et al. Science* 224, 500–503 (1984).

5. Institute of Medicine. *Confronting AIDS—Update 1988* (National Academy Press, Washington, DC, 1988).

6. Centers for Disease Control and Prevention. *Morb Mort Weekly Rep* 41 (No. RR17), 1–19 (1992).

7. Duesberg, P. H. *Pharmacology & Therapeutics* 55, 201–277 (1992).

8. Duesberg, P. H. *Int. Arch. Allergy Immunol.* 103, 131–142 (1994).

9. Murray, H. W., Scavuzzo, D. A., Kelly, C. D., Rubin, B. Y. & Roberts, R. B. *Arch. Intern. Med.* 148, 1613–1616 (1988).

10. Spornraft, P., *et al. Br. J. Dermatol.* 119, 1–9 (1988).

11. Friedman-Kien, A. E., *et al. Lancet* 335, 168–169 (1990).

12. Kaldor, J. M., Tindall, B., Williamson, P., Elford, J. & Cooper, D. A. *J. of Acquired Immune Deficiency Syndromes* 6, 1145–1149 (1993).

13. Bacellar, H., *et al. Neurology* 44, 1892–1900 (1994).

14. Blattner, W. A., Gallo, R. C. & Temin, H. M. *Science* 241, 514–515 (1988).

15. Duesberg, P. H. *Science* 241, 514–516 (1988).

16. Piatak, M., *et al. Science* 259, 1749–1754 (1993).

17. Daar, E. S., Moudgil, T., Meyer, R. D. & Ho, D. D. *N. Engl. J. Med.* 324, 961–964 (1991).

18. Clark, S. J., *et al. N. Engl. J. Med.* 324, 954–960 (1991).

19. Duesberg, P. H. *Science* 260, 1705 (1993).

20. Mims, C. & White, D. O. *Viral Pathogenesis and Immunology* (Oxford: Blackwell Scientific Publications, 1984).

21. Freeman, B. A. *Burrows Textbook of Microbiology* (Philadelphia: W. B. Saunders Co., 1979).

22. Weiss, R. A. *Science* 260, 1273–1279 (1993).

23. Fenner, F., McAuslan, B. R., Mims, C. A., Sambrook, J. & White, D. O. *The Biology of Animal Viruses* (New York: Academic Press, Inc., 1974).

24. Gross, L. *Oncogenic Viruses* (Oxford: Pergamon Press, 1970).

· ·

25. Harper, M. E., Marselle, L. M., Gallo, R. C. & Wong-Staal, F. *PNAS* 83, 772–776 (1986).

26. Simmonds, P., *et al. J. Virol.* 64, 864–872 (1990).

27. Shaw, G. M., *et al. Science* 226, 1165–1171 (1984).

28. Weiss, S. H., *et al. Science* 239, 68–71 (1988).

29. Falk, L. A., Jr. *NEJM* 316, 1547–1548 (1987).

30. Ho, D. D., Moudgil, T. & Alam, M. *New Engl. J. Med.* 321, 1621–1625 (1989).

31. Schnittman, S. M., *et al. Science* 245, 305–308 (1989).

32. Ho, D. *New Engl. J. Med.* 322, 1467 (1990).

33. Centers for Disease Control. *HIV/AIDS Surveillance,* year-end edition, 1–23 (1993).

34. Benditt, J. & Jasny, B. *Science* 260, 1219, 1253–1293 (1993).

35. Fields, B. N. *Nature* 369, 95–96 (1994).

36. Swinbanks, D. *Nature* 370, 494 (1994).

37. Rubinstein, E. *Science* 248, 1499–1507 (1990).

38. Karpas, A., Lowdell, M., Jacobson, S. K. & Hill, F. *PNAS* 89, 8351–8355 (1992).

39. Langhoff, E., *et al. J. Clin. Invest.* 84, 1637–1643 (1989).

40. Lemaitre, M., Guetard, D., Henin, Y., Montagnier, L. & Zerial, A. *Res. Virol.* 141, 5–16 (1990).

41. Hoxie, J. A., Haggarty, B. S., Rakowski, J. L., Pillsbury, N. & Levy, J. A. *Science* 229, 1400–1402 (1985).

42. Anand, R., *et al. Lancet* ii, 234–238 (1987).

43. Wain-Hobson, S. *Nature* 373, (1995).

44. Pantaleo, G., *et al. Nature* 362, 355–358 (1993).

45. Cohen, J. *Science* 259, 168–170 (1993).

46. Weiss, R. *Nature* 349, 374 (1991).

47. Embretson, J., *et al. Nature* 362, 359–362 (1993).

48. Weiss, R., Teich, N., Varmus, H. & Coffin, J. *Molecular Biology of RNA Tumor Viruses* (Cold Spring Harbor, New York: Cold Spring Harbor Press, 1985).

49. Cohen, J. *Science* 260, 292–293 (1993).

50. Cao, Y., Quin, L., Zhang, L., Safrit, J. & Ho, D. D. *N. Engl. J. Med.* 332, 201–208 (1995).

51. Raeymaekers, L. *Analytical Biochemistry* 214, 582–585 (1993).

52. Ho, D. D., *et al. NEJM* 328, 380–385 (1993).

53. Duesberg, P. *Science* 260, 1705 (1993).

54. Duesberg, P. H. *N. Engl. J. Med.* 322, 1466 (1990).

55. Seligmann, M., *et al. Lancet* 343, 871–881 (1994).

56. Goedert, J. J., *et al. Lancet* 344, 791–792 (1994).

57. Wells, J. *Capital Gay,* August 20th, 14–15 (1993).

58. Hughes, M. D., *et al. J. Infectious Diseases* 169, 28–36 (1994).

59. Seremetis, S. V., *et al. Lancet* 342, 700–703 (1993).

60. Duesberg, P. *Science* 267, 313 (1995).

61. Haverkos, H. W. & Dougherty, J. A. *Health Hazards of Nitrite Inhalants* (U.S. Dept. Health & Human Services, Washington, DC, 1988).

62. *Physicians' Desk Reference.* Retrovir, pp. 742–746 (Medical Economics Co., Orandell, NJ, 1994).

* The text above incorporates all of our points of response to the following:

Letter from John Maddox to Peter Duesberg

Nature
4 Little Essex St.
London, WC2R 3LF

2 March 1995

Peter H Duesberg
Department of Molecular and Cell Biology
University of California
Berkeley, CA 94720

Dear Peter,

First, the good news: we shall publish the essence of what you have to say. But there are obvious snags. Let me retail my original conversation with Harvey Bialy. What format? he asked. A letter, I said. That's too little, he said; what about 1,000 words. I said I was not prepared to negotiate the length of a letter not yet written. But what you have sent would take at least 3 pages of *Nature*.

Second, I resent the way in which you appear to have alerted the world's press to the existence of your piece. Why do that?

Third, and this may not be such good news, I plan to go through your piece with a fine-tooth comb with the intention of ridding it of repetitions and various misrepresentations.

Let me illustrate the last point by reference to your page 3 and the continuation of the main paragraph on page 4. You start with the phrase "HIV was proposed to follow an entirely unprecedented course of action," you document various misconceptions about the functioning of HIV and then you conclude with the phrase "this HIV-hypothesis." Frankly, that smacks of the old Goebbels technique, that of creating a straw man from a farrago of indefensible propositions and then knocking it down. I know of nobody who, in the past decade, has put forward your points (1) to (5) as a unified statement of the conventional position. (Even you have to assemble the position with 20 references.) On the contrary, the "HIV-hypothesis" is much simpler: "HIV causes AIDS, in some manner not understood; most of those infected will develop the disease."

Nor is it a fair representation of Wei *et al.* and Ho *et al.* to say that they "claim" to resolve the three specific "paradoxes" you list. In truth, they do nothing of the kind. The only conceivable reference to the 10-year latency period, for example, is in Ho *et al.*, and consists of the simile of the tap and drain. To quote from Wei *et al.*, "The kinetics of virus and CD4+ lymphocyte replication" imply "First,... continuous rounds of *de novo* virus infection, replication and rapid cell turnover ... probably represent a primary driving force in HIV pathogenesis ... Second ... a striking capacity of the virus for biologically relevant change. Third ... that virus production *per se* is directly involved in CD4+ cell destruction." Ho *et al.* go further, but only to this extent: "... our findings strongly support the view that AIDS is primarily a consequence of continuous high-level replication of HIV-1, leading to virus and immune-mediated killing of CD4 lymphocytes."

My position as an editor is that straight misrepresentations such as these have no place in a journal like this. You complain at an earlier stage that I have improperly "personalized" this argument. How do you suppose that Wei *et al.* and Ho *et al.* would feel if we were to publish your travesty of what they have said?

My suggestion, therefore, is that you throw away the first four pages of your introduction, and devise a less inflammatory introduction in which you state that the two papers have not changed your view, and go on to give the reasons. Please let me know whether that is acceptable. I have some other less radical comments on the remainder of the text, but there's no point in sending them at this stage if you cannot agree to something along the lines I have suggested.

Yours sincerely,
John Maddox
Editor
cc: Harvey Bialy

Letter from Peter Duesberg to *Nature*

7 March 1995

Sir John Maddox
Nature, Macmillan Publishing
4 Little Essex St., London WC2R 3LF
England

Dear John,
After you have invited us with an editorial "to comment" on "the new view of HIV" (*Nature,* 19 January 1995), we are surprised to learn that you only want to "publish the essence of what [we] have to say."

We have followed your advice that "it should be no longer than it needs to be." Since neither of the two new *Nature* studies nor the two accompanying News and Views by you and Wain-

Hobson have explained the old view of HIV, we had to explain the old view first for the reader of *Nature* to understand our comments on "the new view of HIV." We are not interested in a discussion between experts restricted just to titers of HIV. Therefore we cannot accept your suggestion to "throw away the first four pages" of our commentary.

Moreover, if our commentary comes out to be 3 pages in *Nature*, as you say, that would only be a fourth of the space you have already dedicated to the "new view of HIV"—10 pages for the two papers and 2 pages for the two editorials. A 3-page commentary on 12 pages in *Nature*, supplemented by an international press release, is hardly a convincing argument that "it is longer than it needs to be."

You write that you "resent the way in which [we] appear to have alerted the world press to the existence of [our] piece." However, we are afraid, if alerting the world's press is a reason for resentment, we should resent you. After all, you have alerted the world's press using the power of your office about the "embarrassment for Duesberg" and that you "eagerly awaited" our "comment." But you did not respond to our commentary from February 7 until March 2. As a result of your activities the world's press has called us, and some callers were given our commentary, weeks after you had received it, with the proviso that it may not be published in its present form by *Nature*. Indeed, the exchange of opinions is protected by the free-speech amendment in this country.

Are you aware that both Wei *et al.* and Ho *et al.* gave their papers to John Coffin and David Baltimore prior to publication in *Nature* to write editorials for *Science* (267, 483, 1995) and *NEJM* (332, 259–260, 1995) respectively?

If you plan to meet your published commitment that "his [Duesberg] and his associates' views on the new developments should be made public" by first cutting, and then editing our commentary with a "fine-tooth comb with the intention of ridding it of ... various misrepresentations," we do not see a basis for an open debate with you.

In response to your letter we resubmit our manuscript with some revisions:

1) page 2, third paragraph: Replace "despite these 'new studies'" by "in light of these new studies."

2) page 2, fourth paragraph: Insert after "immunodeficiency syndrome (AIDS)," "if antibody to HIVis present."

3) page 3, item (2): According to Shaw, Ho and their collaborators, HIV activity is "rapidly and effectively limited" by this antiviral activity.[17,18]

4) page 4, second paragraph: Replace the sentence "The new studies claim to resolve ..." by "The new studies are claimed by two News and Views articles from Maddox (ref. 3) and Wain-Hobson (ref. 43) to resolve the paradoxa, (I) How HIV kills T-cells, (II) how HIV causes AIDS, and (III) why HIV needs 10 years to cause AIDS."

5) page 6, end; Insert the following paragraph after "... numerous previous reports (see above)": "Ho and a different group of collaborators just published a paper in which they show that over 10,000 "plasma virions," detected by the "branched DNA signal-amplification assay" used in the *Nature* paper correspond to less than one (!) infectious virus.[50] Thus Wei *et al.* and Ho *et al.* both reported titers of 10^5 biochemical virus-units that really correspond to one or even less than one infectious virus. However, infectivity is the only clinically relevant criterion of a virus."

6) page 11: Insert after "are immunotoxic or carcinogenic?" "Why is it that among 10 long-term (10 to 15 years) survivors of HIV recently described by Ho *et al.*[50] 'none had received anti-retroviral therapy ...'?"

References

17. Daar, E. S., Moudgil, T., Meyer, R. D. & Ho, D. D. *N. Engl. J. Med.* 324:961–964 (1991).

18. Clark, S. J., *et al.*, *N. Engl. J. Med.* 324:954–960 (1991).

50. Cao, Y., Quin, L. Zhang, L., Safrit, J. & Ho, D. D. *N. Engl. J. Med.* 332:201–208 (1995).

Sincerely,

Peter Duesberg, Harvey Bialy (faxed)

On May 18, 1995, *Nature* published a Duesberg-Bialy letter flanked by two editorial comments:

1) "AIDS pathology unknown"

Nature 375: 167, May 18, 1995

HIV infection provokes hyperactivity of the immune system, but the causes of that are far from understood.

The clutch of contributions to *Scientific Correspondence* (page 193) this week deserves a reading, both for its inherent interest and for what it says about the present state of AIDS research. It will be recalled this journal published in January an account of research that showed that the infection of a person by the virus HIV ordinarily evokes not the previously suspected quiescence of the immune system, but a rapid turnover both of the vulnerable lymphocytes and of the virus itself. The then-general opinion that the first reaction of the human body to infection by HIV is a kind of indifference was dramatically and directly challenged. Nothing that has since come to light denies the challenge. But it has also become plain that too little is yet known of the dynamics of the immune system. That is a gap to fill.

The second arresting feature of this correspondence is the letter from Dr. Peter Duesberg and his colleague, Dr. Harvey Bialy, which has been published without change. Sadly, there seems no way in which the authors concerned can be persuaded that "free and fair scientific debate" is ordinarily understood to mean a progressive process, one in which each of two sides learns from what the other says. A restatement of earlier and well-known positions is not that at all. On this occasion, Duesberg and Bialy's citation of Loveday in their cause is especially inappropriate, given Loveday's name among the authors of a letter supporting Wei *et al.* and Ho *et al.* But no further solicitation of Duesberg's opinion is called for.

2) "HIV an illusion"

Letter from Peter Duesberg and Harvey Bialy,
Nature 375:197, May 18, 1995

SIR—In an editorial in the 19 January issue of *Nature,* John Maddox invited "Duesberg and his associates" to comment on the "HIV-1 dynamics" papers published the previous week, indicating that these new results should prove an embarrassment to us. Although we do not think that a scientist should be embarrassed for pointing out inconsistencies and paradoxes in a hypothesis that have only been reportedly resolved 10 years later, we nonetheless prepared a fully referenced, approximately 2,000-word critique of the Ho *et al.*[2] and Wei *et al.*[3] papers that we believed met the criteria of "not being longer than it needs to be, and pertaining to the papers at hand" that Maddox set out in his widely read challenge.

Unfortunately, he did not share our view and agreed to publish only a radically shortened version, and only after he had personally "gone over it with a fine-tooth comb" to remove our perceived misrepresentations of the issues. We found these new conditions so totally at variance with the spirit of free and fair scientific debate that we could not agree to them.

Readers of *Nature* who are interested in these questions, and feel that they do not need to be protected by Maddox from our ill-conceived logic, can find the complete text of our commentary in the monograph supplement to the most recent issue of *Genetica.*[4]

Here we would point out only that the central claim of the Ho *et al.*[2] and Wei *et al.*[3] papers—that 10^5 HIV virions per ml plasma can be detected in AIDS patients with various nucleic-acid amplification assays—is misleading. The senior author of the Wei *et al.* paper has previously claimed that the PCR method they used overestimates by at least 60,000 times the real titer of infectious HIV[5]: 100,000/60,000 is 1.7 infectious HIVs per ml, hardly the "virological mayhem" alluded to by Wain-Hobson.[6] Further, Ho and a different group of collaborators have just shown[7] that more than 10,000 "plasma virions," detected by the branched-DNA amplification assay used in their *Nature* paper, correspond to less than one (!) infectious virus per ml. And infectious units, after all, are the only clinically relevant criteria for a viral pathogen.

Finally, in view of Wain-Hobson's statement[6] that "the concordance of their [Wei and Ho's] data is remarkable," note that Loveday *et al.*[8] report the use of a PCR-based assay and find only 200 HIV "virion RNAs" per ml of serum of AIDS patients—1,000 times less than Ho and Wei. So much for the "remarkable concordance."

Peter Duesberg
Department of Molecular and Cellular Biology,
University of California, Berkeley, California 94720, USA
Harvey Bialy
Bio/Technology, New York, New York 10012, USA

Notes and References

1. Maddox, J. *Nature* 373, 189 (1995).
2. Ho, D. D., *et al. Nature* 373, 123–126 (1995).
3. Wei. X., *et al. Nature* 373, 117–122 (1995).
4. Duesberg, P. & Bialy, H. *Genetica* Suppl. (in the press).
5. Piatak, M., *et al. Science* 259, 1749–1754 (1993).
6. Wain-Hobson, S. *Nature* 373, 102 (1995).
7. Cao, Y., *et al. New Engl. J. Med.* 332, 201–208 (1995).
8. Loveday, C., *et al. Lancet* 345, 820–824 (1995).

3) Editorial Statement

The letter above was followed by the editorial statement: "Peter Duesberg was offered space in *Scientific Correspondence* for 500 words of his own choice, but declined.—Editor, *Scientific Correspondence*."

Letter from Peter Duesberg to John Maddox

(not published in *Nature*)

Sir John Maddox
Editor, *Nature*
Porters South, Crinnan St.
London, England

10 July 1995

Dear John,

Following publication of the Duesberg-Bialy letter on May 18, *Nature* added: "Peter Duesberg was offered space in "Scientific Correspondence" for 500 words of his own choice but declined." Since our letter used up that "space," *Nature*'s comment is erroneous and should be retracted.

Could you please confirm or un-confirm our conclusion. I have faxed to you twice before requesting an answer to this question (June 20 and June 22, 1995) but have not received a reply.

Sincerely,
Peter Duesberg
cc: Harvey Bialy

Letter from *Nature* to Peter Duesberg

Nature
Porters South, 4–6 Crinan Street
London, England

19 July 1995

Dr. P. Duesberg
Department of Molecular and Cell Biology
University of California
Berkeley, CA 94720

Dear Dr. Duesberg,
Thank you for your various faxes. We offered to publish a 500-word version of your response to Ho/Shaw in our issue in which we published other comments on those papers. You declined, and instead sent us a complaint that we would not publish your long manuscript. We published that complaint. As far as we are concerned, the matter rests.

Yours sincerely,
Dr. Maxine Clarke
Executive Editor, *Nature*

4

....

Good Mourning America

"Entrapment is this society's / sole activity"
—Edward Dorn, *Gunslinger*

John was not always as unkind in rejecting Peter's submissions to *Nature* on the subject of HIV and AIDS as he was to become, though reject them he did, and often in the most revealing prose. On November 17, 1988, he wrote Peter the following:

> I am glad you correctly infer from my letter that I am in many ways sympathetic to what you say. I did not ask you to revise the manuscript, however. The danger, as it seems to me, is that the dispute between you and what you call the HIV community will mislead and distress the public in the following way. You point to a number of ways in which the HIV hypothesis may be deficient. It would be a rash person who said that you are wrong, but ... if we were to publish your paper, we would find ourselves asking people to believe that what has been said so far about the cause of AIDS is a pack of lies. Anyway, I am glad that your paper is going to be published (elsewhere).[1]

The story of this manuscript, which would appear in the February 1989 *Proceedings of the National Academy of Sciences (USA),*[2] is almost as tortured as the reasoning—so exactly opposed to the purpose of scientific discourse—with which it was rejected. It would also record the first time Peter discovered he was not bullet-proof.

Although even at this relatively late juncture it might have been possible for *Nature* to become the foil rather than the slave of scientific fashion, with the above letter Maddox put the weight of his journal (which, along with *Science,* shapes the thinking of the vast majority of working biologists) irrevocably behind the virus-AIDS hypothesis. The significance of their backing to this slam-dunk of the scientific method is even more important than their joint advocacy of the nouveau oncogene, and cannot be overemphasized.

The road to the *Proceedings* paper begins with the first notice taken by either of the two heavyweight journals of Peter's *Cancer Research* article and the attendant interest in the possibility that AIDS was not precisely the terrible scourge that it was portrayed to be. It came in the pages of *Science* in March of 1988,[3] shortly before the AmFar ambush. Prototypically, the piece was written by a youthful journalist, not a serious scientist, and accordingly, it mainly addressed the sociology of Peter's challenges rather than their substance. It was entitled "A rebel without a cause of AIDS." Considering the fact that Peter was defending traditional virology, and the virus-AIDS proponents were in reality the rebels, the title seemed odd and slightly offensive then and appears even more so now. Nevertheless, this piece was to set the future mainstream journalistic standard in regard to the kindly professor Duesberg, indelibly coloring his image with scientists who did not personally know him. Its author's well-learned lesson: Sufficiently distort the messenger and no meaningful message can possibly emerge.

Although one can detect a small amount of affection for the "rebel" Duesberg, the overall tone of the article by William Booth is a genuflection to the power of authority and received wisdom, as would be expected from a reporter far beyond his depth of competence. But as with many a "period piece," the article is much more instructive today than when it appeared. *Res ipsa loquitur.* And in this case the thing that speaks for itself most clearly is the headshot. Although worth only about three hundred words in journal space—as it occupies almost a third of the article's opening page—the photo is in fact worth "whole volumes in folio."

Peter has an extremely photogenic visage and is most often captured with a wry grin befitting Booth's otherwise accurate depiction of him as an "immensely quotable gadfly with a sharp sense of humor who does not hesitate to tweak the noses of figures in the biochemical research community whose egos often loom larger than life."[3] But in this remarkable photograph, he is portrayed as the most sinister and shadowy of figures, looking "like an expressionist villain in a Fritz Lang movie," as he was to email immediately when I asked if he knew where Booth obtained that especially ghastly picture.

> *A* Science *photographer took it, and others, in my lab. I was wondering at the time, why in several of them I looked like an expressionist villain in a Fritz Lang movie, like Dr. Caligari. Now I know. (3 March 2000)*

In stark contrast, on the last page of the article we see a most dignified portrayal of David Baltimore, who a few years later would be driven from the presidency of Rockefeller University for his unrelenting commitment to the veracity of fraudulent research findings that were published with his name attached.[4] Booth quoted him in referring to Peter as "irresponsible and pernicious"; Baltimore is pictured in an appropriately-sized quarter-column box, arms crossed confidently, and exuding all his magisterial pomposity.

The accompanying text is full of equally informative contradictions. For example, Booth begins in a reasonable enough fashion by stating: "Basically, Duesberg does not think that HIV is virulent enough to cause AIDS, a conclusion he bases on widely recognized gaps in knowledge about how the virus operates in the body."[3]—although even here he could have more accurately written: "a conclusion he bases on widely recognized gaps between how HIV behaves and the behavior of all other viral pathogens." He then notes quite accurately that Peter had "aroused a great deal of anger and exasperation among AIDS researchers, who insist that an overwhelming body of evidence points toward HIV as the culprit behind AIDS."[3]

But he immediately continues with a gross distortion unlikely to be noticed as such by *Science*'s usual readers, and designed like the photograph to insinuate unmistakably that Duesberg was an extremely marginal character. Booth plays on both their ignorance and their real or imagined conservatism as follows: "At the same time, these remarks have won for their proponent a large amount of media attention, particularly in the gay press where he is portrayed as something of a hero."[3]

All other implications aside, in fact the amount of media attention Peter received had been quite minimal, and more importantly, in the gay press it was only Chuck Ortleb's *New York Native* that supported Peter's position, and he was eventually hounded out of business by an ActUp-sponsored boycott exactly because of his paper's contrarian views. Every other gay activist publication and group was solidly behind the NIH and the virus-AIDS hypothesis. The truth is that Peter was even more their enemy than he was the retrovirologists', whose hypothesis implied that everybody was at equal risk and that homosexuals were just unfortunate "to (along with heroin abusers, Haitian immigrants, and hemophiliacs) be among the populations where the virus first got its footing in the United States,"[3] as Booth quoted their real hero James Curran, director of the CDC's AIDS program. Never mind what became of the Haitian immigrants, an original member of the "4H club" of AIDS risk groups—or for that matter the spate of dire predictions about the impending decimation of the entire island from which they emigrated[5]—except to note that these same completely inaccurate predictions are echoed today in sanctimonious press releases from Geneva regarding sub-Saharan Africa, Brazil, India, Thailand, and other tropical places with endemic public health problems, poor to non-existent epidemiological statistics, and inhabited by people with dark skin.

Booth continues his enlightening presentation by quoting Peter who I can picture quite plaintively and with real bewilderment, asking, "Why won't they respond?" in reference to the deafening silence with which the *Cancer Research* article was received by his peers. Our intrepid investigative reporter might have chorused at this point, "Indeed, why haven't they?" since it is amazing that more than one year after a respected scientific journal published a damning, scholarly critique of a widely held medical hypothesis; a critique that moreover was written by a member of the U.S. National Academy of Sciences whose pioneering work on retroviruses had frequently caused his name to be mentioned in Stockholm, not a single proponent of the hypothesis had seen the need to respond. Instead, Booth merely asks some of these scientists Peter's simple question. Their answers are illuminating, and the fact that Booth lets these examples of scientific demeanor and logic stand without any further remark is even more so.

"I cannot respond without shrieking," says Gallo. "It is absolute and total nonsense," says Anthony Fauci, coordinator of AIDS research at the National Institutes of Health (NIH). "Irresponsible and pernicious," says David Baltimore, director of the Whitehead Institute in Cambridge, Massachusetts, and a chairman of the Institute of Medicine-National Academy of Sciences committee that produced the benchmark report *Confronting AIDS*. Yet Duesberg keeps pressing. "Like a little dog that won't let go," says Gallo."[3]

Booth, Gallo, and Fauci seem particularly fond of this final insulting adjective ("little"), as *Science*'s point man on AIDS quotes Fauci once again, using it to full effect.

"But he likes to talk about expression and pathogenesis and latency and this and that, and then everybody gets confused and says, I don't know what those guys are talking about. They're all confused! So maybe this little guy is right."[3]

Fauci's own considerable scientific intellect is further demonstrated in his reply to Peter's contention that all of the AIDS risk groups have obvious, long-term immunosuppressive lifestyles, or severe health problems. (Nobody receives several units of transfused blood who is not otherwise quite ill; it would be hard to argue that the lifestyles of heroin addicts and the at-risk sector of the gay sub-culture promote good health; and hemophiliacs are a classic case of an iatrogenically immunosuppressed group because of the clotting factor they must receive.) Apparently forgetting that hemophiliacs rarely reach the age expected of those with sixty-year-old wives, and that the case to which he alludes never existed, Fauci—the coordinator of government AIDS research—proclaims: "Is Duesberg trying to tell me that the transfusion cases are caused by life-style?" "How about the 60-year-old wife of a hemophiliac who gets infected? She's out cruising, too?"[3]

Almost as shameful, and much more to the point of this debate manqué, is the following from David Baltimore:

What Duesberg seems to be saying is that "correlations are not causality," says Baltimore. In establishing HIV as the

etiological agent in AIDS, correlations are extremely important. Duesberg is not the only skeptic in the community, as
he likes to think. In the early days of the AIDS epidemic,
Baltimore says that virologists like himself watched the
scientific literature very carefully. When Gallo put forth
the notion that AIDS might be caused by HTLV-I, a retrovirus that has been linked to a rare form of cancer, there
were few converts. In 1983, when Luc Montagnier of the
Pasteur Institute in Paris found a new retrovirus in AIDS
patients, there was keen interest, but still great skepticism,
since Montagnier had failed to prove that HIV was a
causative agent rather than an opportunistic infection. In
a rapid series of papers in 1984, Gallo and colleagues
reported finding antibodies to HIV in almost 90% of a group
of AIDS patients. In 115 healthy heterosexuals, they
detected no anti-HIV activity. The studies were conducted
double-blind. "This was the kind of evidence that we were
looking for. It distinguished between a virus that was a passenger and one that was a cause."[3]

How these epidemiological studies proved anything more than
the antibody test had some specificity remains mysterious to me,
but David's chronological account is otherwise quite informative.
He unintentionally corroborates Peter's damning observation that
when the NIH announced it had discovered the cause of AIDS,
there was hardly sufficient evidence to support such a grandiose
contention. Baltimore is also correct in pointing out that Peter
was saying exactly that correlation is never sufficient to prove
causation. In fact, Duesberg would go on to incorporate that very
phrase in the title of the *Proceedings* article published in 1989.

Near the end of his piece Booth makes an extremely interesting admission, and one that an attentive (even if unsympathetic)
reader might have taken to heart. He writes: "Duesberg has played

the role of the rebel before. After years of working on oncogenes, Duesberg began shooting holes in some of the overblown claims that were made linking genes to cancer."[3] That perhaps some of the claims about HIV were equally overblown, and after working twenty-four years on retroviruses, Peter was only doing the same thing, did not arise.

The month after Booth's article appeared in *Science,* Peter was in England, the recipient of an Oxford University Lichtfield Lectureship, speaking on his "heresy," as the *New Scientist* (a kind of British *Time* magazine of science) already called it that very week.[6] At the close of a talk at Hammersmith College, London, in which he expounded his heretical position to some genuine interest and extremely mild opposition,[7] Duesberg had another conversation with Peter Newmark of *Nature.* Like myself initially, Newmark was not so much persuaded by the HIV arguments as by the far less politically resonant ones against oncogenes. Nonetheless, he agreed to consider a possible review. Duesberg immediately set to work with his usual diligence and a somewhat heightened sense of urgency as he glimpsed a golden opportunity to turn the light fully on.

My own response to Booth's misleading reporting, which in a mangled account of the White House affair had mentioned my name, was a letter to Daniel Koshland, *Science*'s editor at the time, whom I knew a good deal longer and better than John Maddox, since he was one of my teachers in graduate school.

Koshland, unlike Maddox, is not only a scientist but one of considerable professional accomplishment. As I reminded him in my letter, in the late sixties he was the "Duesberg of allostery" when his own hypothesis about the way conformational changes in enzymes came about was almost universally considered to be wrong. I also chided him for allowing Fauci, Gallo, and Baltimore's unbecoming, *ad hominem* attacks and personal insults. According to Peter, as a result of this letter and a few others—

and, I think, a real sense of personal regret for not paying closer attention to what his journal was intending to publish—Koshland, who was commuting between his lab at Berkeley and a second office in DC (which perhaps explains his lapse in properly editing the Booth article), was sympathetic and accommodating when Peter reached him by telephone shortly after returning from the UK. The eventual outcome of their conversation was a "Policy Forum" that ran in *Science* the last week of July 1988 in which Duesberg and some of his principal opponents would finally begin an exchange of scientific arguments. Peter remembers its inception as follows:

> *Having been so "personally" represented by Booth/Science I insisted to Dan that I should be given adequate space to explain that, contrary to Booth, I was not without a cause, and what my "cause" was. Obviously Koshland/Science decided upon receipt of my piece making essentially the points of the later Policy Forum that so much anti-American HIV writing could not be presented to the readers without immediate "balance" by Blattner, Gallo & Temin. And that was Koshland's Salomonic decision—we all could have our cake. I had my right of reply, Gallo had saved HIV for the "honor roll" of American science, and Dan was everybody's friend.*

Koshland told Duesberg that he wanted him to reduce the length of his piece to approximately five hundred words so that it matched the length of a statement making the case that HIV was the cause of AIDS he had received from William Blattner, Robert Gallo, and Howard Temin. Upon receipt of that he would send Duesberg Gallo's piece (and vice versa) for an additional five hundred-word rebuttal, and the entire exchange would be published as a "Policy Forum." Of all the puzzling features concerning Peter's relentless and almost totally unsuccessful attempts to bring his considered and fully documented arguments to a wider scientific audience, the severe space restrictions that *Science* insisted on (and later *Nature,* as we saw in the previous chapter) is one of the more enigmatic, given the magnitude of the concern about AIDS and the fact that the same journals devote literally thousands of pages to the often much less considered words of the HIV orthodoxy.

Nevertheless, Peter complied, and after a certain amount of back and forth, in July "Koshland/*Science*" published what is still the only semblance of a real debate on the cause of AIDS in the scientific literature.[8] That Howard Temin was the senior representative for the virus-AIDS proponents merits special attention, since Temin never worked on HIV, and Peter's failure to do so was often used as a major hammer against him. But as I pointed out in the last chapter, Temin was the untarnished, undisputed champion of "new" when it came to retroviruses, and "new" as we will now see was to be the first line of defense of the virus-AIDS camp. In addition, neither Gallo nor Blattner (nor the two together) had the scientific credentials to stand against Peter unsupported nor, judging from their later writing, the skill to muster unassisted even the weak rebuttals to his five hundred prosecutorial words that appeared. Nobody I spoke to after the fact thought Gallo's side had won. In keeping with the generally non-confrontational temperament of scientists, most were content to call it a draw, go back to their labs, and await further developments.

As in all debates, in the first round each opponent comes out with his or her best rhetorical flourish. And if I were judging, I would have to score the round 10–9 for Team Virus, since I believe Peter made a tactical error in setting an excessively didactic tone in his opening statement, giving the other side opportunities to feint and jab. I favored the "come out swinging," experimental-challenge style of the *Bio/Technology* "Last Word" and the summation paragraphs in *Cancer Research*. But Peter had his own ideas, and ignoring advice from his corner, began as follows: *Human immunodeficiency virus (HIV) is not the cause of AIDS because it fails to meet the postulates of Koch and Henle, as well as six cardinal rules of virology.*[8]

The postulates for microbial disease causation originally formalized by the German microbiologist Robert Koch in the middle of the nineteenth century are familiar to every student of biology. They were established in order to correct a serious, unintended consequence of Pasteur's essential proof of the germ theory of disease. Almost exactly like the mutant gene hunters of today, the new microbe hunters of Pasteur's time were finding disease-causing microbes everywhere, and conditions from headaches to heartaches were being blamed on all sorts of bacteria with no attention whatsoever given to distinguishing a harmless passenger microbe from a pathogenic one. In stepped Peter's hero Koch, who said it is only logical that any microbe proposed as a disease-causing candidate must satisfy the following conditions: It should be present in all cases of the disease from which it should be possible to isolate it in a pure form, and in such a pure form it should be capable of reproducing the disease in a susceptible host.

Whether or not HIV meets these criteria, there is no one who could counter that the postulates themselves are not standard textbook fare. The "six cardinal rules of virology," however, are a different kettle of fish. There is no text that lists the rules of virology. What Peter, in deciding to play "Herr Doktor Professor" to the hilt, now called rules are really no different from the former experimental challenges. But being re-designated, their actual content was somehow diminished, and the Temin team used this dogmatic approach against the apparent iconoclast. Although failing to do any damage to the body, they could at least redden his face a bit by countering that "Biology is an experimental science and new biological phenomena are constantly being discovered."[8]

In what follows, I comment on rounds one and two, combining them since it is only in the second round that a debate has any action. Peter followed his dogmatic one-two punch with a couple of sharp jabs, noting that detection and isolation of the virus from all AIDS cases had hardly been demonstrated as of mid-1988; and further, that isolation of HIV from AIDS patients depended on the laboratory activation of deeply asleep HIV genomes that at best resided in only 10–15% of the body's white blood cells. This is a task that virologists of even the recent past would have found impossible. This second point is an important corollary of the key argument we examined in the previous chapter concerning the absence of sufficient active virus in AIDS patients to account for the collapse of their T-cell immunity. It is not enough to deflect the first punch, as Team Virus would, by saying that newer techniques, like more sophisticated versions of basic PCR, now did or would show that HIV proviral genes are present in "virtually all" AIDS patients, and then pretend that the second blow was never even thrown, let alone landed hard. Detecting a viral gene or genome is not the same as isolating a virus. If there is too little active virus present to be readily isolated, then its role as a causative agent is automatically suspect. As Peter continues to point out: "Even a post-modern virus should do something to get something done. HIV is biochemically so quiet it needs 35 cycles of PCR to hear it."[8]

Kid Heretic followed his two stiff opening jabs with an uppercut that connected with enough force to reverberate loudly even today. Why don't chimpanzees develop AIDS after experimental infection with HIV? They are, after all, our closest genetic relatives, and they are susceptible hosts for every single human virus, including HIV. And yet, today when more than fifty chimpanzees have been successfully infected for more than seventeen years, as demonstrated by their positive "AIDS-tests," not one has developed clinical AIDS. There is no other virus that causes a disease in humans which will not reproduce that disease in chimps. Team Temin could only come back with: "It is true HIV does not cause AIDS in chimpanzees. Most viruses are species-specific in host range and in capacity to produce disease."[8] Host range is not at issue since HIV infects chimps quite all right, but they follow this flay at thin air with a powerful-sounding near miss. "For example, herpes B virus, yellow fever virus, and dengue virus cause serious diseases in humans, but produce no disease symptoms during infection in many species of monkeys."[8] Chimps may be a lot of things, but they are most definitely not monkeys, and every one of these viruses is pathogenic for them.

The virus corner then throws a thunderous boomerang punch. Temin's team invokes the recently discovered simian immunodeficiency virus (SIV) and its equally new disease, Simian AIDS, to preserve Koch's postulates, just as they would later trot forth the new feline immunodeficiency virus (FIV) and its brand-new disease, feline AIDS. Whether these animal models even resemble human AIDS—a topic we will visit in passing later on—the essential point is that we are now asked to believe one of two highly improbable alternatives: Either these latter diseases were present all along in monkeys and cats, and animal retrovirologists, as desperate as their human retrovirologist colleagues to find some clinical relevance for their work, had somehow missed them; or a whole bunch of new deadly retroviruses all evolved at the very same moment. Coincidentally, just in time to butter a lot of stale bread.

Peter flicks a few stinging, Ali-like jabs by asking the other side to reconcile devastating T-cell loss with minimal infectivity, biochemical quiescence, and with the presence of virus-inactivating antibodies. Not on the steadiest of legs, Team Virus shoots back with p24 antigenemia, and chronic herpes—the former to defend the preposterous notion that there were enormous amounts of active virus "hiding" (their word) in the body, and the latter to establish their point that "Many viruses are highly pathogenic after evidence of immunity appears." Neglecting, of course, to mention that reactivated viral diseases like herpes and hepatitis occur only when the immunity gets low, are in step with easily detected virus production, and recede when the immune system responds. Not quite the scenario of HIV and AIDS.

The Duesenberger follows with a hard right to the head: HIV, in common with all other retroviruses, does not kill defenseless cells in culture. Why, therefore, should we imagine that it does so in the body when it is effectively neutralized by the host's immune system and its tiny genome is sleeping peacefully in a highly evolved, complex community of cells that on rare occasions can even win a fight with rabies, until HIV the absolute deadliest of human viruses. This caused Team Temin, which should have been staggering on the ropes, to dig down and come up with an unexpected—and to almost everyone judging, strong—series of counter punches, although to this judge a lot of them seemed more phantom than ferocious.

For example, they claim several times that Peter is requiring the mechanism by which HIV kills cells to be delineated before it is accepted that it does. He is doing no such thing. He is saying, however, over and over again, that while knowing the mechanism by which a virus destroys cells is not necessary to establish causation in the case of a virulent, active virus, it is in the case of a mild-mannered fellow like HIV. Claiming that it kills legions of cells in the absence of a demonstrable mechanism is a lot like accepting the logic behind the story of the lion-killing bird that I heard from one of my Nigerian in-laws 25 years ago. It is well known that in the forests of West Africa there is a terrible yellow bird that can kill even the king of beasts. Although no one has actually observed this amazing feat, each and every time a dead lion is discovered, perched atop its once-proud head is the diabolical avian assassin. This parable, it should be obvious, is told to children as a caution against inferring cause from correlation.

Temin *et al.* go on to argue: "The exact mechanism of CD4 cell depletion in AIDS patients is not known, but several indirect mechanisms are known by which HIV can cause CD4 cell depletion in laboratory studies and could operate *in vivo*."[8] Can and could, not does. But Team Virus now shifts from phantom punches and misleading adjectives like "exact," which implies approximate knowledge not no knowledge at all, to low blows, saying that in fact HIV does directly kill cells in culture, and that Duesberg is as usual all wrong.

The very special kind of cell-killing they conjure is a transient, laboratory artifact called "syncytia formation" that, while relatively unknown to anyone outside the field, is common knowledge among retrovirologists. Because it appeared often in the defense of HIV between the years 1987 and 1993, and still surfaces on occasion when the asserter thinks he can get away with it, we will expend a little effort to examine it now.

When a retrovirus productively infects a cell—that is, actively directs the synthesis of new virus particles from its residence within the nucleus, which it can do maximally at about 1000 particles per day—the new viruses leave by insinuating themselves in and through the cell's membrane. If such a virus-producing cell is in close proximity to uninfected ones, the sticky protein of the virus' coat can glom onto the membrane of an adjacent cell, causing them to fuse. If enough cells fuse, a giant cell or syncytium forms, and the entire mass becomes unviable and dissolves. Thus apparent cell-killing by HIV. But this phenomenon depends on having infected and uninfected cells extremely close together, as they are in a tissue culture dish but not in the body, and on having just the right ratio of infected to uninfected cells. Once most of the cells in a population are infected, they are no longer fusible since there are no free surface receptors that can be used to make the virus cross-linked giant cell. And perhaps most damningly, fusion is only observed in the laboratory for the simple reason that it is completely inhibited by the antibodies present in the blood of infected people.

Peter would go on to deal with *in vitro* cell-killing by HIV, or more accurately the lack thereof, at much greater detail in the *Proceedings* review, but by then it was clear that no matter what holes were to be punched in the fabric of HIV-AIDS, it would magically heal itself and continue to wrap the entire globe in its satisfying warmth, a kind of medical Linus' blanket for everybody.

The graying, middle-aged heretic delivered his last punch, a Joe Frazier left hook just as the bell sounded. It was effective then, and given the passage of time, even more so now when the genomic revolution has reenergized the biotechnology stock exchange. Thus finding similarities between genes in two organisms, which are taken to imply they do the same thing, or finding large differences between two gene sets, which means they are not likely to do the same things, can be worth mega-bucks. Peter connected solidly with: "It is now claimed that at least two viruses, HIV-1 and HIV-2, are capable of causing AIDS, which allegedly first appeared on the planet only a few years ago (20). HIV-1 and HIV-2 differ 60% in their nucleic acid sequences (24)."[9]

A wobbly Team Virus could only respond to this by reasserting the premise and waving their hands. "It is true that there are two viruses that cause human AIDS, HIV-1 and HIV-2. The origin of these HIVs is an interesting scientific question that is not relevant to whether or not HIV causes AIDS."[8]

Independent of their skill as counter-punchers, in their opening, the defenders of the faith came out cocky and styling. As well they could considering the evidence that HIV caused AIDS was "overwhelming" to the point of not even needing to respond to Dr. Duesberg, who while a "brilliant chemist, is out of his depth when it comes to biology and the complex interplay of the human immune system, which is still very much a black box in persons with AIDS," according to an unspecified number of anonymous AIDS researchers quoted by Bill Booth in his provocative *Science* portrait.[3] But curiously, as sharply as they posture, they do not produce the substance expected of eminent virologists tuned into the "complexities of the human immune system." Quite the contrary, this hastily assembled A-team argues just like their poor-relation epidemiologists, who no matter what they would like to claim are glorified pollsters, not experimental scientists, and cannot prove functional hypotheses.

Kibbitz aside, Team Virus opens with: "AIDS, a new disease, was first recognized in 1981, clustered in male homosexuals, intravenous drug abusers, and hemophiliacs in the United States and among sexually active heterosexuals in some parts of equatorial Africa. Human immunodeficiency virus (HIV) was first discovered in 1983 and was definitively linked in 1984 to AIDS patients and to groups whose members were at high risk for developing AIDS."[8] Quite a feat of recognition. I'm sure our Nobel-carrying and Nobel-aspiring team could have explained, if anyone had bothered other than Duesberg or a few nut-cases who supported his right to ask, exactly how they defined "sexually active heterosexuals in some parts of equatorial Africa," and how they were so different from sexually active heterosexuals in the U.S. that their so-called brand-new AIDS diseases (which had long been present among sexually active and inactive hetero- and homosexuals all over Africa) could be so quickly distinguished, with such precise demography, years before the earliest antibody tests?

Somebody must have asked Cambridge University's eminent virologist Abraham Karpas something similar, however, because not long after the debate, John Maddox (in his continued commitment to "not distress or mislead" but otherwise inform his large scientific readership by withholding and then refusing publication of Peter's review) found he was compelled to publish a full page of "Scientific Correspondence" from Karpas explaining the origin of AIDS in Africa. Consider the ringing words of the distinguished don in which he displays the Sheffield razor-sharp, critical acumen expected after a lifetime in the selfless service of Her Majesty's science:

> The first plausible explanation for the origin of AIDS by cross-species transfer is due to Noireau in 1987 (ref. 11). He referred to a book published by Anicent Kashamura, a member of the Idjwi tribe of the Lake Kivu region in East Zaire. Kashamura deals with the sexual habits of the people of the large African lakes. Noireau quotes the following sentence: "To stimulate a man or a woman and induce them to intense sexual activity, male monkey blood for a man or she-monkey blood for a woman is directly inoculated in the pubic area and also into the thighs and back." (ref. 12) Such practices would constitute an efficient means of trans-species transmission and could be responsible for the emergence of SIV infections of man and thus AIDS.[10]

Forgetting, if we can, this unashamed endorsement of bizarre sado-masochistic fanciful anthropology and racism by Sir John and his journal, and returning to the more refined arena of our interrupted mental boxing match, as a pedantic editor I might have intervened here with my red Pilot Point and eliminated some of the redundant "newness." "Recognized in 1981" and "identified in 1983" are more grammatically correct and factual, if less insistent and evocative. But left unmarked, Team Tuned In lays it on as follows:

The strongest evidence that HIV causes AIDS comes from prospective epidemiological studies that document the absolute requirement for HIV infection for the development of AIDS. It has been shown for every population group studied in the United States and elsewhere that, in the years following the introduction of HIV and subsequent sero-conversion of members of that population, the features characteristic of progressive immunodeficiency emerge in a predictable sequence resulting in clinical AIDS (2–4)."[11]

Only if saying so makes it so, counters Kid Heretic. The references to their first ponderous claim are in fact no more than previous assertions of the same thing, not studies that support it. Actual epidemiological surveys showed, and continue to show, that the occurrence of AIDS based solely on the detection of antibody to HIV is unpredictable in time of onset and in clinical manifestations, which are diverse and constantly changing. The onset of AIDS "varies from almost 0 to over 10%, depending on factors defined by life-style, health, gender, and country of residence (see point 8 of my preceding statement, and references therein)."[8] And one could add now the date of diagnosis, since the CDC has changed the definition of the "disease" several times over the years, just as the incubation period of the virus mysteriously adjusted itself from two to five years to ten to fifteen in order to reconcile epidemiological predictions with the actual numbers of new cases within particular intervals.[12]

Ducking and weaving, the dauntless defenders try to double-up on their next big punch. "Support for the linkage of HIV infection and AIDS comes as well from the results of public health interventions where interruption of HIV infection almost completely prevented the further appearance of AIDS in blood transfusion recipients (4)."[13] And just a hundred words later: "As a result of the decrease in blood transfusion-associated transmission of

HIV, the incidence of blood transfusion-associated AIDS among U.S. newborns showed a decline (4)."[13] Duesberg, looking a little exasperated, resorts to the same quantitative counter: "According to the CDC, transfusion-associated AIDS cases in adults have doubled to 752 cases and pediatric cases tripled to 63 in the year ending May 1988 compared to the previous year (1). This happened 3 years after antibody-positive transfusions were reduced 40-fold with the AIDS test (9),"[14] citing James Ward and a large number of colleagues from the CDC's AIDS Program in the February 1988 *New England Journal of Medicine.*

Having thrown these set-punches, Team Virus lets fly with their best shot:

> Scientists conclude that a virus causes a disease if the virus is consistently associated with the disease and if disruption of transmission of the virus prevents occurrence of the disease. HIV can be detected by culture in most AIDS patients and by culture or polymerase chain reaction in most HIV seropositive individuals (8, 9). Epidemiological data show that transmission of HIV results in AIDS and blocking HIV transmission prevents the occurrence of AIDS. Thus, we conclude that there is overwhelming evidence that HIV causes AIDS.[15]

They finish with a dazzling display of fearless footwork: "Knowing the cause of a disease does not mean that there is complete understanding of its pathology. Discovering the pathogenetic mechanisms of HIV in AIDS is a major focus for research."

After the "Policy Forum" appeared, Peter all but begged Dan to sanction another round, to no avail. And so just when it was getting good, the bout was declared a technical draw on an inexplicable and non-appealable decision of commissioner Koshland. There was never to be a rematch. The failure to extend the discussion in the pages of *Science* was significant. Most scientists have neither time nor inclination to follow specialist literature in fields outside their own. They depend, consequently, on journals like *Science* and *Nature* to tell them what is considered important. Having read, as best they could at the time, the arguments of the Policy Forum, and then seeing nothing more than vulgar anti-Duesberg editorials in the scientific press and worse in the popular media, even a partially persuaded non-specialist could and would eventually concur with the "overwhelming evidence" of Team Virus, although it has become even less overwhelming now than it was in 1988.[12]

But even this highly circumscribed exchange was not exactly what its editors pretended it was. In 1994, Peter received an anonymous fax from someone at the NIH giving a fuller picture of the team effort in *Science*. Among other revealing documents from the word processor of Florence Karlsberg, public relations officer of the NIH, was a memo from December 1987 addressed to top NIH officials stating that: "Alas—in the past few months, inquiries have been mounting. . . . The calls and interest are mounting. Perhaps it's time to review and activate the attached STATEMENT."[16]

The loud statement had a curiously reminiscent title, "HIV: The Cause of AIDS," and bore an uncanny similarity to the words of Team Virus six months later. As well it should since other documents in the fax showed that the statement had been written by William Blattner, months before Koshland received it with Gallo's and Temin's additional signatures. It was apparently composed in response to a request from the PR maven to "create a response team to deal with the controversy." Karlsberg had suggested that "Perhaps the epidemiological approach might be more productive in countering Peter's assertions."[16]. To switch from boxing to another metaphor from the sporting life: Talk about a stacked deck. The memos also explained why the piece in *Science,* despite having Temin as senior author, had none of his style, which was much more Duesberg-like and substantive than the government-ordered fluff to which he added his otherwise excellent name.

While this very peculiar "Policy Forum" was unfolding, Peter engaged in a fruitless attempt to get *Nature* to take action on his review. During the months the paper sat on Maddox's desk, presumably inspiring the brilliant language of the letter that began this chapter, Peter spent more than a few hours readjusting the formatting on his Xerox computer, added material that addressed the unfinished points of the Policy Forum, and sent the manuscript to the *Proceedings of the National Academy.* As an Academy member, and therefore entitled to unfettered access to its journal, Peter thought this would be an easy publication, and while not nearly as visible or influential as either *Nature* or *Science,* it would at least set down his continued analysis for the attention of history, if not that of his apparently uninterested retrovirologist colleagues.

It was, in fact, to be the beginning of what Peter now calls "Duesberg apartheid on the part of the *Proceedings,*" since he would go from a perfect twenty-five-year record of thirty-four first-round acceptances to special reviews and rejections. Over the next months, the manuscript was summarily returned as being "unoriginal" by one editor, Maxine Singer,[16] and then resubmitted with protest to her successor Igor Dawid, where it generated more than sixty pages of correspondence between Dawid, Peter, and three anonymous reviewers before it was finally accepted in November.[16] The point of this chronicle is not to show that Peter was being unfairly treated, which he may have been, but rather to underscore that the paper was published only after the most intensive scrutiny, and therefore its conclusions cannot be flippantly dismissed.

When the review did appear, with the title "Human immunodeficiency virus and acquired immunodeficiency syndrome: Cor-

relation but not causation," it was accompanied by an extraordinary and unprecedented "disclaimer" promising a rebuttal that
was to be prepared by Robert Gallo. But when Peter or I asked
him at various times over the next years how the refutation was
coming, he was always "too busy saving lives to respond."

In the *Proceedings* article, Peter advanced all the unfinished
arguments of the Policy Forum and added a few more. We will
look at some of these now, as they display the finest edge of his
critical thinking, and some of his sparest and best scientific prose.

One of the most often encountered (even to this day), off-the-
cuff refutations of Peter's entire critique runs something like this:
HIV is not nearly as unusual as Duesberg claims—in fact, it is
just like any number of other "lentiviruses," which are very different from the acute oncogenic retroviruses with which he has
worked. The professor's considered response, in full:

> *Considering that HIV replicates within 2 days in tissue cul-*
> *ture and induces antiviral immunity within 1 to 2 months*
> *(19, 23, 69, 130), the inevitably long and seemingly unpre-*
> *dictable intervals, ranging from 1 to 15 years (20, 35, 37),*
> *between the onset of antiviral immunity and AIDS are*
> *bizarre. The average latent period is reported to be 8 years*
> *in adults (21, 33–38) and 2 years in children (21, 36). Indeed,*
> *at least 2 years of immunity is required before AIDS appears*
> *in adults (7, 38). If one accepts that 50–100% of antibody-*
> *positive Americans eventually develop AIDS (7, 20–22,*
> *33–37), the average 1.5% annual conversion corresponds*
> *to grotesque viral latent periods of 30 to 65 years. These*
> *intervals between HIV infection and AIDS clearly indicate*
> *that HIV by itself is not sufficient to initiate AIDS.*
>
> *In an effort to rationalize the long intervals between infec-*
> *tion and AIDS, HIV has been classified as a slow virus, or*
> *lentivirus (40), a type of retrovirus that is thought to cause*

disease only after long incubation periods (129). Yet there are no "slow" viruses. Since viral nucleic acids and proteins are synthesized by the cell, viruses must replicate as fast or faster than cells (i.e., within hours or days) to survive (86, 87).

Nevertheless, as pathogens, viruses may be (i) fast in acute infections that involve many actively infected cells, (ii) slow in subacute infections that involve moderate numbers of actively infected cells, or (iii) asymptomatic and latent. Retroviruses provide examples of each different pathogenic role. Acute infections with the "slow" Visna/Maedi retrovirus of sheep, a lentivirus, rapidly cause pneumonia (131), and those with equine anemia lentivirus cause fever and anemia within days or weeks of infection (132). Such infections typically generate titers of 10^4 to 10^5 infectious units per milliliter or gram of tissue (132, 133). The caprine arthritis-encephalitis lentivirus is also pathogenic within 2 months of inoculation (134). Acute infections with other retroviruses also rapidly cause debilitating diseases or cancers (23). This includes retrovirus infections that are now considered to be animal models of AIDS, termed simian or feline AIDS (12, 23, 30, 111, 135). Unlike HIV in AIDS, these viruses are all very active when they cause diseases, and the respective diseases appear shortly after infection (23). In rare cases, when antiviral immunity fails to restrict Visna/Maedi or other retroviruses, they persist as subacute symptomatic infections (3, 86, 129, 133). Under these conditions, Visna/Maedi virus causes a slow, progressive pulmonary disease (129, 133, 136) by chronically infecting a moderate number of cells that produce moderate titers of 10^2 to 10^5 virus particles per gram of tissue (136). However, in over 99% of all Visna/Maedi or caprine arthritis-encephalitis virus infections, and in most equine anemia *virus infections, the retrovirus is either eliminated or restricted to latency by immunity, and hence asymptomatic, exactly like almost all other retroviruses in mice, chickens, cats, and other animals (23). For instance, 30–50% of all healthy sheep in the U.S., Holland, and Germany have asymptomatic Visna/Maedi virus infections (129, 137, 138), and 80% of healthy goats in the U.S. have asymptomatic caprine arthritis-encephalitis virus infections (133) in the presence of antiviral immunity.*

Thus, the progressive diseases induced by active retroviruses depend on relative tolerance to the virus due to rare native or acquired immunodeficiency or congenital infection prior to immune competence. Since tolerance to HIV that would result in active chronic infection has never been observed and is certainly not to be expected for 50–100% of infections [the percentage of infections said to develop into AIDS (ref. 7 and above)], the rare retrovirus infections of animals that cause slow, progressive diseases are not models for how HIV might cause AIDS. Indeed, not one acute retrovirus infection has ever been described in humans (23).[17]

Your turn, Dr. Gallo.

The following notes some important new experimental observations, which should have cast at least a little doubt on the central biochemical basis of virus-promoted AIDS—HIV's world-famous T-cell tropism—but instead just became more grist for the endlessly churning mill.

The virus-AIDS hypothesis holds that the retrovirus HIV causes AIDS by killing T-cells in the manner of a cytocidal virus (3, 6, 7, 12, 18) and is transmitted by sex and parenteral exposure (3, 7, 12, 19, 22). Early evidence for a T-cell-specific HIV receptor lent support to this hypothesis

(25). Recently, however, the presumed T-cell specificity of HIV has lost ground, as HIV is only barely detectable in T-cells and often is detectable only in monocytes (26–28) and other body cells (23, 29–32), displaying the same lack of virulence and broad host range toward differentiated cells as all other human and animal retroviruses (17, 23).[18]

He continues some several thousand words later with the following interesting information about hypothetical indirect mechanisms of cell-killing and the reality of latent human pathogens:

Regrettably, the hasty acceptance of the virus as the cause of AIDS (16), signaled by naming it HIV (18), has created an orthodoxy whose adherents prefer to discuss "how" rather than "whether" HIV causes AIDS. They argue that it is not necessary to understand HIV pathology, or how a latent virus kills, in order to claim etiology (7, 14, 32, 51). Therefore, many different mechanisms, including ones in which HIV is said to depend on cofactors to cause AIDS, have been discussed (6, 12, 31, 32, 35, 61, 91) to explain how the virus supposedly kills at least 10,000 times more T-cells than it actively infects (26–28, 71–74). Yet all speculations that HIV causes AIDS through cofactors cast doubt on HIV as a cause of AIDS, until such factors are proven to depend on HIV.

If latent viruses or microbes were pathogenic at the level of activity of HIV, most of us would have Pneumocystis pneumonia (80–100%) (167), cytomegalovirus disease (50%) (88), mononucleosis from EBV (50–100%) (see above; ref. 88), and herpes (25–50%) (88) all at once, and 5–10% also would have tuberculosis (168), because the respective pathogens are latent, immunosuppressed passengers in the U.S. population at the percentages indicated. Since we can now, through molecularly cloned radioactive probes, detect latent viruses or microbes at concentrations that are far below those required for clinical detectability and relevance, it is necessary to reexamine the claims that HIV is the cause of AIDS.

In response to this, it has been argued that a biochemically inactive HIV may cause AIDS indirectly by a mechanism(s) involving new biological phenomena (12, 14, 31, 32), even though HIV is like numerous other retroviruses studied under the Virus-Cancer Program during the last 20 years (17, 140), which are only pathogenic when they are biochemically active (23).[19]

It seemed then like a reasonably balanced assessment, certainly not the ravings of a "discredited microbiologist," which was soon to become one of the favorite journalistic epithets attached to Peter almost as religiously as "the virus that causes AIDS" was to his tiny, nine-kilobase nemesis. Like Julio Cortázar's lyrical cronopios,[20] whose sons are genetically predetermined to detest and turn on them at some unspecified moment, there is a certain whimsical, poetic irony here. Imagine, one of his own children doing this, a full-blooded sibling of the viruses that had been so good to him all his professional life. And so Peter vented a little paternal spleen in the following especially dense paragraph. The thought of Gallo actually trying to reply to this is laughable, and will make a great scene in the movie.[21]

HIV Is a Conventional Retrovirus, Without an AIDS Gene.
The virus-AIDS hypothesis proposes that HIV is an unorthodox retrovirus (6, 12, 14, 31, 32) containing specific suppressor and activator genes that control the 2- to 15-year intervals between infection and AIDS (12, 37,188). However, the two known HIVs (see below) are profoundly conventional retroviruses. They have the same genetic complexity of about 9150 nucleotides, the same genetic structure, including the three major essential retrovirus genes linked in the order gag-pol-env, *the same mechanism of replica-*

tion, and the same mutation frequency (3, 7, 17, 90, 125, 126, 148) as all other retroviruses (17, 127, 128, 149, 150). Humans carry between 50 and 100 such retroviruses in their germ line, mostly as latent proviruses (151). The presumably specific genes of the HIVs (12, 188) are alternative reading frames of essential genes shared by all retroviruses (3, 7, 12, 23, 90, 148). Their apparent novelty is more likely to reflect new techniques of gene analysis than to represent HIV-specific retroviral functions. Indeed, analogous genes have recently been found in other retroviruses, including one bovine and at least three other human retroviruses that do not cause AIDS (23, 152, 188). Because HIV and all other retroviruses are isogenic, the newly discovered genes cannot be AIDS-specific. Moreover, it is unlikely that these genes even control virus replication. In vivo, HIV lies chronically dormant, although the presumed suppressor genes are not expressed. In vitro, HIV is propagated at titers of about one million per ml in the same human cells in which it is dormant in vivo, although the presumed suppressor genes are highly expressed (23, 188). Therefore, I propose that antiviral immunity rather than viral genes suppress HIV in vivo, as is the case with essentially all retroviruses in wild animals (23). Further, I propose that the multiplicity of AIDS diseases are caused by a multiplicity of risk factors (see below), rather than by one or a few viral activator genes, since viral gene expression in AIDS is just as low as in asymptomatic carriers. Also, the extremely low genetic complexity of HIV can hardly be sufficient to control the inevitably long times between infection and AIDS, and the great diversity of AIDS diseases. Thus, there is neither biochemical nor genetic evidence that HIV genes initiate or maintain AIDS.[22]

These very powerful but difficult-sounding arguments concerning genetic complexity and the like are actually much more accessible now than they were in 1989 because of the emergence of an entire field of biology and biotechnology called genomics that we have alluded to before and will now look at a little more closely. The genomics revolution, one of several in biotech's ongoing revolutionary history, brought its stocks at least transiently into the giddy world of dotcoms 2000 and made the early days of taking a fling on Genentech or Biogen or Cetus seem tame. Helped by an endless amount of media-supported, NIH-instigated hyperbole about the amazing medical benefits that will come with deciphering the coding sequences of all 35,000 human genes,[23] private DNA sequencing companies multiplied almost as rapidly as oncogenes, which of course are among the big-ticket items in their portfolios. Genomics companies are all founded on the same idea, and it is quite a good one on several levels, although not the one that claims completely new, totally specific, no-side-effect drugs, and promises genetic disease susceptibility profiling (completely private, of course) will be available soon along with gene medicines to allow people with sufficient where-with-all to live to ripe old ages without becoming overly ripe.

The concept is this: Since all the proteins in a human body are derived from specific genetic blueprints, knowing the blueprints will enable us to figure out the structures of the corresponding proteins. Once we have this complete parts catalog we will have access to intervention and repair of every imaginable bodily disturbance, since we are our genes. The first part of this reasoning is impeccable, and is the natural extension of one of the formative principles of molecular biology—the idea of fundamental biochemical universality from which diversity in living systems derives by endless mutations and shuffling. The same genes, distributed the same way, give identical functions; divergent genes or varying distributions of the same genes lead to different functionalities.

A tiger and a pussycat have at least some significant genetic differences. But what Peter argued is that the tiger HIV is essentially genetically identical to all its pussycat relatives, and so it is in reality a *tyger* belonging to the genus Blake, burning brightly but only in the mind.

The whimsical cronopios of Cortázar's fables, who are not easily characterized since they are often simultaneously miserable and joyful, share their world with a few rich and powerful "famas" and many "esperanzas" (hopefuls), who hope of course to become famas. It is ironic, though not in this case whimsically so, that one of the more financially successful of the current genomic famas, William Haseltine (yes, the same Honest Dollar Bill we encountered in the previous chapter at the *AmFar* affair) substantially increased his personal fortune by obtaining a patent on the genetic sequence of a particular receptor protein called CCR5—one of an apparently never-ending series of proteins whose understanding is going to lead to newer, more potent, and more expensive talismans against the phantom tiger HIV.

"Shares" in Haseltine's Rockville-based company, "Human Genome Sciences Inc. roared into record territory yesterday after the company said it landed a patent on a gene that regulates a key doorway that the AIDS virus uses to infect cells," according to the *Baltimore Sun* of February 17, 2000.[24] And *muy pronto,* the famas set to feuding over the immediate and future riches in terms that are quite funny, at least to me. The *Sun* article continues: "But one of the nation's leading AIDS researchers said Human Genome Sciences might have a patent fight on its hands. Despite Wall Street's enthusiasm, Dr. Robert C. Gallo, co-discoverer of the human immunodeficiency virus, said yesterday that he believes the patent might be challenged because so many other researchers had played key roles in uncovering how the AIDS virus enters and infects immune system cells." At the very end of his piece, the reporter tells all his esperanza readers what is really so, or what my thesis advisor, Rich Calendar, likes to call "the true truth." "The market for new treatments for AIDS and AIDS-related disorders is potentially large. Worldwide more than 33 million people are estimated to be infected with the virus that causes acquired immune deficiency syndrome, the majority of them in Africa and other developing countries that lack strong health care." Details like continents and countries aside, today's market-wise investors need to keep their eyes on tomorrow.

Peter may have miscalculated how easily and quickly the *Proceedings* article for posterity would be published. He was dead-on, however, regarding its negligible impact. Unlike the two cancer reviews, which were carefully studied by their important target readers and whose ideas continue to be discussed in private, even if largely ignored in the journals (although as we will see in subsequent chapters, this is changing), it is doubtful that the *Proceedings* review was then, or subsequently, even cursorily read by most of its intended audience of retrovirologists or by too many others. This, in spite of the assistance of Peter's personal representative, Bill Booth, who told the readers of *Science* all they needed to know in the title of a brief story that appeared simultaneously with the rebel's latest publication in the thick and much less well thumbed journal of the Academy, which does not travel nearly as conveniently as its more illustrious cousin from the lab to the lavatory. Booth's helpful advertisement was called: "AIDS Paper Raises Red Flag At Pnas"[25.]

The *Proceedings* article has only been referenced a handful of times by any of Peter's prominent scientific adversaries. And only once have its arguments been addressed directly in a relatively unblemished scholarly context.[26] This response does not, however, represent an acceptable replacement for the promised refutation by the entrepreneurial ex-government scientist who was too busy saving livelihoods to respond in person. While its author, Alfred Evans, is a distinguished scientist and educator, he is very

much a classical not a molecular microbiologist. Most of the eru-
dite arguments presented in the five-page article entitled "Does
HIV Cause AIDS? An Historical Perspective" in the second volume of the *Journal of Acquired Immune Deficiency Syndrome* in
1989 concern interpretations of what it means to satisfy the postulates of Koch. Peter's response, an in-kind one-page letter, was
published a few issues later.[27]

JAIDS was the latest in a series of for-profit publications from
Bio/Technology's fierce competitor for the biotech advertising
dollar, Mary Ann Liebert, who launched new journals at every
opportunity. By 1987, the numbers of AIDS papers had multiplied so mightily there were hardly enough outlets to accommo-
date them all, and a new journal for the new disease seemed a
money-maker. I have no idea what its bottom line looks like today,
but given the general intellectual quality of the papers it has published since, reflected in its impact factor,[28] the brief, inconclusive exchange between professors Evans and Duesberg may
represent a high-water mark for the journal.

In 1996, Peter's one-time friend Stephen O'Brien published a
similar paper, "HIV Causes AIDS: Koch's Postulates Fulfilled,"
in *Current Opinion in Immunology.*[29] Whether or not the text jus-
tifies the title, it is nonetheless a straightforward admission that
Koch's Postulates were not quite as irrelevant as the trio of virological heavyweights contended in the pages of *Science* some
years earlier. The circumstances behind this *"Current" Opinion,*
which is also the last time the *Proceedings* article was cited by
any of Peter's critics, are so extraordinary that they are reserved
for the next chapter.

But really, why should anybody take the trouble to assemble a
detailed rebuttal to the Berkeley professor? There was such "overwhelming evidence," who could be bothered reading, let alone
replying to all of the "molecular minutiae" and "miasmal" thinking of the "flat-earther" Duesberg? Or so said Robin Weiss and

Harold Jaffe in the editorial pages of *Nature* in 1990,[30] echoing with a bit more style but equal incoherence the sentiments of Anthony Fauci ranting in the pages of *Science* two years earlier about "confusing everybody." Their "Duesberg, HIV and AIDS" came with the now-requisite, page-dominating portrait, this time a not totally unflattering cartoon caricature that actually looked a little like Maddox and went very well with the surreal picture of Peter and his "theories" that they painted in two full pages of diatribe masquerading as discourse.

This harsh and personal assessment of the intellectual quality of the Weiss and Jaffe piece is not contradicted by the fact that even though the two names belong to high-ranking bishops in the AIDS church, and their pronouncements were given the most prominent of displays by a leading ecclesiastical publication, it has only been cited a handful of times over the past decade. (One of these *is* noteworthy, however, as we will see in Chapter 5.) Weiss' foray in *Science* a few years later[31] fared a bit better, and has been referenced in the vast AIDS literature almost 200 times.

Although somewhere deep within the idiosyncratic bundled reference style of *Science,* Weiss' article does cite Duesberg, P.H., *PNAS,* 1989, and its own citation numbers are semi-impressive, it does not qualify as even a fractionally adequate response to the *Proceedings* article, and we need spend little space considering it. I write this with no more fear than I already anticipate of accusations of "distorted historiography" from predictable quarters, for two reasons: Weiss' commissioned article "How Does HIV Cause AIDS?" for the Koshland/*Science* 1993 AIDS special (which set a record for display advertising revenues) was almost immediately, forcefully challenged by Maddox/*Nature* when they presented David Ho's entirely "new view" to massive media attention only a few months later. And as we saw in painful detail in the previous chapter, between then and now this all important question is still no closer to being resolved. The second reason is that Weiss' own best answer, boldly presented in the article's first figure, "Schematic course of HIV infection," is nothing other than Robert Redfield's wishful thinking of 1988, unchanged from when William "Clinton" Haseltine flashed its numberless axes on the screen at George Washington University for the edification of 17 'privileged' and mostly important journalists and 100 selected PhDs and medical practitioners five years earlier.

To be fair to Weiss, there had been an effort or two to put some numbers on the graph that was supposed to demonstrate, empirically not poetically, an increasing viremia in phase with a drop in T-cells and the development of clinical AIDS. Certainly had any of the numbers held up, he would have relished the opportunity to use their data to rid the field, once and for all, of the "little dog who wouldn't let go." The most cited of these came in the *New England Journal of Medicine* in December 1989.[32] Its first author is David Ho, and the paper represents the beginning of his journey into "Twilight Zone" virology where PCR viral loads play the parts of infectious viruses. It is also noteworthy for other reasons.

For one, Ho's mentor David Baltimore trumpeted his protégé's accomplishment in an editorial that accompanied the publication. I was a little surprised and deeply disappointed by this at the time. Despite Booth's embarrassing attributions in *Science,* and the "Imanishi-Kari Affair" that led to his resignation as the President of Rockefeller University, I had continued to try to think highly of Baltimore's critical intelligence for the reasons mentioned earlier. But here was the same person who taught me the importance of the single-hit kinetics of viral pathogenicity almost a quarter-century earlier arguing in a citable scientific forum[33] much as he ad-libbed to Booth when he claimed that correlations were good enough. And in this case, the correlation that Ho demonstrated was not even a perfect one. It was instead the imperfect correlation that is the shaky but unmistakable signature of the passenger virus, and which had always before served to distinguish the imposter from the real pathogen, whose signature is firm and reproducible. Peter put it this way:

> *Ho et al. and Baltimore and Feinberg (Dec. 14 issue) suggest that "residual" or "lingering" doubts about the virus-acquired immunodeficiency syndrome (AIDS) hypothesis are now resolved by new evidence of viremia in patients with AIDS. A paper of mine is cited as the source of those doubts (PNAS 89). For the following reasons, my doubts remain unresolved. The data of both Ho et al. and Coombs et al. included patients with AIDS with very low or no titers of the human immunodeficiency virus (HIV) ranging from 0 to 10 infectious units per milliliter, just as low as in asymptomatic carriers. It follows that HIV viremia is not necessary for AIDS.*[34]

He goes on to list another couple of reasons for being unpersuaded by their data and concludes his three-hundred-word letter to the journal's editor thus:

> *Considering that all latent parasites, pathogenic or not, are activated in the setting of immunodeficiency, HIV viremia may well be the consequence rather than the cause of acquired immunodeficiency.*[34]

And that is the other noteworthy aspect of this Ho *et al.* paper. Peter was allowed a response, although it was not published until May of 1990, five months later—a rather long wait for a weekly journal. Even so, and minimal as it is, this exchange represents the best example of normal scientific process in the entire professional literature relating to the *Proceedings* article.

One important exception to my earlier assessment of the contemporaneous attention with which *PNAS* 89 was read is also worth noting here. A scientist who did take this paper very seriously is Harvard's Walter Gilbert, best known today for being the first person to decipher a piece of DNA and for teaching everybody else how to do it—a feat of molecular linguistics for which he shared a Nobel Prize in 1981 with another biochemical wizard, Cambridge, England's, two-time winner, Fred Sanger. What is less well known by today's molecular biology graduate students is that Gilbert was also one of an illustrious assemblage to demonstrate, in 1961,[35] that the short-lived RNA species present in cells were the postulated "messenger molecules," thus completing the proof of molecular biology's central hypothesis—DNA makes RNA makes Protein.

Given even these few facts, the additional one—that for several years he used Peter's *Proceedings* '89 review as the basis of a graduate seminar in critical analysis in molecular biology—should not "escape notice," to recall a phrase from the pages of *Nature* in its better days[36] that is familiar to every molecular biologist reading this. Even more to the point, although Gilbert had no motivation to prepare a critical appraisal of Peter's analysis, each of the brainy grad students that took the seminar sure did. As another Nobelist, Kary Mullis, is fond of noting, even a half-way defensible rebuttal of *PNAS* '89 would have received expedited publication in either the Hertz or Avis of journals, and made an instant fama of its author. That none was ever forthcoming is probably an accurate measure of the task that Gallo, with typical braggadocio, had set himself.

Unlike his close friend at the NIH, Anthony Fauci was neither too busy nor reluctant to take on Peter, but it was not in the pages of a scientific journal. Fauci chose instead the *AAAS Observer* of September 1, 1989.[37] The *Observer* is the newsletter of the approximately 100,000-member American Association for the Advancement of Science, the society of which *Science* is the journal, and traveling even more conveniently than its big sister, is even more widely perused.

Fauci used this forum to discourse on the role of the non-scientific media in dealing with Peter's questioning of the experimental bases that supported the enormous edifice of AIDS. He titled his piece "Writing for my Sister Denise," and its first sentence is a silver dagger to the heart: "AIDS has created a whole new interaction between scientists and the press." If only such perceptive writing continued. But just a few sentences later he degenerates to a more usual peevishness, describing his pet peeve at that moment in a way that a decade's-plus distance puts in sobering perspective. "One crucial area of AIDS research is our attempts to understand the regulatory genes of HIV. It is magnificent science, and it is not only going to tell us things about HIV, but also about how the cell is controlled by viral genes and how the virus is controlled by cellular genes. Yet rarely does it get coverage." Apart from recalling a certain phrase about eating words, this complaint actually speaks favorably about the journalistic nose that on occasion sniffed something other than the Bethesda flake being dished out by Flo and her fellow traffickers in truth at the NIH.

He continues his theatrical, high-toned umbrage: "The media are no place for amateurs, particularly when talking about a public health problem of the magnitude of AIDS. I remember the sinking feeling I got when a writer asked me how to spell 'retrovirus.' Someone who does not know that has not read anything significant on AIDS, and should automatically be disqualified from doing an AIDS story." It gets better. Attend the reasoned words of the twenty-year chief of the War on AIDS as he makes his next points and tells us why we are supposed to believe that this is really written for his smarter-than-himself sounding sister:

The media are great equalizers in science, which is most
disturbing to us scientists. Any scientist quoted in the media
becomes an "expert." We know reporters must consult more
than a single source and make room for dissenting opinions. But many people consider what is in the media to be
true by definition.

One striking example is Peter Duesberg's theory that HIV
is not the cause of AIDS. I laughed at that for a while, but
it led to a lot of public concern that maybe HIV was a hoax.
The theory has extraordinary credibility just on the basis
of news coverage. My barometer of what the general public
is really thinking is my sister Denise. My sister Denise is an
intelligent woman who reads avidly, listens to the radio,
and watches television, but she is not a scientist. When she
calls me and questions my integrity as a scientist, there
really is a problem. Denise has called me at least ten times
about Peter Duesberg. She says, "Anthony"—she is the only
one who calls me Anthony—"are you sure he's wrong?"
That's the power of putting someone on television or in the
press, although there is virtually nothing in his argument
that makes scientific sense. People are especially confused
when they see divergent reports about the same thing.[37]

He closes with a sharper dagger than he wielded at the opening, and this time there is no humorous double entendre possible, and no way to avoid its ominous intent. "Journalists who
make too many mistakes, or who are too sloppy, are going to find
that their access to scientists may diminish."

Fauci was so determined not to allow people to become confused that he personally took it upon himself to prevent or pre-
empt Peter's appearances on more than a few major news
programs during these years.[38] One *Larry King Live* displace-
ment is particularly memorable because of what the telegenic

doctor said, and because Peter and I shared the experience live via telephone, him in Berkeley, me in New York.

The *Larry King Live* interview with Peter Duesberg was scheduled for August 6, 1992. We had been joking the day before about what excuse would prevent the broadcast, how close to air time it would come, and who Peter's stand-in would be. The cancellation came only hours before he was to be at the CNN studio in San Francisco. Peter called the show's producer to make sure it was worth the drive, and she told him she was very sorry, but something about the elections had come up, and they would have to reschedule. So much for what and when. That evening we would simultaneously discover who as we clicked on our bicoastal televisions. Whatever Bush and Bubba or their littermates were up to that summer night, it wasn't chatting with Larry. But there was Anthony (only his sister calls him that) Fauci in his best TV doctor bedside manner, telling a long-term, asymptomatic HIV antibody-positive who had called in that sadly, hard as they were trying, there was not yet a cure and it was just a matter of time before the deadly virus got him, along with everyone else unfortunate enough to be infected—a message that happily has not been taken to heart by Magic Johnson and many thousands of other American HIV-positives living largely normal, nucleoside analog-free, protease inhibitor-free lives fifteen years into their death sentence.[12]

Although Peter is a lot like his favorite TV detective, not doctor—the rumpled, disarming Lieutenant Colombo, who always has "just one more little question" for the inevitable fama felon—his reply to Fauci in *The AAAS Observer* is more like the earlier-generation, much darker LA cop, Sergeant Joe "just the facts" Friday. The inclusion of an autobiographical reference at the end of this list of "charges" that recalls a Germany where thought control was a state-practiced art is, however, quite poignant and human.

Fauci, like many of his peers from the AIDS establishment, relies on media popularity rather than on facts and scientific proof to promote the hypothesis that AIDS is caused by HIV. If Fauci could prove that scientifically, he would not have to promote it with the many powers of his office, including even direct intimidation.

For example, last year I was invited by "Good Morning America" to explain my arguments for why HIV cannot be the cause of AIDS. But after I was flown to New York, I was informed that the show had been canceled. The next morning I woke to see Fauci on "Good morning America," speaking on behalf of the virus-AIDS hypothesis—to Joan Lunden—instead of me.

Fauci also appears unsure of his convictions that science is intrinsically self-correcting and that "it is important for scientists to be wrong." When he reviewed my paper "HIV and AIDS: Correlation but not causation" (PNAS 86: 755, 1989), he recommended rejection based only on many pages of his own opinions, none of which were substantiated by a scientific reference.

He warns journalists to do their homework, declaring that someone who does not know how to spell retrovirus should be disqualified from doing an AIDS story. Perhaps poor spelling is just a metaphor for those who question the virus-AIDS hypothesis.

Since "the media are no place for amateurs, particularly when talking about a public health problem of the magnitude of AIDS," Fauci recently took direct action. Last October a national AIDS-education pamphlet including Fauci's picture was sent to every household in the U.S., at a cost of $17 million. Its message overlapped with the education program that was provided free to me decades ago by my grandmother, who could not spell retrovirus.[39]

But perhaps it was not the powers of Fauci's office that reporters feared as much as the unspeakable horror of the thing itself, to invoke the final literary figure of this chapter in Joseph Conrad's mythic imperialist—an image, if not a text, that a majority of Americans know from its apocalyptic Hollywood transformation. It is hard to remember now—when the pervasive fear of AIDS has receded and been shipped to Africa, a continent portrayed exclusively in recycled, indiscriminant television footage of its continuing miseries—what it was like then. Do you, for example, remember what came in the $17 million mailing? (Other than the sound advice that not too many appear to have taken, given that the incidence of chlamydia infections, first reported to the CDC as a sexually transmitted disease in 1984 with 7000 cases, increased to 380,000 new cases in 1991, and 500,000 in 1998.[40]) Yet fifteen years ago, enmeshed in the general terror and confronted with an apparently enormous responsibility, it might have seemed preferable to err (one supposed) on the side of caution. Better safe than sorry—a very human homily—if not necessarily a prescription for incisive reporting. Beyond these few observations, I have no idea why the things recounted here came to pass. But like all things if we let them, *res ipsae loquentur,* they speak sufficiently for themselves.

Chapter 4 Notes

1. *Per. comm.,* John Maddox to Peter Duesberg, preserved in the *Peter H. Duesberg Archive* of the Bancroft Library of the Univ. of California, Berkeley.

2. Duesberg, P. H. 1989. Human immunodeficiency virus and acquired immunodeficiency syndrome: Correlation but not causation. *Proc. Natl. Acad. Sci. USA* 86:755–764.

3. Booth, W. 1988. A rebel without a cause of AIDS. *Science* 239:1485–1488.

4. Anderson, C. 1991. Imanishi-Kari affair. Baltimore resigns. *Nature* 354:341.

5. Chan, L. C. 1987. The AIDS pandemic: an internationalist approach

to disease control. *Daedalus* (Spring):181–195.

6. Connor, S. 1988. The story behind the Duesberg heresy. *New Scientist* (April):35.

7. *Per. comm.* from Prof. Beverley Griffin, Hammersmith College, to Peter Duesberg, preserved in the *Peter H. Duesberg Archive* of the Bancroft Library of the Univ. of California, Berkeley.

8. Duesberg, P. H. HIV is Not the Cause of AIDS; and Blattner, W., Gallo, R. C., and Temin, H. M. HIV is the Cause of AIDS. 1988. *Science* 241:515–517.

9. *Ibid.* References therein:

20. R. Baum, "AIDS: The molecular biology," *Chem. Eng. News* (November 23, 1987):14–26.

24. F. Clavel et al., *Nature* 324, 691 (1986).

10. Karpas, A. 1990. Origin and spread of AIDS. *Nature* 348:578.

11. Noireau, F. *Lancet* 1(8548):1498–1499. 1987.

12. Kashamura, A. *Famille Sexualite et Culture.* Paris, 1973.

11. Blattner, W., Gallo, R. C., and Temin, H. M. HIV is the Cause of AIDS. 1988. *Science, 241*:515–517. References therein:

2. J. W. Curran et al., *Science* 239, 610 (1988).

3. P. Piot et al., *ibid.,* p. 573.

4. J. J. Goedert and W. Blattner, in *AIDS: Etiology, Diagnosis, Treatment, and Prevention,* V. T. DeVita, S. A. Rosenberg, S. Hellman, Eds. (Lippincott, Philadelphia, 1988). This decline in pediatric AIDS became evident before that in adult AIDS because of the shorter latent period for AIDS in infants.

12. Duesberg, P. H., Koehnlein, C., and Rasnick, D. 2003. The chemical bases of the various AIDS epidemics: recreational drugs, anti-viral chemotherapy and malnutrition. *J. Biosci.,* 28:383–412.

13. Blattner, W., Gallo, R. C., and Temin, H. M. HIV is the Cause of AIDS. 1988. *Science* 241:515–517.

4. J. J. Goedert and W. Blattner, in *AIDS: Etiology, Diagnosis, Treatment, and Prevention,* V. T. DeVita, S. A. Rosenberg, S. Hellman, Eds. (Lippincott, Philadelphia, 1988). This decline in pediatric AIDS became evident before that in adult AIDS because of the shorter latent period for AIDS in infants.

14. Duesberg, P. H. HIV is Not the Cause of AIDS. 1988. *Science* 241:515–517. *References within the Duesberg response:*

1. Centers for Disease Control, *AIDS Weekly Surveill. Rep.* (May 2, 1988).

9. J. W. Ward et al., *N. Eng. J. Med.* 318, 473 (1988).

15. Blattner, W., Gallo, R. C., and Temin, H. M. HIV is the Cause of AIDS. 1988. *Science* 241:515–517.

8. S. Z. Salahuddin et al., *Proc. Natl. Acad. Sci. USA* 85, 5530 (1985).

9. C.-Y. Ou et al., *Science* 239, 295 (1988).

16. Duesberg, P. H. 1996. *Inventing the Aids Virus.* Regnery Publishing, Inc., Washington, DC.

17. Duesberg, P. H. 1989. Human immunodeficiency virus and acquired immunodeficiency syndrome: Correlation but not causation. *Proc. Natl. Acad. Sci. USA,* 86:755–764.

19. Friedland, G. H. & Klein, R. S. (1987) *N. Engl. J. Med.* 317, 1125–1135.

23. Duesberg, P. H. (1987) *Cancer Res.* 47, 1199–1220.

69. Albert, J., Gaines, H., Sonnerborg, A., Nystrom, G., Pehrson, P. O., Chiodi, F., von Sydow, M., Moberg, L., Lidman, K., Christensson, B., Asjö, B. & Fenyo, E. M. (1987) *J. Med. Virol.* 23, 67–73.

130. Kessler, H. A., Blaauw, B., Spear, J., Paul, D. A., Falk, L. A. & Landay, A. (1987) *J. Am. Med. Assoc.* 258, 1196–1199.

20. Rees, M. (1987) *Nature* (London) 326, 343–345.

35. Anderson, R. M. & May, R. M. (1988) *Nature* (London) 333, 514–519.

37. Liu, K.-J., Darrow, W. W. & Rutherford, G. W. (1988) *Science* 240, 1333–1335.

21. Eyster, M. E., Gail, M. H., Ballard, J. O., Al-Mondhiry, H. & Goedert, J. J. (1987) *Ann. Int. Med.* 107, 1–6.

33. Moss, A. R., Bacchetti, P., Osmond, D., Krampf, W., Chaisson, R. E., Stites, D., Wilber, J., Aliain, J.-P. & Carlson, J. (1988) *Br. Med. J.* 296, 745–750.

34. Goedert, J. J., Biggar, R. J., Weiss, S. H., Eyster, M. E., Melbye, M., Wilson, S., Ginzburg, H. M., Grossman, R. J., DiFiola, R. A., Sanchez, W. C., Giron, J. A., Ebbsen, P., Gallo, R. C. & Blattner, W. A. (1986) *Science* 231, 992–995.

35. Anderson, R. M. & May, R. M. (1988) *Nature* (London) 333, 514–519.

36. Medley, G. F., Anderson, R. M., Cox, D. R. & Billard, L. (1988) *Nature* (London) 333, 505.

37. Liu, K.-J., Darrow, W. W. & Rutherford, G. W. (1988) *Science* 240, 1333–1335.

38. Osmond, D.H. & Moss, A.R. (1989) The prevalence of HIV

infection in the United States: a reappraisal of the Public Health Service estimate, in *AIDS Clinical Review*, 1–17, 1989.

7. Institute of Medicine (1988) *Confronting AIDS-Update 1988* (N.A.S., Washington, D.C.).

22. Curran, J. W., Jaffe, H. W., Hardy, A. M., Morgan, W. M., Selik, R. M. & Dondero, T. J. (1988) *Science* 239, 610–616.

40. Gonda, M., Wong-Staal, F., Gallo, R., Clements, J., Narayan, O. & Gilden, R. (1986) *Science* 227, 173–177.

129. Haase, A. T. (1986) *Nature* (London) 322, 130–133.

86. Mims, C. & White, D. O. (1984) *Viral Pathogenesis and Immunology* (Blackwell, Oxford, U.K.).

87. Fenner, F., McAuslan, B. R., Mims, C. A., Sambrook, J. & White, D. O. (1974) *Animal Viruses* (Academic, New York).

131. Lairmore, M. D., Rosadio, R. H. & DeMartini, J. C. (1986) *Am. J. Pathol.* 125, 173–181.

132. Perryman, L. E., O'Rourke, K. J. & McGuire, T. E. (1988) *J. Virol.* 62, 3073–3076.

12. Gallo, R. C. & Montagnier, L. (1988) *Sci. Am.* 259 (4), 41–48.

30. Baum, R. M. (1988) *Chem. Eng. News* 66 (13), 29–33.

111. Baum, R. M. (1987) *Chem. Eng. News* 65 (47), 135. Lackner, A. A., Rodriguez, M. H., Bush, C. E., Munn, R. J., Kwang, H.-S., Moore, P. F., Osborn, K. G., Marx, P. A., Gardner, M. B. & Lowenstine, L. J. (1988) *J. Virol.* 62, 2134–2142.

3. Institute of Medicine (1986) *Confronting AIDS* (N.A.S., Washington, D.C.).

133. Narayan, O. & Cork, L. C. (1985) *Rev. Infect. Dis.* 7, 89–98.

136. DeBoer, G. F. & Houwers, J. (1979) in *Aspects of Slow and Persistent Virus Infections*, ed. Tyrrell, D.A.J. (ECSC, Brussels-Luxembourg), pp. 198–220.

137. DeBoer, G. F., Terpstra, C. & Houwers, D. J. (1978) *Bull. Off. Int. Epizoot.* 89, 487–506.

138. Cutlip, R., Lehmkuhl, H. D., Brodgen, K. A. & Sacks, J. M. (1986) *Vet. Microbiol.* 12, 283–288.

18. *Ibid.* References therein:

3. Institute of Medicine (1986) *Confronting AIDS* (N.A.S., Washington, D.C.).

6. Fauci, A. (1988) *Science* 239, 617–622.

7. Institute of Medicine (1988) *Confronting AIDS-Update 1988* (N.A.S., Washington, D.C.).

12. Gallo, R. C. & Montagnier, L. (1988) *Sci. Am.* 259 (4), 41–48.

18. Coffin, J., Haase, A., Levy, J. A., Montagnier, L., Oroszlan, S., Teich, N., Temin, H., Toyoshima, K., Varmus, H., Vogt, P. & Weiss, R. (1986) *Science* 232, 697.

19. Friedland, G. H. & Klein, R. S. (1987) *N. Engl. J. Med.* 317, 1125–1135.

22. Curran, J. W., Jaffe, H. W., Hardy, A. M., Morgan, W. M., Selik, R. M. & Dondero, T. J. (1988) *Science* 239, 610–616.

25. Sattentau, Q. J. & Weiss, R. A. (1988) *Cell* 52, 631–633.

26. Gartner, S., Markovits, P., Markovitz, D., Kaplan, M., Gallo, R. & Popovic, M. (1986) *Science* 233, 215–219.

27. Popovic, M. & Gartner, S. (1987) *Lancet* ii, 916.

28. Ho, D. D., Pomerantz, R. J. & Kaplan, J. C. (1987) *N. Engl. J. Med.* 317, 278–286.

23. Duesberg, P. H. (1987) *Cancer Res.* 47, 1199–1220.

29. Khan, N. C., Chatlynne, L. G. & Hunter, E. (1988) *Am. Clin. Proc. Rev.* 7 (5), 12–19.

30. Baum, R. M. (1988) *Chem. Eng. News* 66 (13), 29–33.

31. Levy, J. (1988) *Nature* (London) 333, 519–522.

32. Booth, W. (1988) *Science* 239, 1485–1488.

17. Weiss, R., Teich, N., Varmus, H. & Coffin, J. (1985) *RNA Tumor Viruses* (Cold Spring Harbor Lab., Cold Spring Harbor, NY), 2nd Ed.

19. *Ibid.* References therein:

16. Connor, S. (1987) *New Sci.* 113 (1547), 49–58.

18. Coffin, J., Haase, A., Levy, J. A., Montagnier, L., Oroszlan, S., Teich, N., Temin, H., Toyoshima, K., Varmus, H., Vogt, P. & Weiss, R. (1986) *Science* 232, 697.

7. Institute of Medicine (1988) *Confronting AIDS-Update 1988* (N.A.S., Washington, D.C.).

14. Blattner, W., Gallo, R. C. & Temin, H. (1988) *Science* 241, 514–517.

32. Booth, W. (1988) *Science* 239, 1485–1488.

51. Liversidge, A. (1988) *Spin* 3 (11), 56–57, 67, 72.

6. Fauci, A. (1988) *Science* 239, 617–622.

12. Gallo, R. C. & Montagnier, L. (1988) *Sci. Am.* 259 (4), 41–48.

31. Levy, J. (1988) *Nature* (London) 333, 519–522.

35. Anderson, R. M. & May, R. M. (1988) *Nature* (London) 333, 514–519.

61. Schwartz, K. F. (1988) *Ærtztliche Praxis* 45, 1562–1563.

91. Abramson, P. R. & Rothschild, B. (1988) *J. Sex Res.* 25 (1), 106–122.

26. Gartner, S., Markovits, P., Markovitz, D., Kaplan, M., Gallo, R. & Popovic, M. (1986) *Science* 233, 215–219.

27. Popovic, M. & Gartner, S. (1987) *Lancet* ii, 916.

28. Ho, D. D., Pomerantz, R. J. & Kaplan, J. C. (1987) *N. Engl. J. Med.* 317, 278–286.

71. Harper, M. E., Marselle, L. M., Gallo, R. C. & Wong-Staal, F. (1986) *Proc. Natl. Acad. Sci. USA* 83, 772–776.

72. Ranki, A., Valle, S.-L., Krohn, M., Antonen, J., Allain, J.-P., Leuther, M., Franchini, G. & Krohn, K. (1987) *Lancet* ii, 589–593.

73. Richman, D., McCutchan, J. & Spector, S. (1987) *J. Infect. Dis.* 156, 823–827.

74. Biberfeld, P., Chayt, K. J., Marselle, L. M., Biberfeld, G., Gallo, R. C. & Harper, M. E. (1986) *Am. J. Pathol.* 123, 436–442.

167. Pifer, L. L. (1984) *Eur. J. Clin. Microbiol.* 3, 169–173.

88. Evans, A. S., ed. (1982) *Viral Infection of Humans: Epidemiology and Control* (Plenum, New York/London).

168. Evans, A. S. & Feldman, H. A., eds. (1982) *Bacterial Infections of Humans: Epidemiology and Control* (Plenum, New York/London).

17. Weiss, R., Teich, N., Varmus, H. & Coffin, J. (1985) *RNA Tumor Viruses* (Cold Spring Harbor Lab., Cold Spring Harbor, NY), 2nd Ed.

140. Tooze, J., ed. (1973) *The Molecular Biology of Tumor Viruses* (Cold Spring Harbor Lab., Cold Spring Harbor, NY).

23. Duesberg, P. H. (1987) *Cancer Res.* 47, 1199–1220.

20. Cortázar, J. *Cronopios and Famas* (tr. Paul Blackburn). Pantheon Books, NY, 1969.

21. *Per. comm.* from Athel Cornish-Bowden, Oct. 22, 2003: "I can't remember if I told you (I certainly told Peter) about Gallo's visit to Marseilles a year or so ago when he gave a lecture about HIV/AIDS. Among various imbecilities he showed a large map of Africa on which he was quite unable to locate Tanzania (even roughly), despite having just given us the benefit of his expert assessment of the health problems there. Some expert!"

22. Duesberg, P. H. 1989. Human immunodeficiency virus and acquired immunodeficiency syndrome: Correlation but not causation. *Proc. Natl. Acad. Sci. USA,* 86:755–764.

6. Fauci, A. (1988) *Science* 239, 617–622.

12. Gallo, R. C. & Montagnier, L. (1988) *Sci. Am.* 259 (4), 41–48.

14. Blattner, W., Gallo, R. C. & Temin, H. (1988) *Science* 241, 514–517.

31. Levy, J. (1988) *Nature* (London) 333, 519–522.

37. Liu, K.-J., Darrow, W. W. & Rutherford, G. W. (1988) *Science* 240, 1333–1335.

188. Haseltine, W. A. & Wong-Staal, F. (1988) *Sci. Am.* 259 (4), 52–62.

3. Institute of Medicine (1986) *Confronting AIDS* (N.A.S., Washington, D.C.).

7. Institute of Medicine (1988) *Confronting AIDS-Update 1988* (N.A.S., Washington, D.C.)

17. Weiss, R., Teich, N., Varmus, H. & Coffin, J. (1985) *RNA Tumor Viruses* (Cold Spring Harbor Lab., Cold Spring Harbor, NY), 2nd Ed.

90. Baum, R. M. (1987) *Chem. Eng. News* 65 (47), 14–26.

125. Preston, B. D., Poiesz, B. J. & Loeb, L. A. (1988) *Science* 242, 1168–1171.

126. Takeuchi, Y., Nagumo, T. & Hoshino, H. (1988) *J. Virol.* 62, 3900–3902.

148. Clavel, F. (1987) *AIDS* 1, 135–140.

127. Coffin, J. M., Tsichlis, P. N., Barker, C. S., Voynow, S. & Robinson, H. L. (1980) *Ann. N.Y. Acad. Sci.* 54, 410–425.

128. Temin, H. M. (1988) *Cancer Res.* 48, 1697–1701.

149. Duesberg, P. H., Vogt, K., Beemon, K. & Lai, M. (1974) *Cold Spring Harbor Symp. Quant. Biol.* 39, 847–857.

150. Wang, L.-H., Galehouse, D., Mellon, P., Duesberg, P., Mason, W. S. & Vogt, P. K. (1976) *Proc. Natl. Acad. Sci. USA* 73, 3952–3956.

151. Martin, M. A., Bryan, T., Rasheed, S. & Khan, A. S. (1981) *Proc. Natl. Acad. Sci. USA* 78, 4892–4896.

23. Duesberg, P. H. (1987) *Cancer Res.* 47, 1199–1220.

152. Weiss, R. A. (1988) *Nature* (London) 333, 497–498.

23. The number of human genes initially advertised was 100,000. When the human genome sequencing project was "nearing completion," it had shrunk to 35,000. This caused a bit of embarrassment for several biotech companies that were suddenly far short of the number of genes they were selling in their portfolios. We will return to this numerical discrepancy and its biologic, not economic, implications in Chapter 7.

An excellent account, by Tom Bethell, of the press conference at which this reduction was announced can be found in the *American Spectator* of April 2001 under the title, "A Map to Nowhere: The genome isn't a code and we can't read it." The quotation below is from its introductory paragraphs:

> The principal actors had appeared in the White House last June—Francis Collins of the National Human Genome Research Institute, and J. Craig Venter of Celera Genomics. Now they were back with a supporting cast and a more detailed analysis, in the Capital Hilton Hotel, with the TV lights glinting off the ballroom chandeliers, 250 journalists packed into the hot room, and James Watson of DNA fame on hand to take a bow. There would be one more blaze of publicity about the project to decipher the human genome. The new findings were about to be published in long articles, with a comical abundance of co-authors, in the journals *Nature* and *Science*.
>
> New Mexico's Sen. Pete Domenici, an early and eager supporter of the project on Capitol Hill, received a vigorous round of applause. He was sitting next to Watson, and in his remarks Domenici said that Watson had just whispered to him, "You must say that this project was congressionally driven." The senator added, "And that's true.... This project, in terms of the U.S. government, was truly started in the Congress." One of the new buildings going up on the "campus" of the National Institutes of Health will surely be named after Domenici.
>
> One news item was prominently reported. The number of human genes is now believed to be about 30,000, one-third or even one-fourth the number recently estimated. At first this was played as the familiar object lesson in humility for us self-satisfied anthropoids. We thought we were at the center of the universe. Silly old us! Now, our supposedly overweening pride receives another setback. For we have "only twice as many genes as a fruit fly, or a lowly nematode worm," said the ever-so-humble Eric Lander, head of genome research at the NIH-funded Whitehead Institute in Cambridge, Mass. "What a comedown!" The journalists roared on cue. That would be the sound-bite for National Public Radio, you knew, and the *Washington Post* would publish it the next day.
>
> There was, however, a more disturbing implication. It took a few days to sink in. There followed a kind of appalled silence, and then

the alarm bells began to ring, if only faintly. "The way these genes work must therefore be far more complicated than the mechanism long taught," whispered the *Washington Post.* The alarms will grow louder. For if what Craig Venter said is true—and it was accepted by James Watson when I spoke to him immediately after the press conference—the genetics textbooks will have to be rewritten and the therapeutic breakthroughs promised by the map of the genome may not come for decades, if ever. No one at the press conference disputed Venter's claims. That included the editors of *Science* and *Nature,* who made brief remarks.

24. Guidera, M. Md. biotech firm lands patent on AIDS-related gene; Human Genome stock soars; top researcher predicts challenge; Millions in fees at issue. *The Baltimore Sun,* Feb. 17, 2000. Four years later, this protein had not yet noticeably advanced on the road from promise to magic bullet. Its successor, however, was announced in early 2004 in a *Nature* paper (427:848 - 853) that generated "news reports" of the same flavor. For example: McCall, W. *Associated Press,* Feb. 25, 2004. "Study: Monkey's Protein Prevents HIV." Although not telling us in the headline what the monkey protein was supposed to prevent HIV from doing, the first paragraph supplies the missing information. " Scientists say they have discovered why some monkeys are resistant to infection with the AIDS virus—an exhilarating find that points to a new and highly promising strategy for blocking HIV in people."

In this same four year period, Haseltine himself lost some of his glitter while keeping his gold, according to a savage piece by financial writer Christopher Byron that appeared in the Mar. 29, 2004 online edition of the *NY Post.* Among its milder barbs:

> "One thus finds, during the Doc's twelve years at the helm, that *Human Genome Sciences* took in $230.9 million of revenues while spending $1.27 billion to get it. Folks, that's an upside-down ratio of more than $5 of costs for every one dollar of revenues, and to have achieved it not just for a year or two at a time but for more than an entire decade is, I am sure, something of a record.
>
> "It is not easy to keep raising money, year after year, on the promise of spending it to come up with a cure for death. In fact, until Doc Haseltine came along, one would have thought it impossible. But in sum and substance, that is what Doc Haseltine has done.... Meanwhile, the Doc himself made a bundle. Since the launch of the com-

pany in 1992, he has taken home cash compensation of more than $6 million, as well as $26.8 million more from the sale of stock options, plus whatever else he was able to collect from his stock holdings in the company, which at their peak in the summer of 2000 were worth something approaching $400 million. All in all, the math works out to roughly $1 of cash to the Doc for every $27 of shareholders' money he's been able to lose during his years in the corner office."

A final part to this resonant note is a paper that appeared in the Mar. 25, 2004 *PNAS* (Belshaw, R., *et al.,* 101:4894–9). It contains the most powerful new support yet for Peter's old argument that HIV is not different enough at the nucleic acid sequence level from its pussycat relatives to be a tomcat let alone a tiger. In this study the authors examined an abstruse phenomenon that is really of interest to only a handful of remaining non-HIV retrovirologists. The phenomenon in question relates to the mechanisms by which retroviral sequences have spread in the primate lineages for the past thirty million years. But, in the introduction to their investigation the authors tell us that there are presently 98,000 different retroviral DNAs that have been accumulating in the human *germline,* and quietly going along for the ride for quite a long time. What the authors do not tell us is: Faced with 98,000 benign relatives that have undergone all manner of "purifying selection" (their term) over tens of millions of years of primate evolution, a newly evolved sequence variant of a retrovirus that was a serious danger to its host would have no chance of surviving. After all, with close to one hundred thousand genomically stable relatives and a sequence length of nine thousand or so, every possible single-base alteration has been seen by the human germline at least ten times before.

25. Booth, W. 1989. AIDS paper raises red flag at PNAS. *Science* 243:733.

26. Evans, A. S. 1989. Does HIV cause AIDS? An historical perspective. *J. Acquir. Immune Defic. Syndr.* 2:107–113.

27. Duesberg, P. H., 1989. Does HIV Cause AIDS? (letter). *J. Acquir. Immune Defic. Syndr.* 2:514–515.

28. *Nature, Science* and the *PNAS,* the top three journals in ISI's category of Multidisciplinary Science, which ranks 62 journals, had 1998 impact factors of 28.88, 24.39, and 9.82, respectively. *Bio/Technology's (Nature Biotechnology)* 1998 impact factor was 8.05. *JAIDS'* 2.67 brought it in at 26 out of 120 journals in Immunology, and not to put too fine a

point on it, the old *Bioslash,* wrapped two years before in the new *Nature* label, came in that year numero uno of the 118 primary research journals in the category of Biotechnology and Applied Microbiology, a position it continues to maintain, through 2003.

29. O'Brien, S. J., and Goedert, J. J. 1996. HIV causes AIDS: Koch's postulates fulfilled. *Curr. Opin. Immunol.* 8:613–618.

30. Weiss, R., and Jaffe, H. 1990. Duesberg HIV and AIDS; *Nature* 345:659–660.

31. Weiss, R. 1993. How does HIV cause AIDS? *Science* 260:1273–1286.

32. Ho, D. D., Moudgil, T., and Alam, M. 1989. Quantitation of human immunodeficiency virus type 1 in the blood of infected persons. *N. Engl. J. Med.* 321:1621–1625.

33. Baltimore, D., and Feinberg, M. B. 1989. HIV revealed: toward a natural history of HIV-I infection. *N. Engl. J. Med.* 321:1673–1675.

34. Duesberg, P. H. 1990. Quantitation of human immunodeficiency virus in the blood (letter). *N. Engl. J. Med.* 322:1466.

35. Gros. F., Gilbert, W., Hiatt, H. H., Attardi, G., Spahr, P. F., and Watson, J. D. 1961. Molecular and biological characterization of messenger RNA. *Cold Spring Harb Symp Quant Biol.* 26:111–132.

36. Watson, J. D., and Crick, F. H. 1953. Molecular structure of nucleic acids; a structure for deoxyribose nucleic acid. *Nature* 171:737–738. Watson and Crick concluded the letter to *Nature* in which they proposed the double helix structure of DNA with what has been called the coyest sentence in biological science publishing. It has not "escaped our notice that the specific pairing we have postulated immediately suggests a possible copying mechanism for the genetic material."

37. Fauci, A. 1989. Writing for my sister Denise. *The AAAS Observer,* Sept. 1.

38. Duesberg, P. H. 1996. *Inventing the Aids Virus.* Regnery Publishing, Inc., Washington, DC.

39. Duesberg, P. 1989. Duesberg Responds. *The AAAS Observer,* Nov. 3.

40. U.S. Centers for Disease Control. 1998. Cases of STDs reported by State Health Departments in the U.S., 1991–1998, STD Surveillance.

5

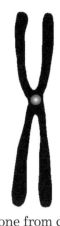

Alpha and Omega

In the fall of 1994, when all his grants had become unworthy of funding, students were warned not to seek his mentorship, he was no longer considered qualified to offer graduate-level classes, and he had gone from chairman of the seminar committee to organizer of the yearly departmental picnic, I received a telephone call from Peter I have always remembered as "A Night at the Opera," even though its humor was as far from the Marx Brothers as imaginable.

In substance, Peter tells me the following: The other afternoon, I hear from my old buddy Steve O'Brien. He is on his way to China on some NIH business and is in the Bay Area for only a brief time. But he has tickets for the SF Opera that night—curiously enough, Susa's *Dangerous Liasons*—and wants to invite me to discuss old times and some important matters. The intrigue is irresistible, so I take an old tux from the closet and we meet. Coincidentally, the silver-bearded J. Michael is also in attendance, and waves hello. Afterwards we go out for a quiet drink, and just like in the movies, Steve surreptitiously pulls out a folded manuscript from the inside of his own tuxedo pocket, and *sotto voce* says, "This has already been accepted at *Nature*. All you have to do is sign."

The manuscript is one that we have already encountered— "HIV Causes AIDS: Koch's Postulates Fulfilled"—except this time the authors were Peter H. Duesberg, Stephen O'Brien, and William Blattner.

Peter told him that he would carefully read the proffered offer at redemption and get back with his response. I said to Peter something like, "Cheer up. It means you are still making big waves and they are so intellectually bankrupt, this is the option of last resort." It did about as much to cheer him as it did me, although any notions we might have retained about the way AIDS science was supposed to operate were in tatters long before this epiphany.

Peter spent more than a few hours rewriting the essay, which was nothing more than a recycling of the well-worn epidemiological arguments we have already examined; his efforts included altering the title to something more appropriate to the facts. And he did this with the urgency that O'Brien had conveyed on his way to the mysterious East. After several international phone calls and faxed revisions between the two, on October 11, Peter received the following:

> I want to bring a personal reflection to your attention because it influenced my decision to approach you with the intention to sign the essay. I was outlining to my post-doc in China the other day some more blatant examples of fraud in science. As I was explaining to him how the scientific community had been thoroughly duped by [here a list of prominent names, including some we have encountered in the previous pages, has been deleted on advice of the publisher's counsel], I realized that there was one striking exception, Peter Duesberg. Your skepticism about oncogenes made skeptics and better scientists of us all, even the 20 plus National Academy Members that oncogenes regalized. But to be honest, Peter, your campaign that HIV does not cause AIDS is not so compelling and I am afraid wrong, just wrong. I am sorry if you think my assessment harsh,

but having said that I believe that you should consider sign-ing the article for your own good.[1]

The piece, of course, never appeared in *Nature*. Minus the Dues-berg recantation it was just another restating of the already mul-tiply-asserted but never proved. It did, however, resurface, essentially unaltered from the draft Peter had rejected, in the much more obscure journal *Current Opinion in Immunology* in 1996.[2] (See previous chapter.) Blattner's name had also disappeared, yet the published version included a note that Peter had declined joint authorship, which must have completely bewildered anyone who bothered to read the article carefully enough to notice.

Nonetheless, in this disingenuous guise, O'Brien's publication became a key citation in *The Durban Declaration*[3] and thus man-aged to sneak into *Nature* via the back door in July of 2000. *The Durban Declaration* is an unprecedented piece of science by con-sensus that came about because the questions Peter had cham-pioned for more than a decade (through all the personal vilification, humiliation, and marginalization) had taken suffi-cient hold to require the equivalent of a Papal edict to put a stop, once and for all, to a potentially dangerous revival of the anti-HIV/AIDS heresy.

The main reason for the revival, and the timing, was that Thabo Mbeki had convened a Presidential Advisory Panel to examine the credibility of all the claims that had been making headlines about the ravages of HIV and AIDS in South Africa since the democratic reforms of a few years earlier. The panel was comprised of about forty-five invitees, two-thirds from the main-stream AIDS establishment and the other one-third most politely referred to by the media as "dissidents," of whom Peter was the most prominent. The Advisory Panel's final formal meeting coin-cided with the annual AIDS international media and pharma-ceutical company circus, scheduled that year for Durban.

Compared to the attacks on Peter, the response to President Mbeki's daring to question the ultra-authoritative proclamations of the World Health Organization (WHO) was, and continues to be, the equivalent of an all-out thermonuclear strike with as much relative effect as lobbing a large firecracker.[4] Mbeki remains unconvinced that sex not poverty and malnutrition is at the root of his country's medical woes.[4] The panel, of which I am a member, still exists, and the South African Minister of Health, Manto Tshabalala-Msimang, once an HIV/AIDS stalwart, has become Mbeki's strong ally in the cabinet[4]—an act that has raised numerous calls in the local, white-controlled press for her resignation if not outright suicide.

That Peter survived long enough for the remarkable resurgence of HIV/AIDS criticism sketched immediately above to even occur is due primarily to the support of three people: Siggi Sachs, David Rasnick, and Robert Leppo. After determining in their own ways that a serious miscarriage of science had taken place, each did what they could to rectify it. Without them, I doubt that there would be anything to write of Peter's scientific life and times other than to depict a noble and tragic fall from fame to obscurity.

Peter and Siggi met in Bonn in 1993, when he was invited to a symposium she had organized on behalf of George Birkmayer, the Secretary General of the International Academy of Tumor Marker Oncology (IATMO) in Vienna. Their relationship began with a characteristically Peter practical joke. Arriving at the symposium's welcome desk, he saw a number of other invited speakers nearby and joined them briefly before registering. Although the others may have been from a lot to a little taken aback by Birkmayer's invitation to Peter, none cancelled their own participation as would Robert Gallo—a "medical emergency" in his family while he was only a short distance away in Hamburg compelling the last-minute "I'm sorry, I can't." At the moment of Peter's arrival, however, Gallo was only mysteriously late, and that of course was the subject of their spirited chat.

Siggi was taking the registrations, and when Peter introduced himself as "Dr. Robert Gallo," she said immediately, "Oh good, we were wondering where you were." But handing him his alter-ego's name tag a few seconds later, she asked with coy bemusement, "Are you sure you're Dr. Gallo? You don't look like his pictures." The relationship advanced much more productively and rapidly than HIV/AIDS research. Not long after, she resigned her position with Prof. Birkmayer to join Peter in Berkeley, and began to organize the mountains of paper and multi-megabytes of electronic files that had accumulated in the time he could not afford highly-skilled administrative assistance. One might correctly surmise there was at least one other element, in addition to a similar playful sense of humor, involved in this decision. Their son Max is now eight.

David Rasnick, a biochemist of my generation who retired at a relatively young age from a South San Francisco biotech company (called at the time Khepri), joined the Duesberg lab in June of 1996, prompted by his own independent reading in the field. He initially took over the majority of the AIDS matters that had consumed Peter for almost ten years and left precious little energy and no resources with which to pursue his lifelong scientifically consuming passion of determining the genetic basis of human cancers. Rasnick was to become, as we will see below, a key player in the formation of Mbeki's panel. He was also to become a true scientific collaborator in the development of a quantitative genetic theory, which as we will also see, has come to rival cellular onco-genes and mutation as an explanation for cancer.

Robert Leppo, a historian and philanthropist, became intrigued by the saga of the once fama now impoverished and despised professor across the bay. After completing his own analysis, Leppo offered sufficient financial support for Peter to restart the laboratory just as the ideas referred to above were beginning to take testable form. Bob has remained a major benefactor of the rejuvenating Duesberg research enterprise, which according to the Institute for Scientific Information produced more papers in the year 2000 that were cited more times than the multimillion-dollar machine of Prof. Gallo.

But for now, let us follow the story that led to *The Durban Declaration* and the American presidential decree that AIDS in Africa is a matter of U.S. national security.[5]

In 1998, Duesberg and Rasnick published an updated, comprehensive review in Volume 104 of *Genetica*, entitled *The AIDS Dilemma: drug diseases blamed on a passenger virus.*[6] Unlike the tortured history of the 1989 *PNAS* article, the time between submission and acceptance was the normal few months, perhaps because while highly respected, *Genetica* is regarded as a specialist journal and does not have the wider circulation of the *PNAS*, for example. Moreover, John McDonald, then its editor, had invited the paper with the express purpose of ending the silence about the still unproved HIV/AIDS hypothesis. He was to more than accomplish his purpose, only not quite as he anticipated. In fact, a readership of one was all that was necessary to restart the stalled AIDS controversy with a resounding roar. The article was among the first pieces of criticism of the virus-AIDS hypothesis that Mbeki read carefully. Mbeki is an economist, and while some of the "molecular minutiae" was at that time beyond his ken, the epidemiological data were completely transparent. And they simultaneously explained and reinforced his bafflement at the basic anomaly that had led him to question the HIV/AIDS epidemic in the first instance. He expressed this puzzle as follows in his welcoming address to the panel, but it was somehow ignored by the large number of TV and print journalists in attendance.

In the years prior to the end of apartheid, all studies on AIDS in South Africa had shown quite clearly that the condition was restricted to the same risk groups as in the United States and Europe—mostly (in South Africa) white, urban drug-abusing male homosexuals and intravenous drug users. Yet somehow in the few years between the end of the '80s and early '90s the demographic profile of the "epidemic" had shifted to predominantly rural, black, heterosexual and impoverished.[7]

That the Western media bought and continues to market this protein-deprived but testosterone-overabundant concoction is hardly surprising considering the "scientific" explanation of the origin of AIDS in Africa provided by Prof. Karpas in the pages of *Nature* a few years earlier.

The part of the *Genetica* review that pertains to a rigorous differentiation between a true pathogen and a harmless passenger or associated virus has been examined sufficiently in the previous chapters to not require further detailed elaboration here. But with regard to the anomaly referred to above, it makes this telling point:

> *The AIDS literature has further shown that HIV is naturally transmitted perinatally* (mother to fetus) *(Duesberg, 1992a; Connor et al. 1994: Duesberg, 1994: Duesberg, 1996c). Indeed, perinatal transmission of HIV is 25 to 50% efficient (Duesberg, 1988; Duesberg, 1992a; Connor et al., 1994; Hallauer & Kupsch, 1997), but sexual transmission is less than 0.1 % efficient (Peterman et al., 1988; Jacquez et al., 1994; Padian et al., 1997). Therefore, HIV depends on perinatal transmission for survival just like all other retroviruses (Duesberg, 1987; Duesberg, I992a).*
>
> *Because pathogenicity during perinatal transmission would he incompatible with the survival of the host, all perinatally transmitted viruses or microbes must be harmless (Duesberg, 1992a; Duesberg, 1996d). It is for this reason*

that antibody against HIV is found in at least 17 million
healthy humans, including 1 million healthy Americans
and 0.5 million healthy Europeans (Figure I) (Merson, 1993;
World Health Organization, 1995; Centers for Disease Con-
trol and Prevention, 1997).[8]

This also explains why the U.S. Armed Forces find that, just as in Africa, the distribution of HIV antibody is gender-neutral among the presumably fit adolescents wanting to enlist.[9] Young men and women who wish to join the armed forces do not in general come from the defined AIDS risk groups, and are unlikely to have had the good luck to have the number of sexual contacts required to acquire their infection the way Africans are said to get theirs.

In South Africa, the only sub-Saharan country that uses a positive HIV antibody test before labeling an otherwise common disease or combination of diseases AIDS, the 1 in 1000 chance of a sexual transmission immediately calls into serious question the testosterone hypothesis. All other African countries rely on the clinical, so-called Bangui definition,[10] which is so general that had it been in place in 1976 when my daughter was born in Ile-Ife, Nigeria, and developed a bad case of thrush as an infant, she would have been designated an AIDS victim by the University's health center and duly reported to the WHO. By contrast, *Pneumocystis* pneumonia—the most common latent pathogen in all of us and whose diagnosis in male homosexuals, along with Kaposi's sarcoma, were the initial inspiration for the epidemic of HIV and AIDS in the U.S. and Europe—are not even included in the Bangui definition. And thrush, unless accompanied by a positive HIV antibody test, is not by itself considered an AIDS-defining disease in the U.S. or Europe.

As antenatal testing is the most used method by which the WHO obtains the numbers on which to base its estimates that are

then, quite incorrectly, linearly extrapolated to entire populations, it is not surprising that HIV/AIDS is said to be evenly distributed between the sexes in Africa.

Yet, as Duesberg and Resnick extensively document, the clus-
tering of HIV infections and AIDS-defining diseases had remained
absolutely non-random in the U.S. and Europe from the first
notice anyone took of the "gay plague" in the early 1980s. This
stubborn refusal of both the virus and the diseases it is said to
indirectly produce to spread into the general population after so
many years is a *prima faciae* reason to consider non-infectious
causes, and to rethink the very idea that AIDS is a singular condition. The major part of the forty-plus-page *Genetica* review is
a painstaking demonstration that chemistry, not a chronically
dormant virus, more plausibly explains the distribution of the
diseases that in the U.S. and Europe are called AIDS, if and only
if they are diagnosed in the presence of antibodies to HIV. It also
explains why HIV is much more common in certain groups than
in the general population, and is therefore in the U.S. and Europe
a surrogate marker for AIDS' risks.

I quote here in full the abstract in which the basic arguments
are enumerated, leaving it to the sufficiently interested reader to
put the necessary flesh on their logic and contentions by undertaking to read the entire article as critically as the President of
South Africa did.

Almost two decades of unprecedented efforts in research
costing US taxpayers over $50 billion have failed to defeat
Acquired Immune Deficiency Syndrome (AIDS) and have
failed to explain the chronology and epidemiology of AIDS
in America and Europe. The failure to cure AIDS is so com-
plete that the largest American AIDS foundation is even
exploiting it for fundraising: "Latest AIDS statistics 0,000,000
cured. Support a cure, support AMFAR." The scientific

basis of all these unsuccessful efforts has been the hypothesis that AIDS is caused by a sexually transmitted virus, termed Human immunodeficiency virus (HIV), and that this viral immunodeficiency manifests in 30 previously known microbial and non-microbial AIDS diseases.

In order to develop a hypothesis that explains AIDS we have considered ten relevant facts that American and European AIDS patients have, and do not have, in common:

(1) AIDS is not contagious. For example, not even one health care worker has contracted AIDS from over 800,000 AIDS patients in America and Europe.

(2) AIDS is highly non-random with regard to sex (86% male); sexual persuasion (over 60% homosexual); and age (85% are 25–49 years old).

(3) From its beginning in 1980, the AIDS epidemic progressed non-exponentially, just like lifestyle diseases.

(4) The epidemic is fragmented into distinct subepidemics with exclusive AIDS-defining diseases. For example, only homosexual males have Kaposi's sarcoma.

(5) Patients do not have any one of 30 AIDS-defining diseases, nor even immunodeficiency, in common. For example, Kaposi's sarcoma, dementia, and weight loss may occur without immunodeficiency. Thus, there is no AIDS-specific disease.

(6) AIDS patients have antibody against HIV in common only by definition—not by natural coincidence. AIDS-defining diseases of HIV-free patients are called by their old names.

(7) Recreational drug use is a common denominator for over 95% of all American and European AIDS patients, including male homosexuals.

(8) Lifetime prescriptions of inevitably toxic anti-HIV drugs, such as the DNA chain-terminator AZT, are another

common denominator of AIDS patients.

(9) HIV proves to be an ideal surrogate marker for recreational and anti-HIV drug use. Since the virus is very rare (< 0.3%) in the US/European population and very hard to transmit sexually, only those who inject street drugs or have over 1,000 typically drug-mediated sexual contacts are likely to become positive.

(10) The huge AIDS literature cannot offer even one statistically significant group of drug-free AIDS patients from America and Europe. In view of this, we propose that the long-term consumption of recreational drugs (such as cocaine, heroin, nitrite inhalants, and amphetamines) and prescriptions of DNA chain-terminating and other anti-HIV drugs, cause all AIDS diseases in America and Europe that exceed their long-established, national backgrounds, i.e. >95%. Chemically distinct drugs cause distinct AIDS-defining diseases; for example, nitrite inhalants cause Kaposi's sarcoma, cocaine causes weight loss, and AZT causes immunodeficiency, lymphoma, muscle atrophy, and dementia. The drug hypothesis predicts that AIDS:

(1) is non-contagious;

(2) is non-random, because 85% of AIDS-causing drugs are used by males, particularly sexually active homosexuals between 25 and 49 years of age; and

(3) would follow the drug epidemics chronologically.

Indeed, AIDS has increased from negligible numbers in the early 1980s to about 80,000 annual cases in the early '90s and has since declined to about 50,000 cases (US figures). In the same period, recreational drug users have increased from negligible numbers to millions by the late 1980s, and have since decreased possibly twofold. However, AIDS has declined less because since 1987 increasing numbers of mostly healthy, HIV-positive people, currently about

200,000, use anti-HIV drugs that cause AIDS and other diseases. At least 64 scientific studies, government legislation, and non-scientific reports document that recreational drugs cause AIDS and other diseases. Likewise, the AIDS literature, the drug manufacturers, and non-scientific reports confirm that anti-HIV drugs cause AIDS and other diseases in humans and animals. In sum, the AIDS dilemma could be solved by banning anti-HIV drugs, and by pointing out that drugs cause AIDS—modeled on the successful anti-smoking campaign.[6]

Substitute chronic malnutrition for heroin or AZT as the chemical cause of immunodeficiency and hence increased susceptibility to otherwise common infections, and one can easily see why Mbeki found this analysis to be so relevant to the unprecedented health crisis that was said to be destroying his beloved country, when after so long it could at last be called his.

By the end of 1999, South Africa's President had read and assimilated as much of the scientific literature on HIV and AIDS as he needed in order to telephone David Rasnick and ask if he and Prof. Duesberg would participate in a panel he was contemplating forming. I was visiting Peter's laboratory at the time of the telephone call in January of 2000, and remember the way he dismissed David's and my enthusiasm, if not elation. Peter had become so pessimistic that all he could say was the powers that be would never let this upstart African upset their carefully constructed and very expensive applecart, and we were once more grasping at mirages masquerading as miracles. I said in rebuttal only that Mbeki had fought and won a much harder and seemingly impossible struggle against an apparently insurmountable and powerful foe, and he was not a person whose commitment should be treated so cavalierly.

The official letters from the government of South Africa inviting each of us to participate in the first panel meeting scheduled for May came a few months later. Peter was obviously pleased to have been mistaken, and the repercussions of those letters continue to destabilize the inner circles of the AIDS power-brokers.

The most unexpected immediate result of the foolish president's decision to flog a dead horse—as non-abusive a summation of the massive media assault that followed the announcement of the panel as I can manage—came from the White House and its outgoing occupant William Clinton, who declared that AIDS in Africa was suddenly of national security concern to the United States. An article from the *Washington Post*[5] explains the reasoning for this as follows: "Authors of one intelligence report said the consequences of AIDS appear to have 'a particularly strong correlation with the likelihood of state failure in partial democracies' and held out the prospect of 'revolutionary wars, ethnic wars, genocides and disruptive regime transitions.' Thus, HIV not only causes poverty and malnutrition in Africa,[11] but it also is a cause of political instability and potential wars. These arguments have been put forth as recently as November 2003, by the shameless, U.S. Secretary of State Colin Powell, who parroted precisely this nonsense to the BBC.[12] When the panel's first meeting convened in Pretoria in May 2000, it was attended by a contingent from the CDC and NIH who were not on the original invitation list.

One might speculate that the actual reasons for this unanticipated attention were two-fold. First, the virus-AIDS hypothesis, formulated on essentially epidemiological arguments, having failed to live up to even one of the epidemiological predictions that had terrorized the US and Europe so effectively between 1984 and the late nineties, was no longer so terrifying. Second, Africa—and South Africa in particular, the only sub-Saharan country with a twenty-first-century infrastructure and an independent, viable economy—could be transformed into a battlefield large enough to require keeping every platoon in the enormous army in the war against AIDS combat-ready 24/7, and even adding a few special forces.

The Panel's formal deliberations consisted of an initial two-day gathering in Pretoria that, a little ironically, was held at the Sheraton Hotel overlooking the South African equivalent of the White House. This was followed by a six-week Internet-based continuation of the "dialog" that was initiated in May 2000. Finally, the Panel reconvened in early July, this time in Johannesburg, and eventually a report of the recommendations was submitted to the President in March of 2001.

Mbeki's decision produced a number of consequences that include the geopolitical, the scientifically substantial, the scientifically shameful, and relative to the preceding, the trivial effect that this appointment as a presidential advisor had on Peter's already demolished professional standing. After years of relative media inattention, during which time he had managed to publish several definitive papers on his now widely recognized alternative genetic theory of cancer, Peter acquired an entirely new, large, and remarkably vitriolic band of enemies to join the prominent, but aging, prior retinue.

Other than the pre-emptive manic response from Washington, the actual content of the live debates (which Mbeki had video-taped from four different angles so he did not miss anything, including Luc Montagnier's afternoon nap) and the written material contained in the Internet exchange served only to reinforce the conviction that he was completely correct in convening the panel and raising exactly the kinds of questions he did. The continuing press coverage in South Africa, almost 100% negative, of this determination and the prominence that government HIV/AIDS policy has taken are well documented and easily available via the Internet.

The scientifically substantial outcome was the clear recom-

mendation that the accuracy of HIV antibody testing in South
Africa be rigorously examined. There is an extensive literature
demonstrating the lack of specificity of these tests when used on
people chronically infected with a variety of pathogens common
to Africa.[13] Since South Africa, as we have noted, is the only
African country to use HIV antibody status as a diagnostic criterion for AIDS, the entire validity of the epidemic rests on the
tests' accuracy. In May of 2003, the first of these studies was begun
at the Medical University of South Africa in Pretoria. To any
reader perplexed by the long time intervals, I can only say that
they represent the obstinacy and mendacious procrastinations of
the South African HIV/AIDS establishment that Mbeki had the
temerity to engage. Eventually these studies may produce sufficient
data to verify empirically the only explanation, other than deep
massage, of the following conundrum. According to the CDC,
between 1985 and 2000, the annual incidence of HIV infection in
the "sexually conservative" United States remained constant at
one million,[14] while according to the WHO, in "sex-obsessed"
Africa during this same period it linearly increased to approximately twenty-five million.[15]

The scientifically shameful outcome of Mbeki's Advisory Panel
was the widely known *Durban Declaration* in which five thousand approved scientists endorsed as the true gospel that there
is only one AIDS and it is caused by HIV. The prime mover of this
let's count-hands-and-degrees version of the scientific method
was Simon Wain-Hobson, an HIV gene sequencer at the Pasteur
Institute. One can only imagine that the poor showing of their
colleagues at the first panel meeting, and their almost complete
silence during the Internet discussion, set enough alarms sounding to instigate the following bulk email that would divert whatever serious attention the substantive undertakings of the Panel
might otherwise have received.

Thu, 22 Jun 2000 04:22:28-0700 (PDT)

Dear——,

You have probably heard about the reappearance of an old myth surrounding the cause of AIDS. Peter Duesberg is back in the columns of *Nature* and *Science*. His thesis is that HIV doesn't cause AIDS, that there is no need to screen blood, or treat patients. The situation has taken a serious turn in that President Mbeki of South Africa is consulting him. The consequences are being felt in Africa and Asia. An international group of scientists and doctors has come up with something called the Durban Declaration to be published in *Nature* on July 6. You will find it at the bottom of this message. As a scientific statement in plain language, it attempts to set the record straight by stating the facts.

The organizing committee of scientists and front-line physicians has 181 members spread over 43 different countries. The list of committee members follows the declaration. Among them you will find David Baltimore, Sir Aaron Klug, President of the Royal Society, Luc Montagnier, Rolf Zinkernagel and many more. The object is to get as many names of scientists and doctors to sign on. Names of signatories will appear on the *Nature* website. If you would like to sign on we would be delighted. Send me an e-mail confirming this. To economise space on the website we have to name people in a single line:

Name, Major degree, One title if necessary, Hospital/University/Institute,

City, Country. The form of the ideal response would be:
Durban Declaration: Agreed

Robin WEISS, PhD, Professor, University College, London, UK

Please note in CAPITALS your name as found in the index of an English-language scientific paper. This is important as we will be listing everyone in alphabetical order. Many of you will say that HIV/AIDS is not your area. However over the years you have heard enough of the arguments to understand the association. Furthermore many of you know well infectious diseases and understand Koch's postulates.

If you have colleagues in the laboratory or in the clinic who you feel would like to sign on please ask them. The more the better. However, please note that in order to be authoritative we feel it necessary to restrict the list to those with major university qualifications. Hence please do not ask students. Apologies for this. We would need email replies as soon as possible and before June 27.

Finally please do not talk to reporters about the Durban Declaration until

Nature publishes it. If you are asked by a member of the press, just say "I'd be pleased to talk to you about this, but I'm afraid I am not at liberty to do so at the moment." Please could you point this out to others who wish to sign on.

Many thanks,
Simon Wain-Hobson
on behalf of the organizing committee

The text of the aptly named "declaration" is provided as an appendix, along with a refutation from Peter's very likely final scholarly review article on this subject, entitled "The chemical bases of the various AIDS epidemics: recreational drugs, antiviral chemotherapy and malnutrition," which appeared in June 2003 in the *Journal of Biosciences*.[16] One piece of quantitative reasoning contained in that review is appropriate to quote here, because it demonstrates the fundamental statistical flaw that underlies all of the WHO-endorsed proclamations about AIDS-related mortality in Africa and the attendant, horrific consequences.

> *According to the US Bureau of the Census International Database, 2001, the population of Sub-Saharan Africa grew at an annual rate of 2.6% between 1980 and 2000, from 378 million to 652 million. Thus Africa has gained 274 million more people, the equivalent of the entire US. According to the WHO, Africa lost to 'AIDS' during this same period a total of "1,093,522" persons. It is statistically impossible to verify this number, unless the African AIDS' diseases are completely distinctive.*[16]

When an in-depth examination of these same points by South African author Rian Malan appeared in the South African investigative monthly *Noseweek* in December 2003, under the title "Apocalypse When?,"[17] the *Mail & Guardian,* a major Johannesburg daily, immediately published an editorial, "Author claims Aids figures based on false surveys." It began: "Rian Malan's crime is not just saying the unsayable, but saying it so well."[18]

Finally, I cannot resist pointing out that in addition to the O'Brien paper, another key citation in this sparsely referenced but definitive declaration is the Weiss and Jaffe caricature of Peter we also encountered in the previous chapter. After abrogating completely any semblance of the proper way in which a scientific journal should operate, *Nature* did allow a brief reply to publication of *The Durban Declaration* from the propagators of "old myths surrounding the cause of AIDS."[19]

Objective confirmation the most recent Duesberg review mentioned above does not omit any important new findings regarding the presumed pathogenicity of HIV is contained in the July 2003 issue of *Nature Medicine* devoted to "20 Years of HIV Science."

In these pages Mario Stevenson from the University of Massachusetts Medical School, in an eerie, persistent echo of the retired John Maddox's words almost ten years previous, writes: "... the reason why HIV-1 infection is pathogenic is still debated and the goal of eradicating HIV-1 infection remains elusive."[20] Exactly how elusive is quite wonderfully described in an article from *The New York Times* of September 23, 2003, entitled "Trying to Kill AIDS Virus by Luring It Out of Hiding."[21]

Perhaps the alternative explanation for the different consortia of diseases that go under the name of AIDS is not as unreasonable a hypothesis as Fauci pronounced fifteen years ago when he ranted in the pages of *Science* about the non-existent risks of non-existent, HIV-infected, sixty-year-old wives of hemophiliacs.[22]

Chapter 5 Notes

1. *Per. comm.* from Stephen O'Brien to Peter Duesberg, preserved in the *Peter H. Duesberg Archive* of the Bancroft Library of the Univ. of California, Berkeley.

2. O'Brien, S. J., and Goedert J. J. 1996. HIV causes AIDS: Koch's postulates fulfilled. *Curr. Opin. Immunol.* 8:613–618.

3. The Durban Declaration. 2000. *Nature* 406:15–16.

4. A sample of articles in the mainstream print media from early 2000 through February 2004. Many similar can easily be found online.

HIV-doctors go ballistic; Doubting Peter Scientists call S. Africa's AIDS policy idiotic. April 19, 2000. By Maggie Fox, Health and Science Correspondent, Washington *(Reuters)*

In South Africa, AIDS and a Dangerous Denial. *The Washington Post Company,* April 20, 2000. Op-ed column by Ronald Bayer and Mervyn Susser.

AIDS skeptic gets boost from South Africa. *San Francisco Examiner,* April 21, 2000, page A-2 (reprinted from: Salopek, P. "Scientific world frustrated at new attention focused on HIV denial," *Chicago Tribune*).

Wilhelm, P. Puppy Fur Gives You AIDS. *Financial Mail (South Africa),* May 19, 2000,

Chicago Tribune, May 23, 2000, p. 16. Headline: South Africa and the AIDS Disaster.

Peterson, A. *Associated Press,* May 25, 2000. S. Africa Head Defends AIDS Policies.

Garrett, L. *Newsday,* July 8, 2002. Rage Over 'Poison' As AIDS Treatment. It begins: *Barcelona, Spain—The minister of health for South Africa yesterday called drugs used to prevent transmission of HIV from mother to child poison.*

Colers, D. *Independent (Johannesburg),* September 26, 2003. This proves Mbeki is an Aids dissident.

Time Europe, November 3, 2003."I knew it needed to be done." Bill Clinton talks to *TIME* about AIDS, aid and aid budgets.

News 24, February 8, 2004. Mbeki questions Aids stats. Jan-Jan Joubert and Willem Jordaan, Edited by Wilmer Muller. A transcript of a television interview with Pres. Mbeki that begins: *Cape Town—President Thabo Mbeki on Sunday questioned the extent of HIV/Aids deaths,* because of the absence of statistics on the causes of death in South Africa. *After Mbeki did not focus on HIV/Aids and Zimbabwe in his State of the Nation address on Friday, he was bombarded with questions on these issues in an interview with the SABC on Sunday.*

Wyndham Hartley writing in *Business Day (Johannesburg)* on February 9, 2004, under the sub-head: Mbeki skirted top three issues. State of the Nation/makes this same point, more pointedly perhaps, but less informatively, when he writes: *And he has tried especially hard to avoid talking about HIV/AIDS, perhaps because he still believes it is a eurocentric invention.*

5. US Makes AIDS Security Threat. *Washington Post,* April 30, 2000.

6. Duesberg, P. H., and Rasnick, D. 1998. The AIDS dilemma: drug diseases blamed on a passenger virus. *Genetica* 104:85–132.

7. An accurate condensation of Pres. Mbeki's remarks as digitally recorded on MD-SA1, track 4, and preserved in the *Peter H. Duesberg Archive* of the Bancroft Library of the Univ. of California, Berkeley. A transcript is available at www.gov.za.

8. Duesberg, P. H. *Op. cit.* References therein:

Duesberg, P. H., 1992a. AIDS acquired by drug consumption and other noncontagious risk factors. *Pharmacology & Therapeutics* 55:201–277.

Connor, E. M., R. S. Sperling, R. Gelber et al., 1994. Reduction of Maternal-Infant Transmission of Human Immunodeficiency Virus Type

I with Zidovudine Treatment. *New Engl. J. Med.* 331(18):1173–1180.

Duesberg, P. H., 1994. Infectious AIDS—stretching the germ theory beyond its limits. *Int. Arch. Allergy Immunol.* 103:131–142.

Duesberg, P. H., 1996c. How much longer can we afford the AIDS virus monopoly? pp. 241–270 in AIDS: virus- or drug induced?, edited by P. Duesberg. Kluwer, Dordrecht, Netherlands.

Duesberg, P. H., 1988. HIV is not the cause of AIDS. *Science* 241:514–516.

Hallauer, J. F. & S. Kupsch, 1997. Die HIV/AIDS-Pandemie. p. 132, in AIDS und die Vorstadien, edited by J. L'age-Stehr & E. B. Helm. Springer Verlag, Berlin, Heidelberg.

Peterman, T. A., R. L. Stonebumer, J. R. Allen, H. W. Jaffe & J. W. Curran, 1988. Risk of human immunodeficiency virus transmission from heterosexual adults with transfusion-associated infections. *J. Am. Med. Assoc.* 259:55–58.

Jacques, J. A., J. S. Koopman, C. P. Simon & I. M. Longini Jr., 1994. Role of the primary infection in epidemics of HIV infection in gay cohorts. *J. Acquired Immune Deficiency Syndromes* 7 (11):1169–1184.

Padian, N.S., S. C. Shiboski, S. O. Glass & E. Vittinghoff, 1997. Heterosexual transmission of human immunodeficiency virus (HIV) in Northern California: results from a ten-year study. *Am. J. Epidemiol.* 146:350–357.

Duesberg, P. H., 1987. Retroviruses as carcinogens and pathogens: expectations and reality. *Cancer Res.* 47:1199–1220.

Duesberg, P. H., 1996d. Inventing the AIDS Virus. Regnery Publishing Inc., Washington, DC.

Merson, M. H., 1993. Slowing the spread of HIV: Agenda for the 1990s. *Science* 260: 1266–1268.

World Health Organization, 1995a. The Current Global Situation of the HIV/AIDS Pandemic. WHO.

Centers for Disease Control and Prevention, 1997. U.S. HIV and AIDS cases reported through December 1997; Year-end edition. 9(2):1–43.

9. Burke, D. S., Brundage, J. F., Goldenbaum, M., Gardner, M., Peterson, M., Visintine, R., Redfield, R., and Walter Reed Retrovirus Research Group. 1990. Human immunodeficiency virus infections in teenagers: seroprevalence among applicants for the U.S. military service. *J. Am. Med. Ass.* 263:2074–2077.

10. WHO. 1986. Acquired Immunodeficiency Syndrome (AIDS) WHO/

. . . .

CDC case definition for AIDS. *Weekly Epidemiology Record* 61:69–76.

11. de Waal, A., and Whiteside, A. 2003. New variant famine: AIDS and food crisis in southern Africa. *Lancet* 362:1234–1237.

12. Secretary Colin L. Powell—Interview on BBC-TV with Owen Bennett Jones, November 6, 2003. United States Department of State (Washington, DC) Released on November 17, 2003.

13. Johnson, C. 1997. Factors known to cause false HIV-antibody test results. *Continuum* 4:5–26, and extensive references therein.

14. Centers for Disease Control and Prevention. 2001. US HIV and AIDS cases reported through December 2001. *HIV/AIDS Surveillance Rep.* 13:1–44.

15. World Health Organization. 2001. Global situation of the HIV/AIDS pandemic, end 2001, Part I; *Weekly Epidemiological Records* 76:381–384.

16. Duesberg, P. H., Koehnlein, C., and Rasnick, D. 2003. The chemical bases of the various AIDS epidemics: recreational drugs, anti-viral chemotherapy and malnutrition. *J. Biosci.* 28:383–412.

17. Malan, R. Apocalypse When? *Noseweek* no. 52 (December 2003).

18. *Mail & Guardian (Johannesburg),* Dec. 21, 2003. Author claims Aids figures based on false surveys.

19. The Durban Declaration is not accepted by all. 2000. *Nature* 407:286.

Sir—In response to recent action by President Thabo Mbeki of South Africa and in advance of the International Conference on HIV/AIDS held in Durban on 9–14 July,the Durban Declaration was prepared by a committee representing a consensus of "181 scientists and front line physicians." Before publication in *Nature,* it was circulated: "To get as many names of scientists and doctors to sign on. Names of signatories will appear on the *Nature* website. If you would like to sign on, we would be delighted. Send me an e-mail confirming this. To economize space on the website, we have to name people in a single line. Many of you will say that HIV/AIDS is not your area. However, over the years you have heard enough of the arguments to understand the association. Furthermore, many of you know well infectious diseases and understand Koch's postulates. If you have colleagues in the laboratory or in the clinic who you feel would like to sign, please ask them. The more the better. However, please note that in order to be authoritative we feel it necessary to restrict the list to those with major university qualifications." This is an extract from the circular distributed on behalf of the organizing committee which included Luc Montagnier, Catherine Wilfert, David Baltimore, Sir Aaron Klug (as President of the UK Royal Society), and many other well-known names and organizations from developing countries as well as from the West.

Briefly, the authors of the declaration state that AIDS/HIV is spreading as a pandemic now affecting 34 million people, of whom 24 million are in sub-Saharan Africa. They say the disease began there as a viral infection of chimpanzees and monkeys conveyed somehow to humans, and is now spreading worldwide by heterosexual and mother-to-infant transmission. The authors consider that their evidence supporting this hypothesis is "clear-cut, exhaustive and unambiguous"; that most people with these infections will develop AIDS within 5–10 years unless treated; and that "there is no end in sight" until research based on their hypothesis leads to a vaccine to supplement safe sex, health education and other, simpler approaches to avoidance and prevention. With no end in sight after 17 or more years of intensive research, priorities and incentives, one might think that this consensus would be open to alternative approaches, but the authors of the declaration are emphatic that this is not needed because the evidence that HIV is the cause of AIDS has met or exceeded the "highest standards of science." By implication, any other evidence is therefore a deception, even less likely to lead to a successful vaccine, curative drug or hypothesis.

Our objection to the Durban Declaration is factual and verifiable from data published in the early 1980s (refs 2–4). We believe that World Health Organization (WHO) figures produced since then can be interpreted to say that AIDS first appeared and spread, not in Africa but in US urban clusters of mainly white, affluent, promiscuous homosexual men and drug addicts, and then spread, on a lesser scale, in Europe and Australasia but hardly at all in Asia. Disastrous epidemics due to heterosexual transmission of HIV were confidently predicted in general populations of developed countries, but they never happened. AIDS has diminished in incidence and severity though it is continuing in female partners of bisexual men and some other communities engaging in or subjected to behaviours which carry high risks of infections, various assaults and misuse of drugs. In sub-Saharan Africa, AIDS was reported later (refs 7,8) with an alarming frequency in mothers and infants not seen in the United States or Europe. Sentinel surveillance by the WHO shows correlation between this frequency and the seroprevalence of HIV, but there are unmeasured overlaps with other major diseases and deprivations which, together with anomalies in classification, distribution, transmission and country-specific pathogenesis, and especially cross-reactions in serological tests (refs 6–9), raise questions about the accuracy of diagnosis and approaches to control. In the absence of satisfactory, or of any, answers from the consensus to his specific questions on this matter, President Mbeki invited us to join other experts with differing viewpoints in a panel to explore the way forward to control AIDS in Africa.

Unlike the signatories to the Durban Declaration, we claim no exhaustive and unambiguous unanimity. There are differences between ourselves and with other panellists, and we are happy to acknowledge possible convergence with certain priorities favoured by the declaration's authors. But we reject as outrageous their attempt to outlaw open discussion of alternative viewpoints, because this reveals an intolerance which has no place in any branch of science. Our viewpoints could also explain the failure to prevent the spread of AIDS in high-risk populations in the West, amounting, in the United States now, to almost 700,000 registrations—an unbeaten score in the global tally of this disease.

Gordon T. Stewart, MD
   (Emeritus Professor of Public Health, University of Glasgow)

   Other signatories to this letter; full addresses available from G.T.S.
   Sam Mhlongo, MB, BS Professor of Medicine, MEDUNSA, Pretoria, South Africa
   Etienne de Harven, MD, Emeritus Professor of Pathology, University of Toronto, Canada
   Christian Fiala, MD, Obstetrician, Vienna, Austria
   Claus Kohnlein, MD, Physician, Stadisches Krankenhaus, Kiel, Germany
   Andrew Herxheimer, MD, Pharmacologist, London, UK
   Peter Duesberg, PhD, Professor of Molecular Biology, University of California at Berkeley, USA
   David Rasnick, PhD, Research Fellow, Dept. of Molecular & Cellular Biology, Univ. of California at Berkeley, USA

Roberto Giraldo, MD, Physician, New York City

Manu Kothari, MD, Pathologist, Seth GS Medical College, Bombay, India

Harvey Bialy, PhD, Resident Scholar, Institute of Biotechnology, National University of Mexico, Cuernavaca, Mexico

Charles Geshekter, Professor of African Studies, California State University, Chico, California

References

1. Durban Declaration, *Nature*406, 15–16 (2000).

2. *Morbidity Mortality Weekly Reports* 30, 250 (US CDC, Atlanta, 1981).

3. *Morbidity Mortality Weekly Reports: Update on Acquired Immune Deficiency Syndrome (AIDS), USA* 31, 507–514 (1981).

4. Gottlieb, M. S. et al. *N. Eng. Med. J.* 305, 1425–31 (1982).

5. *Weekly Epidemiological Records* (WHO, Geneva, 1981–2000).

6. Cox, D., Anderson, R. M., Hillier, H. C. (eds) *Phil. Trans. R. Soc.* 325, 37–187 (1989).

7. *International Classification of Diseases*, 10th revision (WHO, Geneva, 1992).

8. Root-Bernstein, R. *Rethinking AIDS* (MacMillan, New York, 1993).

9. Kashala, O., et al. *J. Inf. Dis.* 109, 296–304 (1994).

20. Stevenson, M., 2003. HIV-1 pathogenesis. *Nat. Med.* 9:853–860.

21. Mcneil, Jr., D. Trying to Kill AIDS Virus by Luring It Out of Hiding. *The New York Times,* September 23, 2003. It begins: *Who knows what evil lurks in the lymph nodes of men? The immunologist knows. But the body may not even suspect it. That evil is the AIDS virus, which has the power to hibernate, virtually forever, even in patients taking their triple-therapy cocktails with religious devotion.*

22. Booth, W. 1988. A rebel without a cause of AIDS. *Science* 239:1485–1488.

Appendix
The Durban Declaration

(*Nature* 406:15–16, 2000)

Seventeen years after the discovery of the human immunodeficiency virus (HIV), thousands of individuals from around the world are gathering in Durban, South Africa, to attend the XIII International AIDS Conference, which starts next week (9 July). At the turn of the millennium, figures released last week reveal that an estimated 34.3 million people worldwide are living with HIV or AIDS, 24.5 million of them in sub-Saharan Africa.[1] Last year alone, 2.8 million people died of AIDS, the highest rate since the start of the epidemic. If current trends continue, southern and Southeast Asia, South America and regions of the former Soviet Union will also bear a heavy burden in the next two decades.

AIDS spreads by infection, like many other diseases, such as tuberculosis and malaria, that cause illness and death particularly in underprivileged and impoverished communities. HIV-1, which is responsible for the AIDS pandemic, is a retrovirus closely related to a simian immunodeficiency virus (SIV) that infects chimpanzees. HIV-2, which is prevalent in West Africa and has spread to Europe and India, is almost indistinguishable from an SIV that infects sooty mangabey monkeys. Although HIV-1 and HIV-2 first arose as zoonoses[2]—infections transmitted from animals to humans—both now spread among humans through sexual contact; from mother to infant; and via contaminated blood.

An animal source for an infection is not unique to HIV. The plague came from rodents and influenza from birds. The new Nipah virus in Southeast Asia reached humans via pigs. Variant Creutzfeldt-Jakob disease in the United Kingdom is identical to "mad cow" disease. Once HIV became established in humans, it soon followed human habits and movements. Like many other viruses, HIV recognizes no social, political or geographic boundaries.

The evidence that AIDS is caused by HIV-1 or HIV-2 is clearcut, exhaustive and unambiguous, meeting the highest standards of science.[3-7] The data fulfill exactly the same criteria as for other viral diseases, such as polio, measles and smallpox:

Patients with acquired immune deficiency syndrome, regardless of where they live, are infected with HIV.[3-7]

If not treated, most people with HIV infection show signs of AIDS within 5–10 years.[6,7] HIV infection is identified in blood by detecting antibodies, gene sequences or viral isolation. These tests are as reliable as any used for detecting other virus infections. People who receive HIV-contaminated blood or blood products develop AIDS, whereas those who receive untainted or screened blood do not.[6]

Most children who develop AIDS are born to HIV-infected mothers. The higher the viral load in the mother, the greater the risk of the child becoming infected.[8]

In the laboratory, HIV infects the exact type of white blood cell (CD4 lymphocytes) that becomes depleted in people with AIDS.[3-5]

Drugs that block HIV replication in the test tube also reduce virus load in people and delay progression to AIDS. Where available, treatment has reduced AIDS mortality by more than 80% (ref. 9).

Monkeys inoculated with cloned SIV DNA become infected and develop AIDS.[10]

Further compelling data are available.[4] HIV causes AIDS.[5] It is unfortunate that a few vocal people continue to deny the evidence. This position will cost countless lives.

In different regions of the world, HIV/AIDS can show altered patterns of spread and symptoms. In Africa, for example, people infected with HIV are 11 times more likely to die within five years,[7] and more than 100 times more likely than uninfected people to develop Kaposi's sarcoma, a cancer linked to yet another virus.[11]

As with any other chronic infection, various factors have a role in determining the risk of disease. People who are malnourished, who already suffer other infections or who are older, tend to be more susceptible to the rapid development of AIDS following HIV infection. However, none of these factors weakens the scientific evidence that HIV is the sole cause of the AIDS epidemic.

In this global emergency, prevention of HIV infection must be our greatest world-wide public-health priority. The knowledge and tools to prevent infection are available. The sexual spread of HIV can be stopped by mutual monogamy, abstinence or by using condoms. Blood transmission can be prevented by screening blood products and by not reusing needles. Mother-to-child transmission can be reduced by half or more by short courses of antiviral drugs.[12,13]

Limited resources and the crushing burden of poverty in many parts of the world constitute formidable challenges to the control of HIV infection. People already infected can be helped by treatment with life-saving drugs, but the high cost of these drugs puts these treatments out of reach for most of the world. It is crucial to develop new antiviral drugs that are easier to take, have fewer side effects and are much less expensive, so that millions more can benefit from them.

There are many ways of communicating the vital information on HIV/AIDS, and what works best in one country may not be appropriate in another. But to tackle the disease, everyone must first understand that HIV is the enemy. Research, not myths, will lead to the development of more effective and cheaper treatments, and, it is hoped, a vaccine. But for now, emphasis must be placed on preventing sexual transmission.

There is no end in sight to the AIDS pandemic. But, by working together, we have the power to reverse its tide. Science will one day triumph over AIDS, just as it did over smallpox. Curbing the spread of HIV will be the first step. Until then, reason, solidarity, political will and courage must be our partners.

The declaration has been signed by over 5000 people, including Nobel prizewinners, directors of leading research institutions, scientific academies and medical societies.

References

1. Joint United Nations Programme on HIV/AIDS (UNAIDS). Report on the Global HIV/AIDS Epidemic, June 2000. (UNAIDS, Geneva, 2000.) www.unaids.org/hivaidsinfo/documents.html

2. Hahn, B. H., Shaw, G. M., De Cock, K. M., Sharp, P. M. AIDS as a zoonosis: scientific and public health implications. *Science* 287, 607–614. (2000).

3. Weiss, R. A., and Jaffe, H.W. Duesberg, HIV and AIDS. *Nature* 345, 659–660 (1990).

4. NIAID (1996). HIV as the cause of AIDS. http://www.niaid.nih.gov/spotlight/hiv00/

5. O'Brien, S. J., and Goedert, J. J. HIV causes AIDS: Koch's postulates fulfilled. *Current Opinion in Immunology* 8, 613–618 (1996).

6. Darby, S. C. et al. Mortality before and after HIV infection in the complete UK population of hemophiliacs. *Nature* 377, 79–82 (1995).

7. Nunn, A. J. et al. Mortality associated with HIV-1 infection over five years in a rural Ugandan population: cohort study. BMJ 315, 767–771 (1997).

8. Sperling, R. S. et al. Maternal viral load, zidovudine treatment, and the risk of transmission of human immunodeficiency virus type 1 from mother to infant. *N. Engl. J. Med.* 335, 1678–80 (1996).

9. Centers for Disease Control and Prevention (CDC). HIV/AIDS Surveillance Report 1999; 11, 1–44 (1999).

10. Liska, V. et al. Viremia and AIDS in rhesus macaques after intramuscular inoculation of plasmid DNA encoding full-length SIVmac239. *AIDS Research & Human Retroviruses* 15, 445–450 (1999).

11. Sitas, F. et al. Antibodies against human herpesvirus 8 in black South African patients with cancer. *N. Engl. J. Med.* 340, 1863–1871 (1999).

12. Shaffer, N. et al. Short course zidovudine for perinatal HIV-1 transmission in Bangkok Thailand: a randomised controlled trial. *Lancet* 353, 773–780 (1999).

13. Guay, L. A. et al. Intrapartum and neonatal single-dose nevirapine compared with zidovudine for prevention of mother-to-child transmission of HIV-1 in Kampala, Uganda: HIVNET 012 randomised trial. *Lancet* 354, 795–802 (1999).

The Duesberg—Koehnlein—Rasnick Refutation

Adapted from: Duesberg, P. H., Koehnlein, C., and Rasnick, D. 2003. The chemical bases of the various AIDS epidemics: recreational drugs, antiviral chemotherapy and malnutrition. *J. Biosci.* 28:383–412, Table 4.

The HIV-AIDS hypothesis: 16 Predictions versus the facts

All quotes are from *The Durban Declaration,* the most authoritative edition of the HIV-AIDS hypothesis to date, which was signed "by over 5000 people, including Nobel prizewinners" and published in *Nature* in 2000 (The Durban Declaration. 2000. *Nature* 406:15–16.). Numbers in parentheses refer to references given at the end of the text.

1.

Prediction: Since HIV is "the sole cause of AIDS," it must be abundant in AIDS patients based on "exactly the same criteria as for other viral diseases."

Fact: But, only antibodies against HIV are found in most patients (1–7). Therefore, "HIV infection is identified in blood by detecting antibodies, gene sequences, or viral isolation." But, HIV can only be "isolated" from rare, latently infected lymphocytes that have been cultured for weeks *in vitro*—away from the antibodies of the human host (8). Thus HIV behaves like a latent passenger virus.

2.

Prediction: Since HIV is "the sole cause of AIDS," there is no AIDS in HIV-free people.

Fact: But, the AIDS literature describes at least 4621 HIV-free AIDS cases according to one survey—irrespective of, or in agreement with allowances made by the CDC for HIV-free AIDS cases (55).

3.

Prediction: The retrovirus HIV causes immunodeficiency by killing T-cells (1–3).

Fact: But, retroviruses don't kill cells because they depend on viable cells for the replication of their RNA from viral DNA integrated into cellular DNA. Thus, T-cells infected *in vitro* thrive, and those patented to mass-produce HIV for the detection of HIV antibodies and diagnosis of AIDS are immortal (9–15)!

4.

Prediction: With a RNA of 9 kilobases, just like polio virus, HIV should be able to cause at most one disease, or no disease if it is a passenger (22).

Fact: But, HIV is said to be "the sole cause of AIDS," or of 26 different immunodeficiency and non-immunodeficiency diseases, all of which also occur without HIV (Table 2). Thus there is not one HIV-specific disease, which is the definition of a passenger virus!

5.

Prediction: All viruses are most pathogenic prior to anti-viral immunity. Therefore, preemptive immunization with Jennerian vaccines is used to protect against all viral diseases since 1798.

Fact: But, AIDS is observed—by definition—only after anti-HIV immunity is established, a positive HIV/AIDS test (23). Thus

HIV cannot cause AIDS by "the same criteria" as conventional viruses.

6.

Prediction: HIV needs "5–10 years" from establishing antiviral immunity to cause AIDS.

Fact: But, HIV replicates in 1 day, generating over 100 new HIVs per cell (24, 25). Accordingly, HIV is immunogenic, ie. biochemically most active, within weeks after infection (26, 27). Thus, based on conventional criteria "for other viral diseases," HIV should also cause AIDS within weeks—if it could.

7.

Prediction: "Most people with HIV infection show signs of AIDS within 5–10 years"—the justification for prophylaxis of AIDS with the DNA chain terminator AZT (Section 4).

Fact: But, of "34.3 million ... with HIV worldwide" only 1.4% (= 471,457 [obtained by subtracting the cumulative total of 1999 from that of 2000]) developed AIDS in 2000 (28). Likewise, in 1985, only 1.2% of the 1 million US citizens with HIV developed AIDS (29, 30). Since an annual incidence of 1.2–1.4% of all 26 AIDS defining diseases combined is no more than the normal mortality in the US and Europe (life expectancy of 75 years), HIV must be a passenger virus.

8.

Prediction: A vaccine against HIV should ("is hoped" to) prevent AIDS—the reason why AIDS researchers try to develop an AIDS vaccine since 1984 (31).

Fact: But, despite enormous efforts there is no such vaccine to this day (31). Moreover, since AIDS occurs by definition only in the presence of natural antibodies against HIV (Section 3), and since natural antibodies are so effective that no HIV is detectable in AIDS patients (see Table 4,1), even the hopes for a vaccine are irrational.

9.

Prediction: HIV, like other viruses, survives by transmission from host to host, which is said to be mediated "through sexual contact."

Fact: But, only 1 in 1000 unprotected sexual contacts transmits HIV (32–34), and only 1 of 275 US citizens is HIV-infected (29, 30) (Fig. 1b). Therefore, an average un-infected US citizen needs 275,000 random "sexual contacts" to get infected and spread HIV—an unlikely basis for an epidemic!

10.

Prediction: "AIDS spreads by infection" of HIV.

Fact: But, contrary to the spread of AIDS, there is no "spread" of HIV in the US. In the US HIV infections have remained constant at 1 million from 1985 (29) until now (30) (see also *The Durban Declaration* and Fig. 1b). By contrast, AIDS has increased from 1981 until 1992 and has declined ever since (Fig. 1a).

11.

Prediction: Many of the 3 million people who annually receive blood transfusions in the US for life-threatening diseases (51), should have developed AIDS from HIV-infected blood donors prior to the elimination of HIV from the blood supply in 1985.

Fact: But there was no increase in AIDS-defining diseases in HIV-positive transfusion recipients in the AIDS era (52), and no AIDS-defining Kaposi´s sarcoma has ever been observed in millions of transfusion recipients (53).

12.

Prediction: Doctors are at high risk to contract AIDS from

patients, HIV researchers from virus preparations, wives of HIV-positive hemophiliacs from husbands, and prostitutes from clients—particularly since there is no HIV vaccine.

Fact: But, in the peer-reviewed literature there is not one doctor or nurse who has ever contracted AIDS (not just HIV) from the over 816,000 AIDS patients recorded in the US in 22 years (30). Not one of over ten thousand of HIV researchers has contracted AIDS. Wives of hemophiliacs don't get AIDS (35). And there is no AIDS-epidemic in prostitutes (36–38). Thus AIDS is not contagious (39, 40).

13.

Prediction: Viral AIDS—like all viral/microbial epidemics in the past—should spread randomly in a population

Fact: But, in the US and Europe AIDS is restricted since 1981 to two main risk groups, intravenous drug users, of which 80% are males, and male homosexual drug users (Sections 1 and 4).

14.

Prediction: A viral AIDS epidemic should form a classical, bell-shaped chronological curve (41–43), rising exponentially via virus spread and declining exponentially via natural immunity, within months (see Fig. 3a).

Fact: AIDS has been increasing slowly since 1981 for 12 years and is now declining since 1993 (Fig. 1a), just like a lifestyle epidemic, as for example lung cancer from smoking (Fig. 3b)

15.

Prediction: AIDS should be a pediatric epidemic now, because HIV is transmitted "from mother to infant" at rates of 25–50% (44–49), and because "34.3 million people worldwide" were already infected in 2000. To reduce the high maternal transmission rate HIV-antibody-positive pregnant mothers are treated with AZT for up to 6 months prior to birth (Section 4).

Fact: But, less than 1% of AIDS in the US and Europe is pediatric (30, 50). Thus HIV must be a passenger virus in newborns.

16.

Prediction: "HIV recognizes no social, political or geographic borders"—just like all other viruses.

Fact: But, the presumably HIV-caused AIDS epidemics of Africa and of the US and Europe differ both clinically and epidemiologically (Section 1, Table 2). The US/European epidemic is highly nonrandom, 80% male and restricted to abnormal risk groups, whereas the African epidemic is random.

References:

1. Marx, J. 1984. Strong new candidate for AIDS agent. *Science* 224:475–477.

2. Gallo, R. C., Salahuddin, S. Z., Popovic, M., Shearer, G. M., Kaplan, M., Haynes, B. F., Palker, T. J., Redfield, R., Oleske, J., Safai, B., White, G., Foster, P. and Markham, P. D. 1984. Frequent detection and isolation of cytopathic retrovirus (HTLV-III) from patients with AIDS and at risk for AIDS; *Science* 224:500–503.

3. Altman, L. K. 1984. Researchers believe AIDS virus is found. *The New York Times*, April 24, pp. C1, C3.

4. Duesberg, P. H. 1987. Retroviruses as carcinogens and pathogens: expectations and reality. *Cancer Res*. 47:1199–1220.

5. Duesberg, P. H. 1988. HIV is not the cause of AIDS. *Science* 241:514–516.

6. Duesberg, P. H. 1994. Infectious AIDS–stretching the germ theory beyond its limits. *Int. Arch. Allergy Immunol*. 103:131–142.

7. Duesberg, P., and Bialy, H. 1996. Duesberg and the Right of Reply According to Maddox–*Nature;* in *AIDS: Virus- or drug-induced?* (ed.) P. H. Duesberg (Dordrecht: Kluwer) pp. 111–125.

8. Levy, J. A., Hoffman, A. D., Kramer, S. M., Landis, J. A., and Shimabukuro, J. M. 1984. Isolation of lymphocytopathic retroviruses from San Francisco patients with AIDS. *Science* 225:840–842.

9. Hoxie, J. A., Haggarty, B. S., Rakowski, J. L., Pillsbury, N., and Levy, J. A. 1985. Persistent noncytopathic infection of normal human T

lymphocytes with AIDS-associated retrovirus. *Science* 229: 1400–1402.

10. Anand, R., Reed, C., Forlenza, S., Siegal, F., Cheung, T., and Moore, J. 1987. Non-cytocidal natural variants of human immunodeficiency virus isolated from AIDS patients with neurological disorders. *Lancet* 2:234–238.

11. Langhoff, E., McElrath, J., Bos, H. J., Pruett, J., Granelli-Piperno, A., Cohn, Z. A., and Steinman, R. M. 1989. Most CD4+ T cells from human immunodeficiency virus-1 infected patients can undergo prolonged clonal expansion. *J. Clin. Invest.* 84:1637–1643.

12. Duesberg, P. H. 1996b. *Inventing the AIDS Virus* (Washington, DC: Regnery Publishing, Inc.).

13. Weiss, R. 1991. Provenance of HIV strains. *Nature* 349:374.

14. Cohen, J. 1993. HHS: Gallo guilty of misconduct. *Science* 259:168–170.

15. McCune, J. M. 2001. The dynamics of CD4+ T-cell depletion in HIV disease. *Nature* 410:974–979.

16. Harper, M. E., Marselle, L. M., Gallo, R. C., and Wong-Staal, F. 1986. Detection of lymphocytes expressing human T-lymphotropic virus type III in lymph nodes and peripheral blood from infected individuals by *in situ* hybridization. *Proc. Natl. Acad. Sci. USA* 83:772–776.

17. Schnittman, S. M., Psallidopoulos, M. C., Lane, H. C., Thompson, L., Baseler, M., Massari, F., Fox, C. H., Salzman, N. P., and Fauci, A. 1989. The reservoir for HIV-1 in human peripheral blood is a T cell that maintains expression of CD4. *Science* 245:305–308.

18. Hazenberg, M. D., Hamann, D., Schuitemaker, H., and Miedema, F. 2000. T cell depletion in HIV-1 infection: how CD4+ T cells go out of stock. *Nature Immunol.* 1:285–289.

19. Duesberg, P. H. 1988. HIV is not the cause of AIDS. *Science* 241:514–516.

20. Blattner, W. A., Gallo, R. C., and Temin, H. M. 1988. HIV causes AIDS. *Science* 241:514–515.

21. Enserink, M. 2001. Old guard urges virologists to go back to basics. *Science* 293:24–25.

22. Fields, B. 2001. *Field's Virology* (Philadelphia: Lippincott Williams & Wilkins).

23. Centers for Disease Control 1992/1993 revised classification system for HIV infection and expanded surveillance case definition for AIDS among adolescents and adults. *Morb. Mortal. Weekly Rep. 41* (No. RR17) 1–19.

24. Duesberg, P. H., and Rasnick, D. 1998. The AIDS dilemma: drug diseases blamed on a passenger virus. *Genetica* 104:85–132.

25. Duesberg, P. H. 1992. AIDS acquired by drug consumption and other noncontagious risk factors; *Pharmacol. Therapeutics* 55:201–277.

26. Clark, S. J., Saag, M. S., Decker, W. D., Campbell-Hill, S., Roberson, J. L., Veldkamp, P. J., Kappes, J. C., Hahn, B. H., and Shaw, G. M. 1991. High titers of cytopathic virus in plasma of patients with symptomatic primary HIV-infection. *N. Engl. J. Med.* 324:954–960.

27. Daar, E. S., Moudgil, T., Meyer, R. D, and Ho, D. D. 1991. Transient high levels of viremia in patients with primary human immunodeficiency virus type 1 infection. *N. Engl. J. Med.* 324:961–964.

28. World Health Organization. 2001b. Global situation of the HIV/AIDS pandemic, end 2001, Part I. *Weekly Epidemiological Records* 76 (49):381–384.

29. Curran, J. W., Morgan, M. W., Hardy, A. M., Jaffe, H. W., Darrow, W. W., and Dowdle, W. R. 1985. The epidemiology of AIDS: current status and future prospects. *Science* 229:1352–1357.[[search me]] Daar, E. S., Moudgil, T., Meyer, R. D., and Ho, D. D. 1991. Transient high levels of viremia in patients with primary human immunodeficiency virus type 1 infection. *N. Engl. J. Med.* 324:961–964.

30. Centers for Disease Control and Prevention. 2001. U.S. HIV and AIDS cases reported through December 2001. *HIV/AIDS Surveillance Rep.* 13:1–44.

31. Cohen, J. 2003. HIV/AIDS: Vaccine results lose significance under scrutiny. *Science* 299:1495.

32. Jacquez, J. A., Koopman, J. S., Simon, C. P., and Longini Jr., I. M. 1994. Role of the primary infection in epidemics of HIV infection in gay cohorts. *J. Acquir. Immune Defic. Syndr.* 7:1169–1184.

33. Padian, N. S., Shiboski, S. C., Glass, S. O., and Vittinghoff, E. 1997. Heterosexual transmission of human immunodeficiency virus (HIV) in Northern California: results from a ten-year study. *Am. J. Epidemiol.* 146:350–357.

34. Gisselquist, D., Rothenberg, R., Potterat, J., and Drucker, E. 2002. HIV infections in sub-Saharan Africa not explained by sexual or vertical transmission. *Int. J. STD AIDS* 13:657–666.

35. Duesberg, P. H. 1995c. Foreign-protein-mediated immunodeficiency in hemophiliacs with and without HIV. *Genetica* 95:51–70; Hoots, K., and Canty, D. 1998. Clotting factor concentrates and immune function in haemophilic patients. *Haemophilia* 4:704–713.

36. Mims, C., and White, D. O. 1984. *Viral pathogenesis and immunology* (Oxford: Blackwell).

37. Rosenberg, M. J., and Weiner, J. M. 1988. Prostitutes and AIDS: A health department priority? *Am. J. Public Health* 78:418–423.

38. Root-Bernstein, R. 1993. *Rethinking AIDS: The tragic cost of premature consensus* (New York: Free Press).

39. Hearst, N., and Hulley, S. 1988. Preventing the heterosexual spread of AIDS: Are we giving our patients the best advice? *JAMA* 259:2428–2432.

40. Sande, M. A. 1986. Transmission of AIDS: The case against casual contagion. *N. Engl. J. Med.* 314:380–382.

41. Bregman, D. J., and Langmuir, A. D. 1990. Farr's law applied to AIDS projections. *J. Am. Med. Assoc.* 263:50–57.

42. Anderson, R. M. 1996. The spread of HIV and sexual mixing patterns. In *AIDS in the World II* (Oxford: Oxford University Press), pp. 71–86.

43. Fenner, F., McAuslan, B. R., Mims, C. A., Sambrook, J., and White, D. O. 1974. *The biology of animal viruses* (New York: Academic Press).

44. Blattner, W. A., Gallo, R. C., and Temin, H. M. 1988. HIV causes AIDS. *Science* 241:514–515.

45. Duesberg, P. H. 1988. HIV is not the cause of AIDS. *Science* 241:514–516.

46. Blanche, S., Rouzioux, C., Moscato, M. L. G., Veber, F., Mayaux, M. J., Jacomet, C., Tricoire, J., Deville, A., Vial, M., Firtion, G., de Crepy, A., Douard, D., Robin, M., Courpotin, C., Ciran-Vineron, N., Le Deist, F., Griscelli, C., and The HIV Infection in New-borns French Collaborative Study Group. 1989. A prospective study of infants born to women seropositive for human immunodeficiency virus type 1. *N. Engl. J. Med.* 320:1643–1648.

47. Rogers, M. F., Ou, C.-Y., Rayfield, M., Thomas, P. A., Schoenbaum, E. E., Abrams, E., Krasinski, K., Selwyn, P. A., Moore, J., Kaul, A., Grimm, K. T., Bamji, M., Schochetman, G., and the New York City Collaborative Study of Maternal HIV Transmission and Montefiori Medical Center HIV Perinatal Transmission Study Group. 1989. Use of the polymerase chain reaction for early detection of the proviral sequences of human immunodeficiency virus in infants born to seropositive mothers. *N. Engl. J. Med.* 320:1649–1654.

48. European Collaborative Study. 1991. Children born to women with HIV-1 infection: natural history and risk of transmission. *Lancet* 337:253–260.

49. Connor, E. M., Sperling, R. S., Gelber, R., Kiselev, P., Scott, G., O'Sullivan, M. J., VanDyke, R., Bey, M., Shearer, W., Jacobson, R. L., Jimenez, E., O'Neill, E., Bazin, B., Delfraissy, J.-F., Culnane, M., Coombs, R., Elkins, M., Moye, J., Stratton, P., Balsley, J., and Pediatric AIDS Clinical Trials Group Protocol 076 Study Group. 1994. Reduction of Maternal-Infant Transmission of Human Immunodeficiency Virus Type 1 with Zidovudine Treatment. *N. Engl. J. Med.* 331:1173–1180.

50. World Health Organization. 2000. Global AIDS surveillance, Part I. *Weekly Epidemiological Records* 75 (26 November):379–383.

51. Duesberg, P. H. 1992. AIDS acquired by drug consumption and other noncontagious risk factors. *Pharmacol. Therapeutics* 55:201–277.

52. Ward, J. W., Bush, T. J., Perkins, H. A., Lieb, L .E., Allen, J. R., Goldfinger, D., Samson, S. M., Pepkowitz, S. H., Fernando, L. P., Holland, P. V., Kleinman, S. H., Grindon, A. J., Garner, J. L., Rutherford, G. W., and Holmberg, S. D. 1989. The natural history of transfusion-associated infection with human immunodeficiency virus. *N. Engl. J. Med.* 321:947–952.

53. Haverkos, H. W., Drotman, D. P., and Hanson, D. 1994 (May). Surveillance for AIDS-related Kaposi's sarcoma (KS): update. *NIDA/CDC*, Rockville, MD/Atlanta, GA.

54. Simmonds, P., Balfe, P., Peutherer, J. F., Ludlam, C. A., Bishop, J. O., and Leigh-Brown, A. J. 1990. Human immunodeficiency virus-infected individuals contain provirus in small numbers of peripheral mononuclear cells and at low copy numbers. *J. Virol.* 64:864–872.

55. Duesberg, P. H. 1993d. The HIV gap in national AIDS statistics. *Bio/Technology* 11:955–956.

A point-by-point, fully referenced, interlinear refutation of *The Durban Declaration* is available at www.thedurbandeclaration.org.

6

The Phoenix Almost Rises

In early summer 2003, I received another unforgettable phone call from Peter. We had each, along with a very large number of others, recently seen an extremely flattering photograph of him on a timeline depicting the most significant advances in cancer genetics in the last century. But the point on the timeline was not 1970 and the note was not for describing the first viral oncogene. Rather it was 1999, and the attribution was for publishing a detailed theory that explained cancer in the absence of oncogenes entirely. The photograph was part of a feature article in the July 2003 *Scientific American*[1] entitled, somewhat misleadingly (but in fair enough popular scientific journal prose, which must always hold out promise), "Untangling the Roots of Cancer." And the latest among the major competing genetic explanations of these tangled roots, according to W. Wayt Gibbs, a senior writer for the magazine, belongs to Peter H. Duesberg, whose theory actually inspired the title of the article. Gibbs' metaphor derives from the numerical chromosomal abnormalities, termed aneuploidy, that are correlated 100% with malignant tumors, and as late as 1966 were still a major focus of cancer geneticists.[2] Twenty-five years later, even the term "aneuploidy" had completely disappeared from the subject indices of all the major textbooks in molecular and cell biology, although the number of pages devoted to oncogenes increased substantially. But the newest editions will not contain such discrepancies, because between 1996 and 2003, Peter created a modern version of this explanation for cancer that was just too good to be ignored by enough of the high-profile cancer geneticists that influence the editorial directors of *Scientific American,* if not the dean of his own department at Berkeley.

It was this incongruity, and not the apparently surprising turn of events above, that made the call so memorable. But as we have seen repeatedly, in the scientific life of Prof. Duesberg, irony rises to bewildering heights.

Peter was phoning to tell me that he had just been denied his ordinary professorial merit increase, after months of fruitless written appeal. The final sentences of the letter containing this news from W. Geoffrey Owen, the Dean of Biological Sciences, read:

> In summary, reviewers judge that Peter Duesberg continues to enjoy high visibility, and performs adequate classroom teaching. His supervision and/or teaching of graduate students and postdoctoral scholars is light. His service is also light, especially for someone at his level. Finally, they note that the research contributions in the review period are small in number and not of high significance. Although he has the support of experts toward his goal of exploring the aneuploidy-cancer link, reviewers believe we must await the results of these studies before awarding them merit.[3]

Had these same standards before awarding merit been applied to oncogenes, there would be two less Nobel laureates, and others that had been "regalized" by them might not find themselves in the U.S. National Academy. There is no need to speculate on what really lay behind this incongruity on the reviewers' and Owen's parts. But given the apparent total marginalization of both Peter and his work, how in the world did this mainstream recognition in *Scientific American* come about?

The remainder of this book is devoted to a detailed answer to this question. For now I restrict myself to the following observation and suggestion. New technologies that were allowing massive gene sequencing projects, and their corresponding complicated analyses, were also permitting scientists to determine how simultaneously active in a cell thousands of genes were at any given time. One of the first uses of these large-scale biochemical comparisons was to examine the gene expression profiles of cancer cells compared to their normal progenitors. Essentially all versions of the oncogene-mutation hypothesis predicted that cancer cells would produce abnormal amounts (either significantly more or less) of at least some of the oncogene messenger RNA molecules that were widely accepted to be at the genetic core of the cancer. In this case, technology came to Peter's rescue. From the very first of these studies until today, not a single laboratory has been able to demonstrate that cancer cells significantly and reproducibly "over- or under-express" the products of any of the 100-plus "enemies within" they are supposed to contain. A rigorous explanation of this severe experimental difficulty for oncogene-mutation cancer was lying in the scientific literature thanks to Duesberg and Rasnick, and it was now impossible to ignore it.

By 1992, Peter was down to his last successful Ph.D. student, any others foolish enough to want to study with the iconoclast professor having been advised by the same reviewers who note their under-abundance in the letter from Owen that getting a degree with Peter was no longer a good career move. Nonetheless, he and the incorrigible Jody R. Schwartz published a 65-page review article in the prestigious *Progress in Nucleic Acids Research and Molecular Biology*,[4] examining all the evidence that had to that time accumulated regarding the role of oncogenes, anti-oncogenes, chromosomal translocations, and the various other epicycles devised to keep the highly problematic mutation-oncogene hypothesis profitably afloat. It also contained in its final paragraphs the essence of the aneuploidy-based hypothesis that Peter was unable to pursue productively until 1996 because he had not yet learned how to raise funds from private sources for the unfundable aneuploidy experiments. Having relied exclusively on the NIH between 1968 and 1992, he was not prepared for thirteen consecutive, rejected grant applications.

Before we can understand the prescience, power, and elegance of these ideas that emerged from the persistent questioning of "specific genes via mutation are the causes of cancers," we need to fill in some of the background between 1985—when Peter published his review of "activated oncogenes" in *Science*—to 1992 when the fully comprehensive *Progress* article appeared. Fortunately, W. Wayt Gibbs provides us with the necessary landmarks in his illustrated and illuminating timeline. I write "fortunately" because between 1985 and 1992 there are only two advances in oncogene-based cancer genetics deemed important enough to be included. One is attributed to Robert Weinberg, and like the inclusion of Peter, does not refer to a piece of scientific work that we already know about. The absent annotation is the demonstration that a *ras*-containing piece of DNA, activated by a point mutation in a particular position, is sufficient to transform primary cells in tissue culture. The reason it is not included, as we have seen, is Peter had put that particular point to its everlasting rest in a 1986 *PNAS* article.[5] Or so he thought.

Weinberg, however, was not to be dissuaded, and the point mutation-activated *ras* hypothesis retained too much importance among the majority of cancer molecular biologists to let it quietly pass to the ghostly realms of scientific hypotheses that are for a time fashionable and then fade without formal retraction. In 1999, he published a paper in *Nature*[6] claiming to have at last satisfied the Duesberg challenge of transforming primary, human, embryonic cells. However, its resurrected form now required a trinity of synthetic oncogenes, including of course an "activated" *ras*. Curiously, this accomplishment—much trumpeted at the time—is also not on the timeline between 1992 and 2000 that includes two other contributions. One does involve *ras,* but neither Weinberg nor the *Nature* paper. The other refers to Duesberg. We will return to this anomaly in the next chapter because its appreciation requires that we become familiar with the crucial differences between the assorted varieties of gene-mutation hypotheses and the aneuploidy explanation of cancer. We begin now.

The accomplishment of Robert Weinberg deemed of sufficient importance to be noted, although not photographically illustrated, on the *Scientific American* timeline involves a term I have used before without much explanation. But we can no longer avoid encountering the "dreaded"[7] anti-oncogene, or as it is more properly known among cancer molecular biologists, the tumor suppressor gene. It is for isolating the first of this type of "cancer gene" in 1986 that Weinberg gets credit.

Unlike the anti-particles of sub-atomic physics, anti-oncogenes did not arise as a necessary requirement to satisfy abstract symmetry rules, although there is a peculiar logic to their conception. If cells contain dominant oncogenes, like *ras, abl, myc,* and scores of others, named and unnamed, that can be activated by "statistically cheap mutations"[4] as Peter calls them, then they should also contain genes whose function is to suppress this potential cellular holocaust. Loss of these anti-oncogenes and their corresponding proteins would therefore be the mutational cause of the cancer they were said to suppress. Such mutations would be, in the language of genetics, recessive, as opposed to dominant because the absence rather than the presence of their protein is responsible for the observed property of the cell.

The more empirical reasons for the anti-oncogene idea go back to the early 1970s, when Alfred Knudson, whose picture is also on the *Sci. Am.* timeline, made his initial observations concerning the heritability of a cancer of the retina called retinoblastoma. Duesberg and Schwartz comment on them as follows:

> There are heritable and spontaneous retinoblastomas (45). Cytogenetic analyses of both have observed that chromosome 13 is either missing or deleted in 20 to 25% (311, 312). In addition, other chromosome abnormalities have been observed in all retinoblastomas (311, 312). On this basis, it was proposed that retinoblastoma arises from the loss of a tumor suppressor or an anti-oncogene, now termed rb, that is part of chromosome 13 (45). In the familial cases, the loss of one rb allele would be inherited and the second one would be lost due to spontaneous mutation. In the spontaneous cases, somatic mutations would have inactivated both loci. In the retinoblastomas with microscopically intact chromosomes 13, submicroscopic mutations were postulated.
>
> This anti-oncogene hypothesis predicts that normal cells would constitutively (continuously) express oncogenes that render the cell tumorigenic if both alleles of the corresponding suppressor are inactivated. The hypothesis further predicts that the suppressor genes must be active at all times in normal cells.[8]

In 1986, Weinberg and co-workers[9] cloned a human DNA sequence that was missing or altered in about a third of 40 retinoblastomas and in 8 osteosarcomas. The gene encoded in this sequence, with the rapidity characteristic of modern-day molecular biology, was termed the *rb* gene. Initially, *rb* was reported to be unexpressed in all retinoblastomas and osteosarcomas, even in those without deletions.[9,10] Further, it was also demonstrated that if the *rb* gene was inserted into a retroviral vector, transfection by this artificial construction inhibited the growth of a retinoblastoma cell line.[11] Neither of these impressive initial results withstood further scrutiny, however. It was subsequently shown that genetic alterations (either deletions or point mutations) of *rb* were present in the cells of only 13 out of 21 tumors.[12] Remember, all retinoblastomas have chromosomal abnormalities, and 75% of these do not involve the chromosome containing *rb*. Moreover, two other studies[13,14] were to show that using a much better functional test than cell lines in culture, an intact, synthetic *rb* gene did not inhibit the formation of tumors in especially tumor-susceptible mice (termed nude because they lack a functioning immune system) when they were injected with retinoblastoma cells that contained and abundantly expressed it.

Weinberg himself expressed doubts about the relevance of using artificial genetic constructions that produced thousands of times the normal amounts of protein and cell lines as reliable ways to experimentally infer the normal role of the transfected gene in the cell.

> . . . many genes . . . will antagonize growth when they are forced on a cell by . . . gene transfer, but this provides no testimony as to whether these genes are normally used by the cell to down-regulate its own proliferation. . . .[15]

But with or without these reservations, what Weinberg did was take Knudson's original gene deletion hypothesis and wrap it in the still not "fully woven fabric" of mutation oncogenetics. If the NIH 3T3 assay made it possible for scores of oncogenes to be discovered, the potential to uncover even more cancer genes was now gargantuan. Any gene in a cancer cell with any mutation in one or both copies was now a potential anti-oncogene that worked by suppressing the cancer-causing effects (whatever they might be) of some already known or unknown oncogene; and it was just waiting to fall into the "broad net" that could now be cast, and had already "revolutionized the research field." The quotations are from the same article cited above in which Weinberg presented very Duesberg-sounding second thoughts about the holes that might be present in this net.

Peter and Jody summarize what they perceive as the most serious shortcomings of the tumor suppressor gene hypothesis in a turgid analysis that computes the probabilities of point mutations and other genetic alterations of the *rb* gene that should be cancerous. They conclude that one would expect at least 20% of humans to develop such a tumor per year.

> *A recent review on tumor suppressor genes reports exactly the same probabilities for* rb *mutations as we do (287a). Thus, all persons with an inherited* rb *deletion should develop retinoblastomas and other cancers. Since this is not the case (45), point-mutation or deletion of both* rb *alleles cannot be sufficient for carcinogenesis. Since neither deletion nor minor mutation of* rb *genes is observed in all retinoblastomas or other specific tumors,* rb *deletion or mutation is not necessary for tumorigenesis.*[16]

Exactly as with Peter's arguments over the years concerning HIV as a viral pathogen, these problems for tumor suppressor genes remain as problematical now as they did a decade ago. And exactly like the challenges to HIV, have apparently gone unheeded, in this case by the large number of onco and anti-onco molecular biologists they keep busy. A Pub. Med. search shows that the *rb* gene has been the subject of more than 12,000 scientific publications as of September 2003, half as many as Weinberg's other favorite cancer gene, *ras,* but not close to the 130,000 on HIV, whose sum contribution is to have cured exactly 0.0000 AIDS patients.

But if the *rb* anti-oncogene was to become so popular so quickly, another tumor suppressor gene, called *p53,* would surpass it with astounding swiftness, and even achieve "Molecule of the Year" status in *Science* in 1992. The number of publications attributed to *p53* since 1988, when it reversed its spin and went from an oncogene to an anti-oncogene, is 20,000, one-third the number for *rb, ras, myc,* and *abl* combined.

Like dominant oncogenes, the *p53* gene and protein have their early history in tumor virus biology, when they were studied because of their relationship with the carcinogenic product of a kind of cancer virus that uses DNA instead of RNA as its genetic material. These DNA-tumor viruses, the best known being SV40, are not nearly as efficient carcinogens as their RNA-containing and much simpler retroviral relatives, but the oncogenic protein of SV40 was known to bind to cellular DNA. When a cellular protein *(p53)* with a nuclear location that bound both DNA and the oncogenic protein of SV40 was discovered in the early 1980s, it became a molecule worth the attention of oncogene molecular biologists. Its cloning in 1988 was reported in a paper entitled "Nucleotide sequence of a cDNA encoding the rat *p53* nuclear oncoprotein,"[17] attesting to the fact that for some years *p53* was considered an onco not an anti-onco gene.

Despite an obviously impressive amount of experimentation, the *p53* tumor suppressor gene hypothesis still retains essentially all of the difficulties of its predecessor *rb*. Additionally, there was one more problem that struck Peter as particularly damaging.

In 1992, Alan Bradley and colleagues published a paper in *Nature* in which they reported successfully breeding mice that were missing both copies of the king of anti-oncogenes.[18] The very fact that a mouse embryo could go through the large number of cell divisions and precise differentiations between fertilization and birth completely lacking the "guardian of the genome"[19] is an extremely strong argument against the relevance of this gene to cancer.

Nonetheless, approximately 75% of these mice do develop

tumors, a fact that has kept them around to be used in thousands of inconclusive experimental studies. The reason this 75% number is not taken seriously by Peter is that the anti-oncogene hypothesis makes the very strong prediction that the cancers in these mice (leaving aside the much more difficult question of how they were even born) should be systemic because every cell lacks the postulated tumor suppressor. Instead, these cancers are sporadic, and thus their more frequent occurrence is more like the enhanced transformation conferred upon preneoplastic 3T3 cells by "activated" *ras* than it is a manifestation of an early, critical event in the generation of the tumors.

Influenced, but not fundamentally altered by the sorts of difficulties sketched above, gene-mutation cancer marched along to the other major advance between 1986 and 1992 that is noted on the *Sci. Am.* timeline—the so-called sequential gene mutation hypothesis of colon cancer, and it is attributed to Bert Vogelstein. The reason the sequential mutation model was initially proposed is it could resolve the contradiction that the frequency of mutation is orders of magnitude too high to reconcile with the actual incidence of cancer based on one or two onco or anti-oncogenes. By postulating multiple mutations that accumulated over time because they conferred unspecified growth advantages to the cells harboring them, mutation and cancer frequencies could be brought into the same ballpark. The hypothesis also derived legitimacy from a long known but side-lined publication of Armitage and Doll[20] in 1954, demonstrating the greater than 1000-fold age bias of cancer from birth to 70. The shape of this curve was taken to imply that an accumulation of mutations (or as they called them, "events") is necessary for cancer. When Vogelstein's laboratory provided what passed for an adequate demonstration of this hypothesis in 1988,[21] it quickly reified into textbook dogma. Naturally, Peter had another way of looking at these same results.

In the case of colon cancer, it has been postulated that point-mutated Kirsten and N-ras genes depend on the mutation of at least three tumor suppressor genes for transforming function (28, 46, 272). Yet the incidence of these mutations in colon cancers is not convincing proof for their postulated function for the following reasons.

Among primary colon cancers, about 40% carry point-mutated Kirsten ras genes (28, 263, 264) and some others contain point-mutated N-ras genes (28). In addition 70% of all carcinomas carry deletions or mutations in the presumed tumor suppressor gene DCC (deleted in colon cancer) located on chromosome 18, 75% in the presumed suppressor gene p53 located on chromosome 17, and 30% in the presumed suppressor gene APC (adenomatous polyposis coli) on chromosome 5 (28). Thus, only about 6% (0.4 x 0.7 x 0.75 x 0.3) of the colon cancers studied carry the genetic constellation postulated for colon cancer. About 87% carry various combinations of these mutations, and 7% carry none of the mutations (28). In addition, recent evidence indicates that mutations on chromosome 5 are scattered over several hypothetical suppressors or anti-oncogenes (296). Despite these radical mutational differences among colon carcinomas, the carcinomas do not differ from each other in any known histological or biological properties. In addition, all of these mutations alone, and even together, are also observed in benign colon adenomas (28). Other tumors with point-mutated proto-ras genes are also histologically and morphologically indistinguishable from counterparts without these mutations (262, 297).[22]

In the face of the abundant logical and experimental contradictions recounted above, as well as the others we have seen, why do the majority of cancer molecular biologists continue to cling to the idea that mutations of specific genes are sufficient for cancer? The scientific explanation returns us to the earliest days of modern cancer genetics, when Duesberg and Vogt isolated the first viral oncogene. If such a piece of nucleic acid, whose origin was cellular, could so efficiently transform primary cells in the laboratory when it was carried by a retrovirus, then some or another version of it must function similarly in its human host. And as complicated as the explanations might become, there was apparently no other universe of discourse.

In fact, another way of looking at the ferocity of viral *onc* genes was possible. As Peter had shown, the reason these genes are such good carcinogens is because their products are produced hundreds to thousands of times more than their corresponding cellular homologs due to the strong promoter elements that retroviruses contain.[23] If it could be similarly shown that cells contain promoters as strong as those of retroviruses, then it is conceivable that a rare genetic exchange could place a proto-oncogene under the control of one of these, thus making a real *onc* gene. To date no such super-promoter has been identified in cells. In their absence, it is next to impossible that a gene whose expression had been optimized by hundreds of millions of years of evolution could become 100-fold more active by spontaneous point mutations.

> *The rare, accidental recombinants with imported retroviral promoters, which in turn have been optimized during virus evolution to override cellular controls, are as yet the only known examples of oncogenic mutations.*[4]

Thus after a scientific lifetime studying the transformation potential of retroviruses, Peter was left with no satisfactory molecular explanation for the properties that made them relevant to human cancer. With a certain despondency he quotes from Peyton Rous, the guy who started it all, writing in *Science* in 1967: "A favorite explanation has been that oncogens [Rous' term for car-cinogens] cause alterations in the genes of the ordinary cells of the body . . . somatic mutations as these are termed. But numerous facts, when taken together, decisively exclude this supposition."[24] It was at this juncture, and in the classical tradition to which he belongs, that Peter revisited the earliest scientific literature for new insights.

The last of the quotations from the Duesberg-Schwartz mono-graph concerns aneuploidy and presents Peter's thinking by the time he became as convinced as Peyton Rous, and with much more available evidence, that specific genes were not at the center of the dysfunctional cancer cellular system, no matter how many epicycles were cleverly constructed to make the hypothesis match the facts.

> *But if there are no cellular genes that are converted to can-cer genes by somatic mutations, cancer would have to be caused by normal cellular genes. Perhaps a cell could become transformed by gross numerical imbalances of nor-mal genes, e.g., via chromosome abnormalities, just as a computer could be rendered uncontrollable by deleting, duplicating, and misplacing intact chips.*
>
> *Indeed, chromosome abnormalities are the oldest, and, as yet, the only consistent observation made on cancer cells. It was postulated by Boveri in 1914, prior to the discovery of DNA and point-mutations, that cancer would be caused by abnormal chromosomes (194, 336). The clonal origin of tumors, the stemline concept predicted by Boveri and defined by Winge in 1930 (336), is the strongest support for the view that clonal chromosome abnormalities are the causes, rather than consequences, of carcinogenesis.*
>
> *This abnormal chromosome-cancer hypothesis would explain why chromosome abnormalities are consistently*

*found in tumors with or without mutated cellular onco-
genes and with or without latent viruses. The hypothesis
predicts that diploid cancers that differ from normal cells
only in mutated oncogenes or anti-oncogenes are not
observed, because certain chromosome abnormalities instead
of somatic mutations of specific genes are carcinogenic.
Tumor progression would be a consequence of further dis-
continuous chromosome abnormalities. The hypothesis
would readily resolve the paradox that all "viral" tumors
have clonal chromosome abnormalities. By contrast, all
virus-cancer hypotheses would have to make the odd
assumption that only cells with pre-existing chromosome
abnormalities are transformed by these "tumor" viruses.*

*This hypothesis also explains why "... despite intensive
efforts to transform normal human fibroblasts or epithelial
cells with varying combinations of activated cellular oncogenes, the results have been uniformly negative" (269). In
addition, the hypothesis explains why mutated proto-onc
genes and anti-oncogenes do not distinguish tumors by their
presence. According to this hypothesis, accidental somatic
mutations generated by chromosome translocations, such
as rearranged proto-myc or proto-abl genes, would be as
irrelevant to carcinogenesis as other mutations of specific
genes, such as point-mutated ras genes. Further, the hypothesis would explain why transgenic mice with activated
oncogenes are breedable and why retinoblastoma cells
remain carcinogenic for mice, even if they are infected by
a retrovirus that overexpresses its presumed suppressor, rb
anti-oncogene. The hypothesis would also resolve the discrepancy between the rather high probability and incidence
of mutation or "activation" of proto-onc genes compared
to the much lower probability and incidence of cancer (37,
337).*[25]

As a reconciliation of many of the contradictions, aneuploidy would appear to be an explanation worth serious attention. In its 1992 form, however, it suffered from several major defects, not the least of which was the lack of any functional demonstration that alterations in chromosome number were sufficient to induce cancer (a proof that Peter correctly demanded for oncogenes). Additionally, and the main reason aneuploidy had faded to almost complete transparency by 1992, was that despite repeated attempts over the years, there were no reports of specific chromosomal combinations that correlated even moderately well with specific cancers. Thus aneuploidy was widely viewed as a secondary effect and not an initiating one in the genetic evolution of a cancer cell.[26]

Between 1997 and 2002, Peter and his coworkers would provide experimental proof that aneuploidy was necessary for, and 100% functionally correlated with, malignant transformation; they would also provide an elegant mathematical treatment that explained this functional correlation in an extremely satisfying manner. Additionally, they and others were able to demonstrate for the first time impressive correlations between specific numerical chromosomal abnormalities and key early events on the multistep path to cancer.

These accomplishments were acknowledged in the following unpersuasive letter from Bert Vogelstein to Dean Owen in October of 2002, in which he wrote, in part:

Dr. Duesberg has played a pivotal role in the emerging recognition of the importance of aneuploidy in neoplasia. Though he and I differ on some issues pertinent to this research, I agree with him that aneuploidy is an essential part of cancer. Oncogenes and tumor suppressor genes play key roles in these diseases, but it will be impossible to adequately understand their nature until the causes and ramifications of aneuploidy are better known. Dr. Duesberg has championed this aspect of malignancy. Aneuploidy is perhaps the final frontier involving cell autonomous events underlying neoplasia. Dr. Duesberg continues to have a major impact on this burgeoning area of research, through his careful experimental observations as well as through his thoughtful reviews and critiques of the subject. There is no question that he is a world leader in this field of investigation.[27]

How such recognition came about is the subject of the last chapter of this *in media res* sketch.

Chapter 6 Notes

1. Gibbs, W. W. 2003. Untangling the Roots of Cancer. *Sci. Am.* July 2003, pp. 56–65.

2. Atkin, N. B., and Baker, M. C. 1966. Chromosome abnormalities as primary events in human malignant disease: evidence from marker chromosomes. *J. Natl. Cancer Inst.* 36:539–557.

3. *Pers. comm.* from W. Geoffrey Owen to Peter H. Duesberg, July 7, 2003, preserved in the *Peter H. Duesberg Archive* of the Bancroft Library of the Univ. of California, Berkeley.

4. Duesberg, P. H., and Schwartz, J. R. 1992. Latent viruses and mutated oncogenes: No evidence for pathogenicity. *Progress in Nucleic Acid Research and Molecular Biology* 43:135–204.

5. Duesberg, P. H., and Cichutek, K. 1986. Harvey *ras* genes transform without mutant codons, apparently activated by truncation of a 5' exon (exon-1). *Proc. Natl. Acad. Sci. USA* 83:2340–2344.

6. Hahn, W. C., Counter, C. M., Lundberg, A. S., Beijersbergen, R. L., Brooks, M. W., and Weinberg, R. A. 1999. Creation of human tumor cells with defined genetic elements. *Nature* 400:464–468.

7. As in: "The dreaded batter pudding hurler of Bexhill-on-Sea." Goon Show Classics, BBC Radio Collection, 1988.

8. Duesberg, P. H. and Schwartz, J. R. 1992. Latent viruses and mutated oncogenes: No evidence for pathogenicity. *Progress in Nucleic Acid Research and Molecular Biology* 43:135–204. References therein:

45. A. Knudson, Jr., *Cancer Res.* 45, 1437 (1985).

311. W. F. Benedict, A. Banerjee, C. Mark and A. L. Murphree. *Cancer Genet. Cytogenet.* 10, 311 (1983).

312. H. A. Gardener, B. L. Gallie, L. A. Knight and R. A. Phillips, *Cancer Genet. Cytogenet.* 6, 201 (1982).

9. Friend, S. H., Bernards, R., Rogelj, S., Weinberg, R. A., Rapaport, J. M., Albert, D. M., and Dryja, T. P. 1986. A human DNA segment with properties of the gene that predisposes to retinoblastoma and osteosarcoma. *Nature* 323:643–646.

10. Horowitz, J. M., Yandell, D. W., Park, S. H., Canning, S., Whyte, P., Buchkovich, K., Harlow, E., Weinberg, R. A., and Dryja, T. P. 1989. Point mutational inactivation of the retinoblastoma antioncogene. *Science* 243:937–940

11. Bookstein, R., Shew, J. Y., Chen, P. L., Scully, P., and Lee, W. H. 1990. Suppression of tumorigenicity of human prostate carcinoma cells by replacing a mutated RB gene. *Science* 247:712–715.

12. Dunn, J. M., Phillips, R. A., Zhu, X., Becker, A., and Gallie, B. L. 1989. Mutations in the RB1 gene and their effects on transcription. *Mol. Cell Biol.* 9:596–604.

13. Xu, H. J., Sumegi, J., Hu, S. X., Banerjee, A., Uzvolgyi, E., Klein, G., and Benedict, W. F. 1991. Intraocular tumor formation of RB reconstituted retinoblastoma cells. *Cancer Res.* 51:4481–4485.

14. Muncaster, M. M., Cohen, B. L., Phillips, R. A., and Gallie, B. L. 1992. Failure of RB1 to reverse the malignant phenotype of human tumor cell lines. *Cancer Res.* 52:654–561.

15. Weinberg, R. A. 1991. Tumor suppressor genes. *Science* 254:1138–1146.

16. Duesberg, P. H., and Schwartz, J. R. 1992. Latent viruses and mutated oncogenes: No evidence for pathogenicity. *Progress in Nucleic Acid Research and Molecular Biology* 43:135–204. References therein:

45. A. Knudson, Jr., *Cancer Res.* 45, 1437 (1985).

287a. R. A. Weinberg, *Science* 254, 1138 (1991).

17. Soussi, T., Caron de Fromentel, C., Breugnot, C., and May, E. 1988. Nucleotide sequence of a cDNA encoding the rat *p53* nuclear oncoprotein. *Nucleic Acids Res.* 16:113–184.

18. Donehower, L. A., Harvey, M., Slagle, B. L., McArthur, M. J., Montgomery, C. A. Jr., Butel, J. S., and Bradley, A. 1992. Mice deficient for *p53* are developmentally normal but susceptible to spontaneous tumours. *Nature* 356:215–221.

19. Lane, D. P. 1992. Cancer. *p53*, guardian of the genome. *Nature* 358:15–16.

20. Armitage, P., and Doll, R. 1954. The age distribution of cancer and a multi-stage theory of carcionogenesis. *Br. J. Cancer* 8:1–12.

21.Vogelstein, B., Fearon, E. R., Hamilton, S. R., Kern, S. E., Preisinger, A. C., Leppert, M., Nakamura, Y., White, R., Smits, A. M., and Bos, J. L. 1988. Genetic alterations during colorectal-tumor development. *N. Engl. J. Med.* 319:525–532.

22. Duesberg, P. H., and Schwartz, J. R. 1992. Latent viruses and mutated oncogenes: No evidence for pathogenicity. *Progress in Nucleic Acid Research and Molecular Biology* 43:135–204. References therein:

28. B. Vogelstein, E. R. Fearon, B. A. Stanley, R. Hamilton, S. E. Kern, A. C. Preisinger, M. Leppert, Y. Nakamura, R. White, A. M. M. Smits, and J. L. Bos. *N. Engl. J. Med.* 319, 525 (1988).

46. E. Stanbridge. *Science* 247, 12 (1990).

272. J. Marx. *Science* 251, 1317 (1991).

263. J. L. Bos, E. B. Fearon, S. B. Hamilton, M. Verlaan-de Vries, J. H. van Boom, A. J. van der Eb, and B. Vogelstein, *Nature* 327, 293 (1987).

264. K. Forrester, C. Almoguera, K. Han, W. Grizzle, and M. Perucho. *Nature* 327, 298 (1987).

296. I. Nishisho, Y. Nakamura, H. Miyoshi, Y. Miki, H. Ando, A. Horii, K. Koyama, J. Utsunomiya, S. Baba, P. Hedge, A. Markham, A. J. Krush, G. Petersen, S. R. Hamilton, M. C. Nilbert, D. B. Levy, T. M. Bryan, A. C. Preisinger, K. J. Smith, L.-K. Su, K. W. Kinzler, and B. Vogelstein. *Science* 253, 665 (1991).

262. M. Barbacid, *ARB* 56, 779 (1987).

297. F. McCormick, *Cancer Cells* 1, 56 (1989).

23. Duesberg, P. H. 1987. Cancer genes: Rare recombinants instead of activated oncogenes. *Proc. Natl. Acad. Sci. USA* 84:2117–2124, and with complete precision a decade later in: Hua, V. Y., Wang, W. K., and Duesberg, P. H. 1997. Dominant transformation by mutated *ras* genes *in vitro* requires 100 times higher expression than is observed in cancers. *Proc. Natl. Acad. Sci. USA*, 94:9614–9619.

24. Rous, P. 1967. The challenge to man of the neoplastic cell. *Science* 157:24–28 (as quoted in Duesberg and Schwartz, *op. cit.*).

25. Duesberg, P. H., and Schwartz, J. R. *Op. cit.* References therein:

194. J. German (ed.). *Chromosomes and Cancer* Wiley, New York, 1974.

336. S. Heim and F. Mitelman. *Cancer Cytogenetics*. Liss, New York, 1987.

269. E. J. Stanbridge. *ARGen* 24, 615 (1990).

37. P. H. Duesberg. *PNAS* 84, 2117 (1987).

337. W. Lijinsky. *Environ. Mol. Mutagen.* 14, 78 (1989).

26. Bialy, H. 1998. Aneuploidy and cancer: Vintage wine in a new bottle? *Nat. Biotechnol.* 16:137–138.

27. *Per. comm.* from Bert Vogelstein to W. Geoffrey Owen (cc: Peter Duesberg, July 7, 2003), preserved in the *Peter H. Duesberg Archive* of the Bancroft Library of the Univ. of California, Berkeley. Further evidence of this incongruity, as well as indication of a turning tide, is contained in the following email that Peter received from the office of undergraduate research in late January 2004. Perhaps undergraduates can afford to be a bit more adventuresome than graduate students.

Tue, 27 Jan 2004 14:44:24-0800

To: Peter Duesberg
From: Terry Strathman
Subject: Your list of URAP applicants' e-mail addresses

Dear Professor Duesberg,
I'm sure you will have mixed feelings on learning that your project (on cancer and aneuploidy) has been the most popular ever listed at the URAP website. We received 104 applications for your project, which I believe is almost double our previous record. I know that this will make the task of selecting an apprentice a bit daunting.

Terry Strathman
Program Director
Office of Undergraduate Research

7

The Idea Whose Time Had Come

To a very recent Ph.D., looking up from his notebook to discover Max Delbrück sitting across from him at a rustic lunch table of the Cold Spring Harbor Laboratory was like seeing the burning bush. Delbrück was the generally acknowledged father of molecular biology and an almost godlike figure to every young person in the field. Leaning forward to fix me squarely with his gaze, he said, "They tell me you are a poet. Does poetry have the answers?" My eyes became a little moist and I stammered something I can't remember, although the incident was the start of a warm relationship that lasted until a cancer claimed his life in 1981 at the age of seventy-five.

In asking this poignant question, Delbrück was expressing something very similar to the conclusions Peter had sadly reached after a life of studying retroviral *onc* genes. Maybe it was just "molecular minutiae" after all, with no real relevance. Philosophical and poetic implications aside, the specific import of this somber reflection has become the defining characteristic of the crossroads biology finds itself at the beginning of the 21st century.

By the year 2000, the tools and associated technologies that molecular biologists had at their disposal were indeed awesome. Large-scale gene sequencing projects were contemplated and completed, including the massively hyped deciphering of the entire human genome. Computer sciences and other electronic engineering disciplines were incorporated into the armory and even more data were generated. Now comparisons between the genetic blueprints, their primary products (mRNAs), and their ultimate protein products were possible in any and all combinations. Each of these "revolutionary" types of analyses naturally acquired its own special name and commensurate clique of biotech start-ups. Thus biology and biotechnology are now replete with "functional genomics," "proteomics," "micro-arrays," and the all-encompassing but almost meaningless and exceptionally ugly term, "metabolome," which is supposed to signify the entire, integrated collection of chemical reactions occurring in a cell at a particular time and under particular conditions.

The problem of course is transforming data into information, and information finally into knowledge. Contrary to expectations, the more data that became available, the clearer it became to genetic reductionists—even those as die-hard as Jim Watson[1]—that the problem of interpretation was becoming harder rather than easier. For example, genes predicted to be essential for one or another biological function could be removed from experimental animals without any consequence whatsoever, not even the increased tumor susceptibility of some of the inbred strains of mice without their most important tumor suppressor gene. Other inconsistencies mounted, and now the crossroads is quite clearly defined.[2-7]

Molecular genetic reductionism of the variety practiced by the first generations of molecular biologists was successful beyond all expectations. If the complete parts catalog of the cell is not yet complete, it is only a matter of (a short) time before it is. However, the logic and theory of deconstruction (reduction) are not applicable to reconstruction, any more than the converse of a proposition is logically true.

To the genetic determinists (geno-centrists), the fundamental proposition is we are our genes. That is to say, the properties of cells and multicellular organisms are reducible to complicated sets of biochemical interactions, all with genetic determinants— a view depicted in the colorful metabolic charts adorning the walls of every molecular and cellular biology laboratory in the world. To the growing group of systems biologists, it is the gene resonating with robust harmonics in the entire cellular system that is closer to reality. For the former, treatments void of discontinuities and resembling printed circuits are the norm. For the latter, a branch of mathematics that has become popularly known as chaos theory, or complexity, is more useful. Just as it required only a realization that the circle is a special case of the ellipse to turn hundreds of years of geo-centric epicycles into a more correct and useful view of the Earth's place in the solar system, "it may take only the realization that genes are parameters in networks and not isolated causes in themselves"[8] to persuade the next generation of molecular biologists to take the more productive turn.

In fact, this is already beginning to occur, and the concept of complexity is becoming increasingly popular. So much so, it is even in danger of attaining the dubious status of "hot idea of the moment." However, the actual implications of what it means to seriously consider the cell and the organism as truly connected, interdependent systems are profound and profoundly disturbing to the ideas underlying the way much of biotechnology, particularly in the pharmaceutical sectors, is presently carried out. So disturbing, in fact, it has become common to use "complicated" and "complex" interchangeably in order to mask them. The essence of "complicated" is "hard to figure out." "Complex" is something altogether different.

A complicated system is composed of a large number of interacting components. Importantly, the properties of such a system can be accurately predicted from knowing the properties of each of its components and a complete enumeration of their interactions. In other words, a complicated system is exactly the sum of its parts. Complex, on the other hand, is a term reserved for systems that display properties that are not predictable from a complete description of their components, and that are generally considered to be qualitatively different from the sum of their parts. A spaceship is extraordinarily complicated but is not complex. The degree to which cells, individually or as differentiated collections called higher organisms, are more complicated than even space stations, and the degree to which they are actually complex, is the most important theoretical and practical issue facing biology and biotechnology today.

As suggested previously, all of these developments worked in Peter's favor. Results from the use of the ultra-sophisticated, new analytical, digital toolbox—combined with this incipient shift in fundamental thinking—were to make his reformulation of the genetic bases of cancer attractive enough to warrant serious consideration, even from prestigious oncogeno-centrists like Bert Vogelstein. Of equal importance, as we will see, is the fact that the aneuploidy view of cancer coincided perfectly with a highly evolved form of basic biochemistry called metabolic control analysis, and an associated biotechnology called metabolic engineering, as well as with technological advances in cytogenetics. Thus a large cadre of biologists with no vested interests in one or another hypothesis about cancer could follow the clear, sequential development of the aneuploidy theory as it was published between 1997 and 2002 without adversarial preconception. Something we will do now.

In 1996 I was making the transition from full-time scientific editor of *Nature Biotechnology* (as *Bio/Technology* had by then become known) to my present position as resident scholar at the Institute of Biotechnology of the National University of Mexico, and I was in the New York offices infrequently. A phone call from

Peter caught me at one of those times, and like the others recounted thus far, it was memorable for several reasons.

For one, he was excited and cheerful. Ruediger Hehlmann, Professor and Director of the III Medizinische Klinik of the University of Heidelberg at Mannheim, had invited him for a six-month sabbatical to pursue a new experimental exploration of Boveri's almost century-old theory. These experiments had already begun, thanks to the philanthropic Bob Leppo, but there was only so much Peter could do in a laboratory that was built to study retroviruses not chromosomes. And this was the other reason he was excited. After a long time without any freedom to research the vast literature related to chromosomes and cancer, the relatively brief respite from AIDS after the farce with *Nature* and Maddox described in Chapter 3 gave him sufficient time to answer definitively whether anyone else had ever asked the question he was now prepared to address experimentally.

The question and experiments are simple. Although there was no argument that numerical chromosomal abnormalities were the best correlated genetic markers for cancerous cells, that this was an initiating event and not an epiphenomenon brought about by a mutation or two in some onco or anti-onco gene was vigorously contested by the mutation-oncogene theorists. Peter discovered from his literature search that no one had ever examined how early aneuploidy appeared when individual cells were treated with some carcinogen and then examined at regular and frequent intervals for the earliest signs of morphological transformation. If aneuploidies were a frequent consequence of transformation, and not its cause, then some early transformed colonies should contain a normal set of chromosomes. While not a proof that aneuploidy was the causative event in carcinogenesis, if only aneuploid colonies were detected this would at the least be an encouragement for further experiments. On the other hand, if diploid transformants, i.e., early cancer cells with a normal number of chromosomes, were found this would be the end of aneuploidy, and Peter would have to try and think of something else or, as most of his colleagues at Berkeley would surely prefer, take early retirement.

Since he was still around in 2003 engaging in the merit increase dispute with dean Owen, and appearing on the *Sci. Am.* timeline, we can correctly suppose that the results of these experiments did not falsify the hypothesis. But before we examine this and a few other research manuscripts more closely, I want to make a general point. In science, when a hypothesis is substantial and worth elevation to the status of theory, there is always a small number of experimental papers that can be easily ordered to demonstrate this. When a hypothesis is weak, however, this is not possible because the ground on which it rests is shakier than the San Andreas Fault in California. Therefore, the number of papers published on a topic is not necessarily a measure of its knowledge-generation potential. In fact, the opposite is often true, as is well illustrated by the 130,000+ papers on HIV and AIDS. They may indeed have "told us many things we did not know," as Fauci so insightfully predicted in the letter to his sister in 1989, but among them is not the answer to the all-important question of "how." The number of articles devoted to oncogenes, as of 2003, is 90,000.

With his long-time friend and Berkeley colleague Ruhong Li as lead author, and the new Mannheim allies, Peter published the first of the scientific papers that I propose meet the standard set above in the *PNAS* in 1997. It is entitled "Aneuploidy correlated 100% with chemical transformation of Chinese hamster cells."[9] As we saw, by 1992 the basic functional notion on which the aneuploidy hypothesis was to be constructed maintained that a cell could become schizophrenic enough to be called cancerous much more readily by the alterations in thousands of genes and their products that accompany a gain or loss of chromosomes, than by mutation in a small number. This schizophrenia is defined by a long list of symptoms that quite literally make the cancerous cell a species of its own that eventually consumes the organism from which it evolved. The analogy is not gratuitous since species are defined (in part) by a *specific* number of chromosomes. As we will see, Peter's biological intuition already had a firm biochemical basis that would allow his friend and collaborator, David Rasnick, to take the 100% correlation and adapt the biochemical reasoning and equations to give aneuploidy theory a rock-solid foundation.

Since the 1997 paper was the first time that aneuploidy had been reinvestigated as a cause of cancer in many years, Peter devoted a substantial amount of text to presenting all the problems with mutation theory we have already encountered, plus a few others. One is a particular favorite. The most frequently cited tumor suppressor gene, *p53,* does not appear to offer much protection against cancer, considering that 280 different point mutations were postulated to inactivate it.[10] He goes on to outline the evidence favoring an aneuploidy explanation, and continues with a refined description of the possible mechanisms that could cause it, most of which involve some serious physical disruption of the large network of proteins involved in correct mitosis. We then get the beef.

As I have repeatedly emphasized, in all experimental investigations, the system and conditions used are critical to the confidence that can be placed in their results. In the work that produced the 1997 *PNAS* paper, Peter and his colleagues chose to use Chinese hamster embryo (CHE) cells since they have only 22 chromosomes, making their microscopic examination and identification, called karyotyping, at the metaphase of mitosis relatively easy. Additionally, transformation of these cells can be detected quickly. Third, and very intentionally, as carcinogens they chose the polycyclic aromatic hydrocarbons (PAHs)—benzopyrene, methylcholanthrene, and dimethylbenzanthracene—

which are "not geno-toxic (mutagenic) in most test systems, including CHE cells *in vitro,* and colcemid, which is not even mutagenic after treatment with liver enzymes."[10] This would avoid any interpretation of the results, should they turn out to favor the aneuploidy hypothesis, that some undefined prior mutation caused the aneuploidy. Although mutation-oncogene theory attributes carcinogenic potential to any mutagen, it has always side-stepped the fact that among the very best carcinogens are substances like coal tars (PAHs) and asbestos that are essentially chemically inert.

The results of these studies were unambiguous: "... 38 out of 38 transformed colonies and sub-colonies of carcinogen-treated CHE cells, 2 out of 2 transformed colonies of colcemid-treated CHE cells, and 4 out of 4 spontaneously transformed colonies of CHE cells were 50 to 100% aneuploid. Because 39 of these 44 transformed colonies contained more than 50% of aneuploid cells, the aneuploidy must have originated in the same cell from which the transformed colony originated."[10] When tested in an animal model, 4 out of 4 transformed colonies were strongly tumorigenic.

Thus the revived aneuploidy hypothesis had survived its first crucial test, a success that was not to go unnoticed by Bert Vogelstein as he was rethinking, at least in part, the causative rather than consequential aspects of chromosome imbalances in cancer. Although sequential mutations may have been a landmark, it was not a place to take up permanent residence. By 1997, Vogelstein had committed himself to an essentially chromosomal-based model of cancer that was announced in a paper in *Nature* entitled "Genetic instability in colorectal cancers,"[11] and noted in an entry that immediately precedes Peter on the *Sci. Am.* evolution of cancer theory timeline. Unlike those scientific adversaries who choose to ignore Duesberg publications, in this paper Vogelstein does reference the contemporaneous *PNAS* article, even though he does not discuss it. Nonetheless this simple and, in the not-sobygone days, expected courtesy in scientific discourse demonstrates a major difference between Vogelstein as a collegial opponent and the other illustrious names we have encountered.

What exactly is "genetic instability," and how did it become so important in attempting to understand at least the properties of cancerous cells, even though the underlying cause of the cancer was still thought to be found revolving around one or another mutation? The answer to the second part of the question is easier. Except to onco-geneticists in the pharmaceutical sectors, it was obvious by the late 1990s that no simple biochemical change or three could possibly account for the panoramic dimensions of the deranged cancer cell. It was also obvious, and agreed to by everyone (including Peter), that the progression from a normal cell to a fully malignant one capable of relocation (metastasis) was a multi-step process that at some point generated enough genetic disruption to make the cell cross the boundary and become a real threat to the organism. The key difference between aneuploidy and gene mutation theories had reduced to whether the necessary and sufficient disruptions were mutations in particular genes that eventually generated the boundary conditions or whether aneuploidy in and of itself was the necessary and sufficient anarchist.

Enter genetic instability. Like aneuploidy, a long-recognized property of cancer cells and quite closely related to it, genetic instability was, similarly to its cousin, relegated to the status of epiphenomena until its reappearance center stage in 1997. In this year, Vogelstein and *Nature* elevated it to "the engine that drives tumorigenesis."[11] Normal animal cells have a species-specific (diploid) number of chromosome pairs, and must be genetically stable to guard the identity of the species. Maintaining this balance of chromosomal DNA molecules is so important, an entire complicated series of events called meiosis has evolved to make certain that each parent contributes exactly one half of their chromosome complement to the embryo. In humans, one extra chromosome 21, the smallest of our diploid number of 46, leads to Down's syndrome, and most other chromosomal imbalances spontaneously abort.

Cancer cells, however, are notoriously genetically unstable. The number of chromosomes in each cell of a tumor varies widely, and from one generation to the next there is a high probability that no two daughter cells will be genetically identical. Thus individual cells of a given cancer differ considerably in properties such as metastatic capacity, transplantability, antigenic make-up, drug sensitivity, growth rates, metabolism, and morphology.

In their 1997 *Nature* paper, Vogelstein and his collaborators correctly realized that this genetic instability was at the heart of the cancer.

> It has long been considered that genetic instability is an integral component of human neoplasia, ... but the nature and magnitude of the postulated instability is a matter of conjecture. We show here that colorectal tumours ... exhibit a striking defect in chromosome segregation, resulting in gains or losses in excess of 10^{-2} per chromosome per generation. This form of chromosomal instability reflected a continuing cellular defect that persisted throughout the lifetime of the tumour cell and was not simply related to chromosome number.[11]

This last observation is not quite accurate, as the Duesberg multi-national laboratory was to show to the advantage of aneuploidy theory in their second *PNAS* paper, which we will encounter shortly. But other than that it was a pretty good show that concludes with the suggestion "... persistent genetic instability may be critical for the development of all colorectal cancers."[11]

This key shift in gears would quickly go into overdrive when the same criticality was extended to cancers in general a year later.[12] To many readers, it would appear as though both Duesberg and Vogelstein are finally saying the same thing. Cancer is the result of gross genetic imbalances. But once again, the crucial difference is that in this and subsequent publications, Vogelstein, and others, would attribute the functionally all-important genetic instability to mutations in "mutator" genes (now designated CIN for chromosomal instability) that worked by either increasing the number of chromosomes with "activated oncogenes" or by decreasing those with "tumor suppressor genes."[11,13,14] A large number of candidates, some of whom we have even met before under different names, like *p53,* were auditioned to play the role of this postulated, mutable, master cancer driver. To date, none has been given the part, and the Oscar that would certainly go along with it.

The data from Vogelstein's paper and the perfect correlation that Peter had demonstrated in his own 1997 publication sufficiently intrigued the mathematically inclined biochemist David Rasnick to take time away from "the AIDS wars," as they were known around the laboratory, and begin to derive a theoretical treatment of aneuploidy that explained genetic instability and numerous other properties of the cancer cell. He was helped in this by another contemporaneous publication from the Vogelstein laboratory in which the first of the large-scale comparative analyses of gene expression in cancerous and normal cells was reported.[15] These expensive experiments provided data that the practically penniless Duesberg lab could never hope to generate.

As some of this gets a little heavy going, we will ease into it gently by first seeing how the developing theoretical treatment contributed to the continued cytogenetic experimental investigation of the transformed CHE clones. These studies would explain genetic instability as a direct consequence of aneuploidy without any need to postulate additional mutations, or mutator genes, or even mutator of mutator genes—a criterion that goes under the noble rubric of "Occam's Razor."

Before we examine this next of the papers that made aneuploidy respectable again, and moved its prime mover in a similar direction, I want to emphasize one result of Rasnick's treatment
that is essential to grasping the fundamental difference between
the aneuploidy explanation of cancer and even the newest versions of gene mutation that get very close to it, at least functionally.[16] As we will see, according to the fully developed aneuploidy
theory, it is impossible for even relatively large alterations in one
or several genes to generate enough dynamic disturbance in an
interconnected and robust metabolic system like a differentiated
animal cell to set it on the road to cancer. At best, a particular
mutation might be the final driver in the marathon that began
with the initial aneuploidy, but it cannot be the first.

The paper, which had Rasnick as one of the co-authors, was
published in the *PNAS* the following year (1998).[17] Contrary to
what Vogelstein's laboratory had stated in their genetic instability article quoted earlier, there is a very beautiful correlation
between aneuploidy (chromosome number) and the genetic instability of a given clone. They were correct in noting that it is not a
simple one, however. But while not simple in the sense that those
clones with more chromosomes are more genetically unstable,
i.e., an obvious linear correlation, it is simple to derive from a
perspective that views aneuploidy, rather than some dominant
mutation, as the cause of the genetic instability. The title of the
1998 article reflects this perfectly: "Genetic instability of cancer
cells is proportional to their degree of aneuploidy." The key word
is "degree."

What Peter and his small platoon did, as opposed to what they
thought, was simple and difficult simultaneously. Simple because
the essence of the data generated was to take individual cells
from the clones of as many as practicable of the transformed CHE
cells generated in the first experiments and follow, under the old-
fashioned microscope, the resulting karyotypes as the sub-cloned

cells multiplied and formed colonies of their own. The difficult part is keeping an accurate accounting of these numerous sub-clones and their constantly changing numbers of chromosomes. Moreover, keeping the cells healthy and uncontaminated is not trivial. Peter at the age of sixty-seven still changes the growth media for his experimental babies with his own hands. He would probably do this anyway, even if he could afford the technicians to perform this routine but essential chore impeccably.

What they thought, however, was simply elegant. By intro-ducing a quantitative measure of aneuploidy that they termed "the ploidy factor," the numbers from the eye-straining chromo-some counting became clearly interpretable data. This parameter is just the average chromosome number in a group of daughter cells divided by the normal number of the species. The results from these long divisions would allow them to conclude that trans-formed CHE cells indeed change their chromosome number in proportion to their ploidy factor.

But when this same analysis is applied to the more extensive data set supplied in the Vogelstein group's *Nature* paper, some-thing almost magical occurs, and random noise becomes music. Since the cells examined in this genetic instability study came from clinical colorectal tumors, their chromosome numbers var-ied much more widely than the CHE cells Peter and his colleagues were studying, ranging from around 40 to more than 120. If the members of this number set are divided by 46 and the fraction of stable cells is plotted against the ploidy factor, a sine-like wave pattern emerges in which those cells with ploidy factors close to 1 or 2 are highly stable and form the peaks of the wave. This is exactly what the aneuploidy theory would predict, since cells with multiples of their normal chromosome complement have a balanced number of mitotic genes and mitotic proteins. Those cells with ploidy factors furthest from a multiple form the val-leys, and intermediate ploidy factors fill out the curve.[17] Cells with simply more chromosomes may be more malignant, because their normal metabolism is more confused, but they are not necessarily more genetically unstable.

Recall that Vogelstein *et al.* argued in their *Nature* '97 paper, and continue to maintain, that a dominant mutation causes the genetic instability, turning the wheels of the cancer car. Duesberg *et al.* argue that an initial aneuploidy sets the wheels in motion. In their own words:

> *The existence of a human or animal gene that could be converted to a "dominant" aneuploidy gene is hard to reconcile with the evolution of multi-cellular organisms. Since the normal, spontaneous mutation rates are 1 in 10^9 nucleotides per mitosis even after proof reading, and since human cells contain about 10^9 nucleotides, 1 in 10^9 human cells would contain such a mutation (15, 26, 36). Thus one such mutation would soon kill the organism via carcinogenesis because cancers are clonal.*
>
> *This argument does not call into question the existence of mutations that cause karyotype instability. But unlike those postulated by Vogelstein et al., such mutations would have to be recessive requiring homozygous mutation to destabilize the karyotype. Since the probability of a specific base mutation per cell generation is 1 in 10^9 (see above), the probability of the same mutation in both sister alleles is 1 in 10^{18}. Thus only 1 in 100 average humans would be at risk to develop cancer from such a specific base mutation, because a human lifetime corresponds to approximately 10^{16} cells (2, 15, 37, 38). Indeed there is a rare genetic defect, Bloom's syndrome, that is caused by such a mutation (39). In accord with our hypothesis, persons with Bloom's syndrome do indeed develop colon cancer at young age (40, 41).[18]*

The following quotation is from later in the same paper. In addition to a plain-language explanation of aneuploidy as the mechanism underlying cancer, it also serves as the perfect introduction to the upcoming brief encounter with some history of theory-based, metabolic control.

Since cellular phenotypes are determined by molecules that are assembled by thousands of kinetically linked enzymes (45, 46), aneuploidy can dominantly alter normal phenotypes because it multiplies or divides the diploid, biosynthetic assembly lines of normal cells (32, 33, 47–49). In the light of this hypothesis normal cells are the equivalent of car factories with concerted assembly lines producing appropriate numbers of engines, bodies and wheels, but cancer cells would be equivalent to factories with dis-concerted assembly lines that produce two or more bodies per engine, or more or less than 4 wheels per body. Qualitative changes would be achieved by multiplying or dividing assembly lines that produce regulatory molecules.

Since aneuploidy can readily change the metabolic output, that determines the phenotype of the cell, by adding or subtracting biosynthetic assembly lines, aneuploidy is in fact better suited to generate cancer-specific phenotypes than gene mutation. The reason is that most mutations, both negative and positive, have little effect on the output of a biosynthetic assembly line because enzymes work in vivo only at a small fraction of their capacity, i.e. far below saturation (45, 46). As a result biosynthetic assembly lines resist very efficiently any changes in the activities of their enzymes.... In view of this, it is not surprising that mutated cellular oncogenes and tumor suppressor genes fail to perform dominant transforming functions (51–55), are typically not more active than unmutated counterparts (37, 43,

54–56), and are not consistently present in otherwise identical cancers (13, 15, 37, 53, 55, 57, 58).[18]

The essentials of the arguments above derive from a paper published in 1981 in the journal *Genetics,* entitled "The molecular basis of dominance."[19] Its authors, Henrik Kacser and James Burns, a biochemical geneticist and mathematician, had developed ideas that were so disconcerting to the dogma that was in all the textbooks, their truly landmark work appeared in a genetics journal rather than a biochemical one. What they demonstrate in this 30-page paper, dense with equations, is that the textbook concept of the "rate-limiting enzyme" is only true in the test tube, and that it has almost nothing to do with the actual way enzymes perform in the cell. So-called rate-limiting enzymes are those whose activity is said to control the output of a given pathway. If an enzyme is eliminated completely, then indeed the metabolism of a cell can be drastically affected. Suppose, for example, the enzyme is in a bacterial biochemical pathway that produces the amino acid tryptophan. Eliminating it by mutation will produce a cell that can no longer synthesize its own tryptophan, and will require that it be added to the medium for the cell to grow. But these are recessive mutations, since they involve loss of a protein's activity. Dominant mutations, on the other hand, involve a gain of activity. What Kacser and Burns showed is that in a sufficiently complicated metabolic network, such as a typical bacterial cell, the output of any metabolic pathway is almost completely insensitive to changes in one or a few enzymes, even those thought to be at critical branch points.

The derivation of their final simple, dimensionless (logistical) equation that predicts how the overall carbon metabolism of a cell, which they called flux, is affected by altering the amounts of different numbers of enzymes involves some knowledge of calculus, but one arithmetical fact should suffice to make its point.

Diploid cells are so resistant to changes in enzyme levels that eliminating one allele, or 50% of the potential activity, makes no difference at all to the organism. The converse, increasing the dosage
of an enzyme two-fold, also has no effect, even on a simple genetic
system like a bacteria with only one chromosome.

Had this branch of biochemistry been as popular in the early
eighties as it has become today, a lot of biotechnology company
dollars might have been saved. Because in addition, as Duesberg
and Rasnick note above, Kacser and Burns also demonstrate that
most enzymes are functioning at far below their optimal capacity in a cell. Thus doubling or tripling the amount of an enzyme
by adding extra copies of its gene by recombinant DNA technology is not likely to do much. This was discovered to the great
chagrin of many first-generation "metabolic engineers" who
thought they could make bacteria produce more of a specialty
amino acid, for example, by adding additional copies of some
gene whose product was listed in the textbooks as a "rate-limiting
enzyme."

More directly relevant to the development of aneuploidy theory is that Rasnick was able to convert the equations of Kacser
and Burns, which were derived from considering the entire collection of enzymatic reactions in a cell at any time, into a completely analogous system of equations that now reflected the
collective properties of the genes that produced the enzymes. The
outcomes of this theoretical treatment are straightforward. Among
others, it describes aneuploidy as a self-perpetuating process
without any driver mutations, and moreover it explains why
changing the activity of a small group of genes, even those thought
to be master control genes (just like the enzymes once thought to
be "rate-limiting") cannot perturb the system to a noticeable
degree. It also sets some parameters for aneuploidy thresholds in
order for a cell to become irrevocably committed to a trajectory
leading to a cancerous metabolism that correlate very well with

published cytogenetic analyses of different tumor types.[20,21] These parameters describe a genetic system that is highly sensitive in its final outcomes to the initial aneuploidy. Systems of this general description, displaying extreme dependence on initial conditions, are by definition complex.

Just like the Kacser and Burns treatment of the effect that changes in enzyme levels have on overall metabolism, Rasnick's transformation makes some strong predictions about how many genes are involved and how much their expression will be altered as a cell becomes cancerous. In particular, it says that in a cancerous cell the most frequent changes that will be observed are simultaneous, small alterations in the levels of many thousands of gene products. And most pointedly, it does not follow from the reasoning that the more a gene's expression is altered, the more biological effect it is likely to have.

But one set of moving pictures is in this case worth a thousand equations. Exactly how difficult it would be for a change in one or several proteins to affect something as robust as mitosis can be seen in a time-lapse microscopic study available on the CD that accompanies the latest edition of *Molecular Cell Biology*,[22] and which in my opinion does deserve an Oscar.

As Rasnick was "doing the math," as they say, another paper appeared from the Vogelstein laboratory that gave persuasive experimental support to the emerging theory. This paper, in *Science* (so that the riches of the laboratory could be equally shared), is entitled somewhat innocuously "Gene expression profiles in normal and cancer cells,"[15] and as mentioned before, it is the first of the large-scale, "functional genomic" chip-based studies that have now become commonplace. The reason that I use the adjective "innocuous" is made plain by the authors themselves. Their abstract begins:

As a step toward understanding the complex differences between normal and cancer cells in humans, gene expression patterns were examined in gastrointestinal tumors. More than 300,000 transcripts derived from at least 45,000 different genes were analyzed. Although extensive similarity was noted between the expression profiles, more than 500 transcripts that were expressed at significantly different levels in normal and neoplastic cells were identified.[15]

With so many different genes that were significantly differentially expressed, the authors limited themselves to the approximately 300 showing a ten-fold or greater difference in expression. The reasoning, in their own words, is, "the genes exhibiting the greatest differences in expression are likely to be the most biologically important."[15] And the results of this expectation, also in their own words: "most of the transcripts could not have been predicted to be differentially expressed."[15] More striking even is their honest admission that "two widely studied oncogenes, *c-fos* and *c-erb3*, were expressed at much higher levels in normal colon epithelium than in (colorectal) cancers."[15] Both of these are so-called dominant oncogenes that would be predicted to be much more highly expressed in the cancer cell than the normal one. And what about *ras*, the grandfather of all oncogenes, that became so important as a cooperating factor in the "tumorigenic process" that drives colon cancer? It was "expressed at very low levels in all tissues examined and no significant changes in cancer cells compared with normal cells were detected."[23] Difficult results indeed to reconcile with the gene mutation hypothesis but easily explained by aneuploidy theory, which views changes in the fraction of the genome rather than the number of individual mRNAs as a defining parameter, and which demands that large changes in genomic flux, like cancer, result from the compound effect of small changes in many thousands of genes. I would bet my multilingual, Amazonian parrot Attila, who says, among other things, *Om Mani Peme Hung,* that had any oncogene, tumor suppressor gene, or candidate CIN gene been present in the expected category of highly over- or under-expressed, the title of the paper would have been "C-xyz is the cause of colon cancer," and it would have been reported to at least a hundred TV and print journalists in salivatory anticipation. In 2002, the results of a similar investigation were published from another high-profile laboratory, at Stanford, presided over by David Botstein. This extremely colorful and carefully executed study[24] describes the results of performing a highly normalized correlation between gene copy number and mRNA levels in breast cancer cells and cell lines. Pollack *et al.* confirm that the main differences between normal and transformed cells lie in the number of genes, rather than in the types of genes differentially expressed.

To summarize the main argument to this point: The cancer cell is generally portrayed as a rogue super-cell that somehow manages to "disobey" the environmental signals that should check its growth and determine its function, and also succeeds in colonizing other, sometimes very different, tissue environments. In the view of the aneuploidy hypothesis, the transformed cell is a damaged cell trying to resolve the ever-more-complex, irreversible, and unstable gene dosage it accumulated by self-complicating mitotic asymmetries.

The data from the large-scale expression study above became incorporated in the theoretical treatment David was undertaking. Simultaneously, his "manuscript in preparation" was seen by two of the more influential scientists in the now heavily MCA-based (metabolic control analysis) biotechnology properly called metabolic engineering. One of them, Jay Bailey, was a good friend through *Bio/Technology* and is generally credited with giving the term its first rigorous interpretation and practically useful impetus in an article that appeared in *Science* in 1991.[25] The other was an even older acquaintance from my Bezerkeley daze, Athel Cornish-Bowden, whom I knew slightly when he was a postdoctoral fellow in Dan Koshland's lab; he is now one of the leading lights in MCA theory and practice. Each was so intrigued and impressed by this unforeseen application of the Kacser and Burns equations that they invited Peter and David to participate in a NATO specialist's workshop devoted to MCA and drug discovery, of which Athel was the prime organizer, and at which Jay Bailey was to be the keynote speaker. Through Jay, I wrangled an invitation of my own. I just could not miss the first real test the new theory would receive by being presented to a select gathering of fifty or so mathematically super-sophisticated metabolic control experts who knew nothing about oncogenes, but infinity about complex networks of enzymes.

The workshop was surreal, super, and sad. The surreal aspect is that it was held in a castle outside Budapest while the NATO war against neighboring Yugoslavia was in full-tilt mode. We were all told to keep a low NATO-associated profile while in Hungary. The super part was that Rasnick's presentation was received with riveting attention. The only comments afterwards were one version or another of "Can it really be that simple?" This was because MCA, although a beautiful and mathematically simple (at least to them) general theory, became quite Baroque when it was applied in the laboratory to even small metabolic networks involving only a few dozen enzymes. The participants were noticeably impressed by how easily the fundamental, robust theory could be adapted to networks of genes instead of enzymes. This collective realization was expressed by Athel in a commentary for *Nature Biotechnology* subsequent to the workshop in which he compared the Duesberg-Rasnick theory to continental drift.

The close fit between the continents was obvious to everyone who looked at a world map since accurate maps existed;

similarly, the association between aneuploidy and cancer has been obvious to everyone who studied it for more than 100 years. But just as continental drift was not taken seriously by most geophysicists until plausible mechanisms were worked out, most experts in recent decades have regarded aneuploidy as a side effect of cancer, rather than its cause.

If Peter Duesberg and David Rasnick (University of California, Berkeley) are right, however, aneuploidy is indeed the cause, and metabolic control analysis reveals why. Not only is the association between aneuploidy and cancer so close as to be virtually exact, but the predicted metabolic effect of over-expressing a large and arbitrary set of genes is just the collapse of normal regulation seen in cancer.[26]

The sad component to the sibilant trilogy I used above was that Jay was suffering, although he did not know it then, from a colon cancer that would take him, in his prime, only two years later in 2001. His last published words, composed on his deathbed, appeared in another *Nature Biotechnology* commentary:

Recent publication of analyses of the human genome sequence dramatically signals a turn in biology research from reductionist dissection to systems integration. Mathematical and computational tools, clearly indispensable for genome assembly and sequence comparisons, have otherwise become almost invisible in recent molecular biology. Because systems with only two or three independent variables can exhibit extraordinarily complex behaviors in time and space, there has long been a need for application of mathematics and computation to the understanding and analysis of biological systems. Arrival of the sequenced human genome now makes efforts in these directions imperative.[27]

The refined, triple-checked version of the aneuploidy theory appeared in 1999 in the very hard-edged *Biochemical Journal,* volume 340, with the title "How aneuploidy affects metabolic control and causes cancer."[20] In December 2002, the Vogelstein corps (as distinct from the Duesberg platoon) published their own theoretical treatment of CIN mutations and genetic instability.[28] For this they recruited Martin Nowak, a mathematician from the Institute of Advanced Study at Princeton. I like to imagine Nowak as kind of a mathematical gunslinger for hire, since he also attempted in 2002 to resurrect David Ho's model of HIV-1 dynamics[29] that had "the final nails in its coffin," as we may recall from Chapter 3, hammered in place in 1998.[30] The majority of Nowak's publications prior to 1999 have to do with game theory, which partially explains why he is at Princeton, where John Nash reinvented its basics. And obviously Nowak is a very adroit mathematician. The problem, however, is that a *post hoc* mathematical model can be constructed to "explain" almost any data set. This is qualitatively different from a theory-based explanation that makes predictions. As the authors themselves note, their model will prove difficult to test, and is presented "to hopefully provide a framework"[29] for such future experiments.

The presentation itself is statistical, and unlike the aneuploidy theory, it requires much more than pre-calculus to follow it in any detail. But essentially it assumes that mutations in CIN genes cause genetic instability and then analyzes the various probabilistic scenarios that follow from that assumption. It presents no new data, and cites the second CHE analysis publication in passing, yet curiously makes no reference to the 1999 *Biochem. J.* paper that was its obvious inspiration.

While Vogelstein may be forthcoming to the point of effusiveness in his private regard for Peter, as we saw from his letter to dean Owen, he is publicly much more parsimonious.[31] But since so many scientists who were not cancer biologists had now seen the aneuploidy explanation of cancer presented in a language that made sense to them, it seems to me that Vogelstein was forced to come up with some heavy-duty math of his own with which to dazzle cancer molecular biologists, who generally tend to be simultaneously intimidated and impressed by equations. The one thing the model does specifically address, and for which it provides an explanation, are the quotations earlier in the chapter in which Peter argues that the probabilities for dominant genetic instability mutants are too high, and those for recessive ones too low, to account for the frequency with which cancer occurs. One might notice a certain similarity to the rationale underlying the sequential mutation hypothesis that preceded genetic instability. In any case, the 2002 model is not a place from which one could begin and easily deduce these facts.

Nor could one deduce from it another all-important feature of cancer that until now we have not mentioned. The time between treatment with any carcinogen, mutagenic or not, and the appearance of cancer is extremely long, averaging decades in humans. This presents the equivalent of several Mount Everests for mutation theory, since it is inexplicable how after massive irradiation of an experimental animal, in which every conceivable mutation has been induced, it still takes so many generations for the cancer to develop when the effects of mutations are felt almost immediately by the cell. Aneuploidy theory predicts exactly this, as well as the age bias of cancer mentioned earlier, with the dead-eye aim and smooth draw of a two-gun-toting Billy the Kid.

The evolution of an aneuploid cancer cell from its diploid parent is a self-perpetuating process that begins with its first non-lethal aneuploidy and produces over time cells that are ever more metabolically and genetically perturbed. This initial aneuploidy may be spontaneous or induced by physical substances like asbestos that directly interfere with the mitotic protein network, or by the many non-specific mutations that result from ionizing radiations or certain chemicals, thereby creating sufficient disruptions in the dynamic balance of these same proteins. Independent of the mechanistic cause, such chromosomally destabilized cells proceed step by step, from a tolerable hyperplasia or benign tumor, to full metastatic malignancy without the need of any special mutations in any special genes. It is important to emphasize that not every aneuploid cell is destined to become cancerous. However, every aneuploid cell has the potential to further its own somatic evolution, which over the course of decades in humans may lead to a cancer cell. How improbable such chromosome combinations are can be inferred from the fact that only one in three people develop a cancer over the course of a lifetime of seventy-five years, and cancers derive from a single initially transformed cell.

Whatever the scientific outcome of the Nowak *et al.* framework, Vogelstein has now committed to a final epicycle, continuing the analogy with Copernicus and Ptolemy. It will be much harder to change models than metaphors at this midstream and produce a new and improved version without serious retracing. An alternative would be to abandon the fortress, which he could still do gracefully, and join his considerable forces to those of Peter. One might imagine all sorts of golden scenarios that such an alliance could produce. Stranger things have happened, and "science," after all, "is full of surprises."

One such surprise, albeit not a pleasant one, was waiting for Peter almost immediately upon his victorious return from Budapest, and it distracted him temporarily from completing the third set of experiments with the transformed CHE cells that I consider to prove the aneuploidy hypothesis. The distraction came in the form of a well-advertised paper in *Nature* from the Weinberg laboratory that claimed, "after more than 15 years of trying,"[32] to "define" a set of three genes "sufficient to convert normal human cells into tumorigenic ones."[33] The Weinberg publication will also temporarily divert us from examining the definitive experiments alluded to above. I promise, however, to make the detour brief.

Considering all that has been written here about the robustness of the theoretical treatment of aneuploidy, and the logical and experimental contradictions of gene-mutation hypotheses, if the results of the Weinberg group's experiment were as advertised, all the theory would have to go out the window, and mutation prior to aneuploidization would prevail. To put the last first, they were not. After reading the *Nature* publication, Peter wrote to his old compatriot asking for the tumorigenic cell lines so that he might analyze them for their degree of aneuploidy, something that was not reported in the paper. The brief email exchange between them is filled with grandiose German salutatory flourishes like *Selbstverstaendlich mein Lieber! Es waere meine Ehre! Hochachtungsvoll!,* showing both Weinberg's excellent command of the language and the remaining personal affection between these long-time scientific opponents. Weinberg "dutifully" sent the cells, and immediately upon receiving them on a Saturday morning, Peter equally dutifully began their examination, after which he composed a short "letter to the editor" that he sent to *Nature* and Weinberg simultaneously. The note pointed out that the cell lines were highly aneuploid and that this was not unexpected since it took more than sixty generations from the sequential (not simultaneous) introduction of the first of the synthetic gene trinity before the first clonal (not polyclonal) tumor cells appeared. The letter also called attention to the somehow-overlooked fact that among the three genes was the SV40 transforming protein, long known to be an excellent aneuploidy-inducing agent.[34] Thus the experiments failed to distinguish between aneuploidy as cause or effect of the transformation.

Peter sent the letter in early September 1999; in November he received a curt email from the "Scientific Correspondence" editor at *Nature* saying that Weinberg had rejected its publication.[35] The first part of Dr. Cotter's email is normal procedure with scientific journals. When the results or conclusions of a paper are challenged, the senior author of the paper is always sent the challenge for reply. It is unconscionable, however, for the author whose results are being questioned to be allowed to dismiss the objections out of hand. Any reader who has stuck with the story this far knows that Peter was not going to let this pass quietly. Therefore instead of a brief letter to the editor, Duesberg's laboratory published an extensive analysis of the Weinberg human tumor cells in the *Proceedings of the National Academy of Sciences* in March of 2000.[36] This time the MIT laboratory did respond, but in a paper that curiously did not appear in the *Proceedings* but rather in *Cancer Research* the following year.[37]

All the argument had now condensed to whether any of the tumor cells generated in these experiments were diploid. The *Cancer Research* paper claimed that such colonies did indeed exist and that therefore aneuploidy was consequential and not causal. In 2002, Peter sent a letter to the same journal with a detailed analysis of the "diploid" tumor clones that showed every one of them to be aneuploid.[38] Unlike the editors at *Nature,* those at *Cancer Research* asked Dr. Weinberg if he would care to reply to Dr. Duesberg's comment without the option of rejecting its publication. His response appears directly below Peter's correspondence, and is so similar to his *ad hominem* attack at the Lilly symposium fifteen years previous to deserve the qualifier "typical."

> We have now concluded that the cells that Dr. Duesberg sent back to us were very different from the ones that we had sent him earlier. Those that he returned to us were highly aneuploid, whereas those that we sent to him contained a large percentage of diploid cells.... We can only conclude that it is possible, as has long been known, that

the improper handling of cultured cells, including their thawing and culturing under suboptimal conditions, can encourage and select for the outgrowth of aneuploid variants, and that Dr. Duesberg's observations once again provide testimonial to this long-accepted principle.[39]

End of detour, and scientifically an irrelevant one, since a definitive answer to whether aneuploidy was a necessary initiating condition for tumorigenesis or a secondary consequence was provided in the third of the papers using CHE cells. This appeared as the "Lead Article" in *Cancer Genetics Cytogenetics,* Vol. 119, in June of 2000 with the title "Aneuploidy precedes and segregates with chemical carcinogenesis."[40]

Recall that the first paper in this series reported experiments designed to find early diploid transformants among CHE cells treated with PAHs, and that none were found, suggesting that aneuploidy may be the cause rather than a consequence of transformation. This study directly tested the prediction of the "aneuploidy-is-a-consequence hypothesis" that prior to transformation there is either no aneuploidy, or at least none that exceeds the normal background in untransformed cells. The Berkeley-Mannheim collaborators did this by analyzing whether Chinese hamster embryo cells treated with carcinogenic polycyclic aromatic hydrocarbons become aneuploid before transformation. After subtracting the background of untreated, aneuploid cells, they found that transforming concentrations of PAHs render about 20% of CHE cells aneuploid weeks earlier than the first signs of morphological transformation in a few of them. The high percentage shows that PAHs function as aneuploidogens, and all but rules out any mutational provocation.

However, since only very few of millions of cells that are treated with PAHs ever become transformed, and since oxidized metabolites of PAHs can function as mutagens, it could still be argued that transformation is due to mutation and that aneuploidy is a transformation-unrelated event. To test this argument, Peter and his colleagues computed the odds ratio of aneuploidy in tumors induced in Chinese hamsters by a low dose, one-time treatment with PAHs to that of aneuploidy in the PAH-treated cells from which the tumors originated. Because it is impossible to know exactly how many cells in an animal are exposed to an injected chemical, they used the 20% aneuploidy of the similarly treated CHE cells in culture as an upper-limit approximation. The result was that 14 out of 14 cancers were aneuploid. The chance that the aneuploidy of the 14 cancers was transformation-unrelated is easily calculated to be 0.20 to the power of 14, or approximately 1 in 10 billion. If this improbability is not impressive enough, it is only necessary to add a few more experimental animals to bring the odds ratio into the trillions.

Having provided compelling theoretical and empirical support for the hypothesis that aneuploidy is the genetic determinative of the transformed phenotype, Peter now began to mine the rich vein he had uncovered for all he could. The first gem to come to light was reported in the *Proceeding of the National Academy of Sciences* in 2000,[41] and it has a strong, practical reflection. One of the major distinctions between even a very good hypothesis and an actual theory is that theories are expansive. They make accurate predictions in settings not directly related to those in which they were formulated, and similarly, they explain previously inexplicable findings.

Of all the peculiarities of cancer cells, the extraordinarily high rate at which they become resistant to chemotherapeutic drugs (one in one thousand to one in one million per mitosis) has for almost fifty years remained one of the more difficult for theoreticians to explain and clinicians to confront. As recently as 1995, the eminently respected cancer biologist Henry Harris considered it to be a "major conceptual difficulty to reconcile the very high mutational frequency with genetic theory if two functional alleles are present in the same cell."[42]

Because aneuploidy simultaneously imbalances, through effects in gene dosage, large numbers of balance-sensitive proteins, including those involved in the mitotic spindle apparatus, its occurrence in a cell results in a self-perpetuating chromosomal instability. The average cell in a typically aneuploid tumor is at a 46% risk to gain or lose one chromosome per mitosis.[11,17] Thus, continuous chromosome reassortment (genetic instability) catalyzed by aneuploidy offers a quite plausible way to explain the high mutation rates of cancer cells to chemotherapy. It may reflect more than simple coincidence that this model has an exact precedent in the mechanistic explanation of the influenza virus' exceptionally high mutation rate through reassortment of sub-genomic RNA segments that Duesberg provided in the pages of a 1968 number of the *Proceedings*.[43]

In the 2000 paper, aneuploidy-catalyzed chromosome reassortment as an explanation for the high mutation rates of cancer cells is directly tested by comparing the mutation of aneuploid, tumorigenic cells with those of diploid, normal cells from the same inbred line of Chinese hamsters. As all of the cells studied have an otherwise identical genetic background, any differences in the numbers of drug-resistant colonies that appear must result from their different chromosome numbers. The mutations investigated were to resistance against the anticancer drugs puromycin, cytosine arabinoside, colcemid, and methotrexate. Exactly in accord with a chromosomal reassortment model, the mutation frequencies of aneuploid cells were high, between 1 in 10,000 and 1 in a million, whereas the frequency of resistance in the diploid cells was undetectable.

In addition to the quantitative dilemma that cancer cells pose for gene mutation theories by their high mutation rates to single-drug resistance, it is completely bewildering to these theories that such cells often become simultaneously resistant to a number of functionally and structurally unrelated drugs.[44] But this is precisely what one would expect if chromosomal reassortment was the cause, as large numbers of genes are being affected simultaneously. Experimentally, this means that selection for one phenotype should produce cells possessing novel, unselected properties. As succinctly put in the abstract from Peter's 2000 paper:

> *Mutants selected from cloned (aneuploid) cells for resistance against one drug displayed different unselected phenotypes, e.g., polygonal or fusiform cellular morphology, flat or three-dimensional colonies, and resistances against other unrelated drugs.*[41]

Beyond providing a unifying explanation for both the high mutation rates of cancer cells and the frequent occurrence of multi-drug resistance, the data from this paper immediately suggest using the highly frequent drug resistance of cancer cells in the laboratory diagnosis of pre-cancerous cells in benign lesions. Although culturing human cells is neither cheap nor trivial, and it still takes weeks before the results can be interpreted, it is nonetheless an extremely powerful and straightforward way to determine if a large population of cells contains aneuploidies that are destabilizing enough to generate drug-resistant variants with a high frequency, and therefore well on the road to cancer. And it is considerably less expensive, easier, and more reliable than doing chromosome spreads and counting. Millions rather than a few cells can be tested, and as yet there are no acceptable ways of identifying those specific aneuploidies that might signal cancerous progression.

Because cancer cells are so genetically unstable, and almost all cytogenetic studies in which cancer-specific aneuploidies were sought used cells from highly aneuploid, well-developed tumors, it is not surprising that any underlying, sufficient chromosome combinations, if they were present, would be masked by the genetic turmoil inside their nuclei. But in fact, a careful search of the literature, such as that undertaken by Peter and included in the last of the experimental jewels we will parse, shows that there is quite a bit of evidence that specific aneuploidies significantly correlate with the various stages in the initiation and maintenance of a cancer cell. One such study, reported in 1999, is worth singling out now not only since its senior author, Thomas Ried, is chief of cancer genomics at the NIH, but because it makes use of a new technique that allows subtracting the uncritical redundant chromosomes to reveal possibly meaningful correlations between specific aneuploidies and specific cancers. The paper is entitled "Genomic changes defining the genesis, progression, and malignancy potential in solid human tumors: a phenotype/genotype correlation," and its key conclusion is:

> Subtractive karyograms of chromosomal gains and losses were used to map tumor stage-specific chromosomal aberrations and clearly showed that nonrandom chromosomal aberrations occur during disease progression in colorectal and cervical tumors.[45]

Although the aneuploidy theory in its formal development does not demand that cancer stage-specific or type-specific aneuploidies exist, neither does it exclude them, as it does individual gene mutation. Moreover, the S-shaped (sigmoid) curve, described by its basic equation, does allow the derivation of what are appropriately called "attractor basins" by chaos mathematicians. An attractor basin is almost exactly what it sounds like: a set of solutions to an equation that gets smaller and smaller depending on the previous partial solution. In biological terms this means that among the large number of aneuploidies that could potentially initiate the genetic and metabolic disruption minimally necessary for a cancer phenotype, as the aneuploid cell evolves under the selective pressures of its environment those that continue to divide are likely to maintain particular chromosome combinations that got them that far. It is not at all unreasonable, therefore, to expect to find at least some of those combinations more likely to set the cell on one of these black-hole cancer trajectories. This is what Peter and his colleagues reported in the *PNAS* in May 2002, under the title "Specific aneusomies in Chinese hamster cells at different stages of neoplastic transformation, initiated by nitrosomethylurea."[46]

The paper clearly demonstrates that particular abnormal chromosome combinations (aneusomies) appear in chemically transformed Chinese hamster cells *in vitro,* and in tumors derived from these cells *in vivo,* with a much higher frequency than would be expected based on random chromosome shuffling. For example, 79% of *in vitro*-transformed cells had an extra copy of chromosome 3, and 59% had lost chromosome 10; moreover, 52% of the transformed cells shared this particular combination, much higher than the 0.6% expected if the aneusomies were the result of random chromosomal imbalances. This type of analysis will, with near certainty, be multiplied many-fold over the next years by an ever larger number of cancer cytogeneticists like Ried. Using ever more cutting-edge technologies, it is likely that they will identify unambiguous, sufficient aneusomies for various cancers at their different evolutionary stages. It is even possible that the actual biochemical dynamics that differentiate a cancer cell from its normal progenitor, and one cancer from another, will be fished out from the present morass of expression data once the mathematical and experimental tools with which to connect final effects in complex systems and their initiating causes are firmly in place.[7] In the end, the idea of the onco-chromosome may very well come to replace the onco-gene in the textbooks, scientific journals, and popular press.

But the motherlode for aneuploidy as a theory is that viewing the cancer cell as a species of its own that rapidly evolves in its human host simultaneously opens the window on the much larger panorama of speciation in general, something that happens over long evolutionary time scales. An extremely beautiful and comprehensive illustration of this principle appeared in *Science* in 1999[47] in which a large group from the Laboratory of Genomic Diversity of the National Cancer Institute used the new global computerized toolbox to do a comparative study of mammalian genomes. In brief, their results show that bats and baboons, white whales and white mice, humans and horses all have basically the same 35,000 genes. What make each species distinct are the manner and number of chromosomes in which these genes are distributed.

As I write the final paragraphs of this sketch of the thinking, triumphs, and trials of my friend of almost forty years, the old MBVL where we began both our friendship and the sketch is now a three-story-deep black hole of its own, from which will emerge the new Wendell Stanley Hall. How new the molecular biology practiced within its gleaming laboratories will be is an open question, as is whether Peter will be considered worth a few hundred square feet of its expensive architecture. At the moment, the Duesberg laboratory is located immediately adjacent the crater in the oldest science building on the Berkeley campus, Donner Hall. The bulk of his notebooks, floppy discs, diskettes, hard drives, papers, letters, and photographs are safe in the *Peter H. Duesberg Archive* of the university's Bancroft Library. This distinction is given to only a handful of distinguished professors, among them Wendell Stanley himself, who was still alive and teaching when I arrived in 1966 at the intellectual paradise of the first department of molecular biology in the country. When Peter told me that the Bancroft had asked for his papers, I remarked that the librarian was clearly more perceptive than his dean.

Chapter 7 Notes

1. As quoted in: Bethell, T. A., Map to Nowhere: The genome isn't a code and we can't read it. *American Spectator,* April 2001.

2. Richard Lewontin was among the first to articulate these troubling anticipations in his essay, "The dream of the human genome: doubts about the Human Genome Project." 1992. *The New York Rev. Books* 39:31–40.

3. Strohman, R. C. 1997. The coming Kuhnian revolution in biology. *Nat. Biotechnol.* 15:194–200.

4. Cardenas, M. L., and Cornish-Bowden, A. 2000. Metabolic analysis in drug discovery. *Science* 288:618–619.

5. Palsson, B. 2000. The challenges of *in silico* biology. *Nat. Biotechnol.* 18:1147–1150.

6. Strohman, R. C. 2002. Maneuvering in the complex path from genotype to phenotype. *Science* 296:701–703.

7. Gabor Miklos, G. L. and Maleszka, R. 2004. Microarray reality checks in the context of a complex disease. *Nat. Biotechnol.* 22: 615–621.

8. Stock, R. P., and Bialy, H. 2003. The sigmoidal curve of cancer. *Nat. Biotechnol.* 21:13–14.

9. Li, R., Yerganian, G., Duesberg, P., Kraemer, A., Willer, A., Rausch, C., and Hehlmann, R. 1997. Aneuploidy correlated 100% with chemical transformation of Chinese hamster cells. *Proc. Natl. Acad. Sci. USA* 94:14506–14511.

10. Hollstein, M., Sidransky, D., Vogelstein, B. and Harris, C. C. 1991. *p53* mutations in human cancers. *Science* 253:49–53.

11. Lengauer, C., Kinzler, K. W., and Vogelstein, B. 1997. Genetic instability in colorectal cancers. *Nature* 386:623–627.

12. Lengauer, C., Kinzler, K. W., and Vogelstein, B. Genetic instabilities in human cancers. 1998. *Nature* 396:643–649.

13. Orr-Weaver, T. L., and Weinberg, R. A. 1998. A checkpoint on the road to cancer. *Nature* 392:223–224.

14. Rajagopalan, H., Nowak, M. A., Vogelstein, B., and Lengauer, C. 2003. The significance of unstable chromosomes in colorectal cancer. *Nat. Rev. Cancer* 3:695–701.

15. Zhang, L., Zhou, W., Velculescu, V. E., Kern, S. E., Hruban, R. H., Hamilton, S. R., Vogelstein, B. and Kinzler, K. W. 1997. Gene expression profiles in normal and cancer cells. *Science* 276:1268–1272.

16. Pihan, G., and Doxsey, S. J. 2003. Mutations and aneuploidy: co-

conspirators in cancer? *Cancer Cell* 4:89–94.

In the words of one scientist who read these pages in manuscript, "It might appear, especially to people who read books with references," as though I "have given short shrift to exciting new developments in clinical oncology with drugs such as Gleevec" and to "a large literature that shows specific mutations in genes like *rb, p53* and *BRCA1* and *BRCA2* generate polyclonal tumors and are sufficient for cancer." For those readers, I offer the following by way of explanation.

The efficacy of such drugs is transient and partial (see below), and it is always dangerous to draw genetic and biochemical conclusions from clinical data. With respect to the second point: The relevant mutational data are exceedingly fragile, and this is especially true for tumor suppressor genes. Most genes are functionally described in terms of the biochemical activity of an implicated protein, but tumor suppressors are defined by a process whose phenotype is the output of an entire metabolic network. Since this is the case, genetic background is of extreme importance, as the definition of the endpoint depends on the entire output of that particular genome. By way of example, mutational inactivation, in the well studied case of *PI3Kgamma,* may predispose already perturbed cells to cancer in one genetic background, and not lead to any cancers whatsoever in a different one (Barbier, M., et al. Tumour biology (Communication arising): Weakening link to colorectal cancer? *Nature* 413:796, 2001).

These constantly moving, but never really changing, tepid waters of oncogene-mutation theory are well illustrated by an essay that appeared in *The Scientist* at the end of 2003 entitled. "A Cell-Cycle couple loses its luster" (Steinberg, D., *The Scientist,* Dec. 23, 2003). The piece pointed out, in no uncertain language, that after more than ten years in which cyclinE and cyclin dependent kinase 2 were held to be prime movers in driving cancer cell proliferation, five recent papers totally demolished this (for oncogene theory at least) long-held view. "Everything flows" wrote the philosopher. Or, as it is more often paraphrased, "You never step in the same river twice."

As with the various epicycles devised to make Ptolemaic descriptions of the solar system fit the facts, interest in these single gene entities as *agents provocateurs* of cancer will fade. The Copernican replacement will be a perspective derived from quantitative analyses of network perturbations based largely on the central idea of aneuploidy-catalyzed, continuous genomic rearrangements instead of an endless parade of multi-problematic mutations. This perspective is exemplified in:

Duesberg, P., Stindl, R., and Hehlmann, R. 2001. Origin of multidrug resistance in cells with and without multidrug resistance genes. *Proc. Natl. Acad. Sci. USA* 98:11283–11288.

> *Recent literature provides an ideally controlled example in support of the chromosome reassortment hypothesis. In an attempt to control the diploid and chronically hyperplastic phases of chronic myeloid leukemia as well as the aneuploid and malignant phase, or blast crisis (19), the same cytotoxic drug, STI-571, was developed (66, 67). According to a "News and Views" article in Nature, the "new-age drug" was "rationally designed" to inhibit the putative common cause of the chronic and malignant phases, a tyrosine kinase encoded by the BCR-ABL hybrid gene that "drives the cells ... to become cancerous" (66). But, contrary to expectation, only patients suffering from the diploid chronic phase showed lasting responses, whereas "most" patients suffering from the aneuploid blast crisis "relapsed within a few months, despite continued treatment" (66). In searching for an answer, some investigators have quickly offered several mutations of the BCR-ABL gene that would render the encoded kinase resistant against STI-571 without affecting its putative oncogenic kinase function (67). But, as the "News and Views" article points out, this answer generates at least one new question: "Why do drug-resistant cells emerge from blast crisis and not from the earlier phase?" In addition, one wonders why mutations of the active site of the kinase, which prevent the competitive inhibitor from binding, would not also prevent the kinase from maintaining transforming function. Our hypothesis suggests simple answers to both questions. The blast crisis is caused by aneuploidy rather than by the kinase (19), and aneuploidy also generates drug-resistant variants by chromosome reassortments. Indeed, drug-resistant blast cells without mutations of the active site have already been observed (67). By contrast, the diploid hyperplastic leukemia cells cannot generate drug-resistant variants by chromosome reassortments.*

19. Duesberg, P., and Rasnick, D. (2000) Cell Motil. Cytoskel. 47, 81–107

66. McCormick, F. (2001) Nature (London) 412, 281–282.

67. Gorre, M. E., Mohammed, M., Ellwood, K., Hsu, N., Paquette, R., Rao, P. N., and Sawyers, C. L. (2001) Science 292, 876–880.

17. Duesberg, P., Rausch, C., Rasnick, D., and Hehlmann, R. 1998. Genetic instability of cancer cells is proportional to their degree of aneuploidy. *Proc. Natl. Acad. Sci. USA* 95:13692–13697.

18. *Ibid.* References therein:

15. Strauss, B. S. (1992) *Cancer Res.* 52, 249–253.

26. Li, R., Yerganian, G., Duesberg, P., Kraemer, A., Willer, A., Rausch, C. & Hehlmann, R. (1997) *Proceedings of the National Academy of Sciences (USA)* 94, 14506–14511.

36. Lewin, B. (1994) *Genes V* (Oxford University Press, Oxford).

2. Cairns, J. (1978) *Cancer: Science and Society* (W. H. Freeman and Company, San Francisco).

37. Duesberg, P. H. & Schwartz, J. R. (1992) *Prog. Nucleic Acid Res. Mol. Biol.* 43, 135–204.

38. Koshland, D. (1994) *Science* 266, 1925.

39. German, J. (1974) in *Chromosomes and Cancer,* German, J. ed. (John Wiley & Sons, New York), pp. 601–617.

40. German, J. (1997) *Cancer Genet Cytogenet* 93, 100–106.

41. German, J. (1993) *Medicine* 72, 393–419. *Ibid. References therei*

45. Kacser, H. & Burns, J. A. (1981) *Genetics* 97, 639–666.

46. Fell, D. (1997) *Understanding the control of metabolism* (Portland Press, London).

32. Shapiro, B. L. (1983) *Am. J. Medical Genetics* 14, 241–269.

33. Epstein, C. (1986) *The consequences of chromosome imbalance: principles, mechanisms, and models* (Cambridge University Press, Cambridge, London, New York).

47. Lindsley, D. L., Sandler, L., et al. (1972) *Genetics* 71, 157–184.

48. Sandler, L. & Hecht, F. (1973) *Amer J Hum Genet* 25, 332–339.

49. Papp, I., Iglesias, V. A., Moscone, E. A., Michalowski, S., Spiker, S., Park, Y.-D., Matzke, M. A. & Matzke, A. J. M. (1996) *The Plant J* 10, 469–478.

50. Cornish-Bowden, A., Homeyr, J.-H. S. & Cardenas, M. L. (1995) *Bioorg. Chem.* 23, 439–449.

51. Lijinsky, W. (1989) *Env. Mol. Mutagenesis* 14, 78–84.

52. Stanbridge, E. J. (1990) *Annu. Rev. Genet.* 24, 615–657.

53. Augenlicht, L. H., Wahrman, M. Z., Halsey, H., Anderson, L., Taylor, J. & Lipkin, M. (1987) *Cancer Res.* 47, 6017–6021.

54. Duesberg, P. (1995) *Science* 267, 1407–1408.

55. Hua, V. Y., Wang, W., K. & Duesberg, P. H. (1997) *Proc. Natl. Acad. Sci. USA* 94, 9614–9619.

37. Duesberg, P. H. & Schwartz, J. R. (1992) *Prog. Nucleic Acid Res. Mol. Biol.* 43, 135–204.

43. Bialy, H. (1998) *Nature Biotechnology* 16, 137–138.

56. Zhang, L., Zhou, W., Velculescu, V. E., Kern, S. E., Hruban, R. H., Hamilton, S. R., Vogelstein, B. & Kinzler, K. W. (1997) *Science* 276, 1268–1272.

13. Heppner, G. & Miller, F. R. (1998) *International Review of Cytology* 177, 1–56.

15. Strauss, B. S. (1992) *Cancer Res.* 52, 249–253.

57. Bos, J. L., Fearon, E. R., Hamilton, S. R., Verlaan-de Vries, M., van Boom, J. H., van der Eb, A. J. & Vogelstein, B. (1987) *Nature (London)* 327, 293–297.

58. Cooper, G. M. (1990) *Oncogenes* (Jones and Bartlett Publishers, Boston).

19. Kacser, H. and Burns, J. A. The molecular basis of dominance. *Genetics* 97:639–666.

20. Rasnick, D., and Duesberg, P. H. 1999. How aneuploidy affects metabolic control and causes cancer. 1999. *Biochem J.* 340:621–630.

21. Rasnick, D. 2002. Aneuploidy theory explains tumor formation, the absence of immune surveillance, and the failure of chemotherapy. *Cancer Genet. Cytogenet.* 136:66–72.

22. Harvey F. Lodish (Editor), Arnold Berk, Paul Matsudaira, Chris A. Kaiser, Monty Krieger, Matthew P. Scott, S. Lawrence Zipursky, James Darnell. *Molecular Cell Biology.* W. H. Freeman & Co.; 5th edition, August 2003.

23. *Pers. comm.* from L. Zhang and B. Vogelstein to Peter Duesberg, Nov. 3, 1997, preserved in the *Peter H. Duesberg Archive* of the Bancroft Library of the Univ. of California, Berkeley.

24. Pollack, J. R., Sorlie, T., Perou, C. M., Rees, C. A., Jeffrey, S. S., Lonning, P. E., Tibshirani, R., Botstein, D., Borresen-Dale, A. L., and Brown, P. O. 2002. Microarray analysis reveals a major direct role of DNA copy number alteration in the transcriptional program of human breast tumors. *Proc. Natl. Acad. Sci. USA* 99:12963–12968.

25. Bailey, J. E. 1991. Toward a science of metabolic engineering. *Science* 252:1668–1675.

26. Cornish-Bowden, A. 1999. Metabolic control analysis in biotechnology and medicine. *Nat. Biotechnol.* 17:641–643.

27. Bailey, J. E. 2001. Complex biology with no parameters. *Nat. Biotechnol.* 19:503–504.

28. Nowak, M. A., Komarova, N. L., Sengupta, A., Jallepalli, P. V., Shih, IeM., Vogelstein, B., and Lengauer, C. 2002. The role of chromosomal instability in tumor initiation. *Proc. Natl. Acad. Sci. USA* 99:16226–16231.

29. Wodarz, D., and Nowak, M. A. Mathematical models of HIV pathogenesis and treatment. 2002. *Bioessays* 24:1178–1187.

30. Roederer, M. 1998. Getting to the HAART of T cell dynamics. *Nat Med.* 4:145–146.

31. Two years later, even parsimonious citation disappeared. In three papers published in March 2004, the Vogelstein lab would lapse into the more familiar mode of other fama scientific adversaries and pretend that Duesberg did not exist. After seeing a PDF of one of these papers, I wrote to my friend: "Vogelstein has stopped referencing you and now goes back to Boveri for his inspiration." To which Peter replied:

4 March 2004

I think Vogelstein sees the coming danger of "aneuploidy-only" to the gene mutation theory of cancer. The strategy to save the mutation theory now seems to be: Accept aneuploidy as a historical fact of cancer, "recognized" for "nearly a century," and then turn it into a consequence of a primary gene mutation. According to the latest Nature *paper, "chromosomal instability of cancer cells ... is a direct result of specific genetic alterations." Until recently that primary mutation was the* Apc-*gene for colon cancer, now it is said to be a "ubiquitin ligase activity" of the* CDC4 *gene. However, at this point the only evidence for the new "chief cause of chromosomal instability" of colon cancer is an 11.6 % correlation with "190 colorectal tumors"—88.4% shy of meeting Koch's first postulate of causation, and reflecting no more than the genetic noise predicted by aneuploidy-catalyzed, unselected mutations. All the latest* Nature *paper shows, once more, is that instability and malignancy are proportional to the degree of aneuploidy, despite interpretations in favor of mutations by the authors.*

By the way, we are also not cited in a new PNAS *paper from today (now weekly! soon daily?) in which Vogelstein et al. explain FUDR-resistance by amplification of thymidylate synthase genes á la Schimke—not via reassortments of chromosomes, as we did in the same journal in 2000 and 2001. However, the amplifications were only 3–5x and thus totally compatible with chromosome amplifica-*

tions. Moreover, only 23% of the resistant tumors showed amplification of the enzymes, again compatible with multiple, alternative chromosome combinations generating the same drug-resistant phenotypes via different biochemical pathways.

And Ruhong found yet another brand-new Cell Cycle *paper of Lengauer, "Linear model of colon cancer initiation." This follows last year's "Multistep carcinogenesis, a chain reaction of aneuploidizations" from our lab in the same not so high visibility venue. But again, no collegial reference to its precursor, even in this "less prestigious" journal.*

The three papers referred to above are:

Rajagopalan, H., Jallepalli, PV., Rago, C., Velculescu, VE., Kinzler, KW., Vogelstein, B. and Lengauer, C. 2004. Inactivation of hCDC4 can cause chromosomal instability. *Nature* 428:77–81.

Wang, TL., Diaz, LA Jr., Romans, K., Bardelli, A., Saha, S., Galizia, G., Choti., M., Donehower, R., Parmigiani, G., Shih, IeM., Iacobuzio-Donahue, C., Kinzler, KW., Vogelstein, B., Lengauer, C.and, Velculescu, VE. 2004. Digital karyotyping identifies thymidylate synthase amplification as a mechanism of resistance to 5-fluorouracil in metastatic colorectal cancer patients. *Proc Natl Acad Sci USA*. 101:3089–94.

Michor, F., Iwasa, Y., Rajagopalan, H., Lengauer, C. and Nowak, MA. 2004. Linear Model of Colon Cancer Initiation. *Cell Cycle* 3:358–62.

32. Weitzman, J. B., and Yaniv, M. 1999. Rebuilding the road to cancer. *Nature* 400:401–402.

33. Hahn, W. C., Counter, C. M., Lundberg, A. S., Beijersbergen, R. L., Brooks, M. W., and Weinberg, R. A. 1999. Creation of human tumour cells with defined genetic elements. *Nature* 400:464–468.

34. Ray, F. A., Peabody, D. S., Cooper J. L., Cram, L. S., and Kraemer, P. M. 1990. SV40 T antigen alone drives karyotype instability that precedes neoplastic transformation of human diploid fibroblasts. *J. Cell Biochem.* 42:13–31.

35. *Pers. comm.* from Rosalin Cotter to Peter Duesberg, November 11, 1999, preserved in the *Peter H. Duesberg Archive* of the Bancroft Library of the Univ. of California, Berkeley.

36. Li, R., Sonik, A., Stindl, R., Rasnick, D., and Duesberg, P. 2000. Aneuploidy vs. gene mutation hypothesis of cancer: recent study claims mutation but is found to support aneuploidy. *Proc. Natl. Acad. Sci. USA* 97:3236–3241.

37. Zimonjic, D., Brooks, M. W., Popescu, N., Weinberg, R. A., and Hahn, W. C. 2001. Derivation of human tumor cells *in vitro* without widespread genomic instability. *Cancer Res.* 61:8838–8844.

38. Li, R., Rasnick, D., and Duesberg, P. H. Correspondence re: D. Zimonjic *et al.*, Derivation of human tumor cells *in vitro* without widespread genomic instability. *Cancer Res.* 62:6335–6347.

39. Zimonjic, D. B., Brooks, M. W., Popescu, N., Weinberg, R. A., and Hahn, W. C. 2001. Reply. *Cancer Res.* 62:6347–6349.

40. Duesberg, P., Li, R., Rasnick, D., Rausch, C., Willer, A., Kraemer, A., Yerganian, G., and Hehlmann, R. 2000. Aneuploidy precedes and segregates with chemical carcinogenesis. *Cancer Genet. Cytogenet.* 119:83–93.

41. Duesberg, P., Stindl, R., and Hehlmann, R. 2000. Explaining the high mutation rates of cancer cells to drug and multidrug resistance by chromosome reassortments that are catalyzed by aneuploidy. *Proc. Natl. Acad. Sci. USA* 97:14295–142300.

42. Harris, H. 1995. *The Cells of the Body: a history of somatic cell genetics.* Cold Spring Harbor Lab Press, Plainview, NY.

43. Duesberg, P. H. 1968. The RNAs of influenza virus. *Proc. Natl. Acad. Sci. USA* 59:930–937.

44. Schoenlein, P. V. 1993. Molecular cytogenetics of multiple drug resistance. *Cytotechnology* 12:63–89.

45. Ried, T., Heselmeyer-Haddad, K., Blegen, H., Schrock, E., and Auer, G. 1999. Genomic changes defining the genesis, progression, and malignancy potential in solid human tumors: a phenotype/genotype correlation. *Genes Chromosomes Cancer* 25:195–204.

46. Fabarius, A., Willer, A., Yerganian, G., Hehlmann, R., and Duesberg, P. Specific aneusomies in Chinese hamster cells at different stages of neoplastic transformation, initiated by nitrosomethylurea. 2002. *Proc. Natl. Acad. Sci. USA* 99:6778–6783.

47. O'Brien, S. J., Eisenberg, J. F., Miyamoto, M., Hedges, S. B., Kumar, S., Wilson, D. E., Menotti-Raymond, M., Murphy, W. J., Nash, W. G., Lyons, L. A., Menninger, J. C., Stanyon, R., Wienberg, J., Copeland, N. G., Jenkins, N. A., Gellin, J., Yerle, M., Andersson, L., Womack, J., Broad, T., Postlethwait, J., Serov, O., Bailey, E., James, M. R., Marshall Graves, J. A., *et al.* 1999. Genome maps 10. Comparative genomics. Mammalian radiations. *Science* 286:463–478. (Yes, this is the same Stephen O'Brien of *A Night at the Opera*.)

Curriculum Vitae

Peter H. Duesberg

Prof. of Molecular and Cell Biology, University of California, Berkeley, CA

Born: December 2nd, 1936

Birthplace: Germany

Parents: Mother: Hilde Saettele, MD., Father: Richard Duesberg, Prof. of Internal Medicine

Education:
University of Wurzburg, Germany, 1956–1958: Vordiplom (Chemistry)
University of Basel, Switzerland, 1958–1959
University of Munich, Germany, 1959–1961: Diploma (Chemistry)
University of Frankfurt, Germany, 1961–1963: Ph.D. (Chemistry)

Research & Professional Experience:
Max Planck Institute for Virus Research, Tubingen, Germany,1963: Postdoctoral Fellow
Department of Molecular Biology and Virus Laboratory; Dept. of Molecular & Cell Biology, University of California, Berkeley CA
1964: Assistant research Virologist and Postdoctoral Fellow
1968: Assistant Professor in Residence and Research Biochemist
1970: Assistant Professor
1971: Associate Professor
1973 to present: Professor

Honors:
1969: Merck Award
1971: California Scientist of the Year Award
1981: First Annual American Medical Centre Oncology Award
1986: Outstanding Investigator Award, National Institutes of Health
1986: Elected National Academy of Sciences
1986–1987: Fogarty Scholar-in-Residence at the National Institutes of Health, Bethesda, MD
1988: Wissenschaftspreis, Hannover, Germany
1988: Lichtfield Lecturer, Oxford, England
1990: C. J. Watson Lecturer, Abbott Northwestern Hospital, Minneapolis, MN

1992: Fisher Distinguished Professor, University of North Texas, Denton, TX

1992: Shaffer Alumni Lecturer, Tulane University, New Orleans, LA

1996: Distinguished Speaker, Department of Biology, Univ. Louisville, KY

1997: January-July: Guest professor of the University of Heidelberg at the Medical School in Mannheim (III Med. Klinik, director Prof. R. Hehlmann)

1998: August-December: Guest professor of the University of Heidelberg at the Medical School in Mannheim (III Med. Klinik, director Prof. R. Hehlmann)

2000–03: Recipient of a Mildred Scheel Guestprofessorship at the University of Heidelberg at Mannheim from the Deutsche Krebshilfe.

Publications (through March 2004)

1. An Dehydrogenasen gebundene Umwandlungsprodukte des Diphospho-Pyridin-Nucleotides. Theodor Wieland, Peter Duesberg, Gerhard Pfleiderer, Arthur Stock, and Eberhard Sann, *Arch. Biochem. Biophys.* Suppl. I, 260–263, 1962.

2. Synthese des DL-b-[Indolyl-(5)]-alanins (Isotryptophans). Hans Behringer and Peter Duesberg, *Chem. Ber.* 96, 377–380, 1963.

3. Synthese des DL-Histidins und des DL-2-hydroxy-4 methyl-histidins. Hans Behringer and Peter Duesberg, *Chem. Ber.* 96, 381–384, 1963.

4. Zum Molekulargewicht der Lactat-dehydrogenasen. Studien des Verhaltens bei der Gelfiltration. Theodor Wieland, Peter Duesberg, and Helmut Determann, *Biochemische Z.* 337, 303–311, 1963.

5. Preparative zone electrophoresis of proteins on polyacrylamide gels in 8 *M* Urea. P. H. Duesberg and R. R. Rueckert, *Anal. Biochem.* 11, 342–361, 1965.

6. Isolation of the nucleic acid of Newcastle disease virus (NDV). Peter H. Duesberg and William S. Robinson, *PNAS* 54, 794–800, 1965.

7. Nucleic acid and proteins isolated from the Rauscher mouse leukemia virus (MLV). Peter H. Duesberg and William S. Robinson, *PNAS* 55, 219–227, 1966.

8. Non-identical peptide chains in mouse encephalitis virus. R. R. Rueckert and P. H. Duesberg, *J. Mol. Biol.* 17, 490–502, 1966.

9. Isolation of the nucleic acid of mouse mammary tumor virus (MTV). Peter H. Duesberg and Phyllis B. Blair, *PNAS* 55, 1490–1497, 1966.

10. Inhibition of mouse leukemia virus (MLV) replication by Actinomycin D. Peter H. Duesberg and William S. Robinson, *Virology* 31, 743–746, 1967.

11. On the structure and replication of influenza virus. Peter H. Duesberg and William S. Robinson, *Journal of Molecular Biology* 25, 383–405, 1967.

12. Tumor virus RNAs. William S. Robinson, Harriet L. Robinson, and Peter H. Duesberg, *PNAS* 58, 825–834, 1967.

13. Tumor virus RNA. William S. Robinson and Peter H. Duesberg, *in* Subviral Carcinogenesis, eds. Yohei Ito; Editorial Committee for the 1st International Symposium on Tumor Viruses, Nagoya, Japan, 3–18, 1967.

14. The myxoviruses. W. S. Robinson and P. H. Duesberg, *in* Molecular Basis of Virology, *ACS Monograph* 164, eds. H. Fraenkel-Conrat; Reinhold Book Corp., New York, 255–305, 1968.

15. The chemistry of the RNA tumor viruses. W. S. Robinson and P. H. Duesberg, *in* Molecular Basis of Virology, *ACS Monograph* 164, eds. H. Fraenkel-Conrat; Reinhold Book Corp., New York, 306–331, 1968.

16. The RNAs of influenza virus. Peter H. Duesberg, *PNAS* 59, 930–937, 1968.

17. Physical properties of Rous sarcoma virus RNA. P. H. Duesberg, *PNAS* 60, 1511–1518, 1968.

18. Proteins of Rous sarcoma virus. Peter H. Duesberg, Harriet Latham Robinson, William S. Robinson, R. J. Huebner, and H. C. Turner, *Virology* 36, 73–86, 1968.

19. Structure of Rauscher mouse leukaemia virus RNA. Carol D. Blair and Peter H. Duesberg, *Nature (London)* 220, 396–399, 1968.

20. Structural relationships between the RNA of mammary tumor virus and those of other RNA tumor viruses. P. H. Duesberg and R. D. Cardiff, *Virology* 36, 696–700, 1968.

21. Double-stranded RNA in vaccinia virus infected cells. C. Colby and P. H. Duesberg, *Nature (London)* 222, 940–944, 1969.

22. Distinct subunits of the ribonucleoprotein of influenza virus. P. H. Duesberg, *Journal of Molecular Biology* 42, 485–499, 1969.

23. Proteins of Newcastle disease virus and of the viral nucleocapsid. Ilan Bikel and Peter H. Duesberg, *J. Virol.* 4, 388–393, 1969.

24. On the biosynthesis and structure of double-stranded RNA in vaccinia virus-infected cells. P. H. Duesberg and C. Colby, *PNAS* 64, 396–403, 1969.

25. On the role of DNA synthesis in avian tumor virus infection. Peter H. Duesberg and Peter K. Vogt, *PNAS* 64, 939–946, 1969.

26. On the structure of RNA tumor viruses. P. H. Duesberg, *Current Topics in Microbiology and Immunology* 51, 79–104, 1970.

27. Distinct nucleoproteins of influenza virus. Peter Duesberg, *in* The Biology of Large RNA Viruses: Papers Based on a Symposium, held in Cambridge, England, 21–25 July 1969, eds. Richard D. Barry and Brian W. J. Mahy; Academic Press, New York, 301–323, 1970.

28. Glycoprotein components of avian and murine RNA tumor viruses. Peter H. Duesberg, G. Steven Martin, and Peter K. Vogt, *Virology* 41, 631–646, 1970.

29. Myxovirus ribonucleic acids. Carol D. Blair and Peter H. Duesberg, *Annual Review of Microbiology* 24, 539–574, 1970.

30. Complementarity between Rous sarcoma virus (RSV) RNA and the *in vitro*-synthesized DNA of the virus-associated DNA polymerase. P. H. Duesberg and E. Canaani, *Virology* 42, 783–788, 1970.

31. Differences between the ribonucleic acids of transforming and nontransforming avian tumor viruses. Peter H. Duesberg and Peter K. Vogt, *PNAS* 67, 1673–1680, 1970.

32. Electrophoretic distribution of the proteins and glycoproteins of influenza virus and Sendai virus. Jean Content and Peter H. Duesberg, *J. Virol.* 6, 707–716, 1970.

33. DNA polymerase of avian tumor viruses. P. Duesberg, E. Canaani, and K. v. d. Helm, *in* Nucleic Acid-Protein Interactions—Nucleic Acid Synthesis in Viral Infection: Proceedings of the Miami Winter Symposia, January 18–22, 1971, *Miami Winter Symposia* 2, eds. D. W. Ribbons, J. F. Woessner, and J. Schultz; North-Holland Pub. Co., Amsterdam, 311–327, 1971.

34. Structure and replication of avian tumor viruses. Peter H. Duesberg, Peter K. Vogt, and Eli Canaani, *in* The Biology of Oncogenic Viruses: Proceedings of the 2nd Lepetit Colloquium, held in Paris, November 1970, eds. Luigi C. Silvestri; North-Holland Pub. Co., Amsterdam, 154–166, 1971.

35. Properties of a soluble DNA polymerase isolated from Rous sarcoma virus. Peter Duesberg, Klaus v. d. Helm, and Eli Canaani, *PNAS* 68, 747–751, 1971.

36. Virus interference by cellular double-stranded ribonucleic acid. P. C. Kimball and P. H. Duesberg, *J. Virol.* 7, 697–706, 1971.

37. The specificity of interferon induction. Clarence Colby, Michael

J. Chamberlin, Peter H. Duesberg, and Melvin I. Simon, *in* Biological Effects of Polynucleotides: Proceedings of the Symposium on Molecular Biology, 1970, eds. Roland F. Beers, Jr. and Werner Braun; Springer-Verlag, New York, 79–87, 1971.

38. Comparative properties of RNA and DNA templates for the DNA polymerase of Rous sarcoma virus. Peter Duesberg, Klaus v. d. Helm, and Eli Canaani, *PNAS* 68, 2505–2509, 1971.

39. Base sequence differences among the ribonucleic acids of influenza virus. J. Content and P. H. Duesberg, *Journal of Molecular Biology* 62, 273–285, 1971.

40. The induction of interferon. Clarence Colby, Michael Chamberlin, and Peter Duesberg, *in* Viruses Affecting Man and Animals, eds. Murray Sanders and Morris Schaeffer; Warren H. Green, Inc., St. Louis, 78–88, 1971.

41. The *a* subunit in the RNA of transforming avian tumor viruses: I. Occurrence in different virus strains. II. Spontaneous loss resulting in nontransforming variants. G. S. Martin and P. H. Duesberg, *Virology* 47, 494–497, 1972.

42. Adenylic acid-rich sequence in RNAs of Rous sarcoma virus and Rauscher mouse leukaemia virus. Michael M. C. Lai and Peter H. Duesberg, *Nature (London)* 235, 383–386, 1972.

43. Role of subunits of 60 to 70S avian tumor virus ribonucleic acid in its template activity for the viral deoxyribonucleic acid polymerase. Eli Canaani and Peter Duesberg, *J. Virol.* 10, 23–31, 1972.

44. Distinct oligonucleotide patterns of distinct influenza virus RNAs. J. Horst, J. Content, S. Mandeles, H. Fraenkel-Conrat, and P. Duesberg, *J. Mol. Biol.* 69, 209–215, 1972.

45. Structure of the ribonucleoprotein of influenza virus. Richard W. Compans, Jean Content, and Peter H. Duesberg, *J. Virol.* 10, 795–800, 1972.

46. RNA tumor virus replication: facts and fancy. Peter H. Duesberg, *in* Workshop on Mechanisms and Prospects of Genetic Exchange, Berlin, December 11–13, 1971, *Advances in the Biosciences* 8, eds. Gerhard Raspé; Pergamon Press/Vieweg, New York, 145–157, 1972.

47. Differences between the envelope glycoproteins and glycopeptides of avian tumor viruses released from transformed and from nontransformed cells. Michael M. C. Lai and Peter H. Duesberg, *Virology* 50, 359–372, 1972.

48. On the structure of influenza virus RNA. Jean Content, Jürgen

Horst, and Peter H. Duesberg, *in* RNA Viruses: Replication and Structure. Ribosomes: Structure, Function and Biogenesis: Proceedings of the Federation of European Biochemical Societies Eighth Meeting, Amsterdam, 1972, *FEBS Meeting* 27, eds. Hans Bloemendal; North-Holland/American Elsevier, Amsterdam, 101–119, 1972.

49. Evidence for 30–40S RNA as precursor of the 60–70S RNA of Rous sarcoma virus. E. Canaani, K. v. d. Helm, and P. Duesberg, *PNAS* 70, 401–405, 1973.

50. Studies of the Rous sarcoma virus RNA: Characterization of the 5' terminus. Robert Silber, V. G. Malathi, LaDonne H. Schulman, Jerard Hurwitz, and Peter H. Duesberg, *Biochem. Biophys. Res. Commun.* 50, 467–472, 1973.

51. RNA species obtained from clonal lines of avian sarcoma and from avian leukosis virus. Peter H. Duesberg and Peter K. Vogt, *Virology* 54, 207–219, 1973.

52. The 60–70S RNA of avian sarcoma and leukosis viruses—distribution of class *a* and *b* subunits. P. H. Duesberg, P. K. Vogt, and G. S. Martin, *in* Unifying Concepts of Leukemia: III. Molecular Biology of Leukemia, *Bibl. Haemat.* 39, eds. Ray M. Dutcher and L. Chieco-Bianchi; S. Karger, Basel, Switzerland, 462–473, 1973.

53. Evidence for 30–40S RNA as precursor of the 60–70S RNA of Rous sarcoma virus. P. Duesberg, E. Canaani, and K. von der Helm, *American Journal of Clinical Pathology* 60, 57–64, 1973.

54. Gel electrophoresis of avian leukosis and sarcoma viral RNA in formamide: Comparison with other viral and cellular RNA species. Peter H. Duesberg and Peter K. Vogt, *J. Virol.* 12, 594–599, 1973.

55. Avian tumor virus RNA: A comparison of three sarcoma viruses and their transformation-defective derivatives by oligonucleotide fingerprinting and DNA-RNA hybridization. Michael M. C. Lai, Peter H. Duesberg, Jürgen Horst, and Peter K. Vogt, *PNAS* 70, 2266–2270, 1973.

56. News and views on avian tumor virus RNA. P. H. Duesberg, E. Canaani, K. von der Helm, M. M. C. Lai, and P. K. Vogt, *in* Possible Episomes in Eukaryotes: Proceedings of the 4th Lepetit Colloquium, held in Cocoyoc, Mexico, November 1972, eds. Luigi G. Silvestri; North-Holland Pub. Co., Amsterdam, 142–152, 1973.

57. DNA polymerase of murine sarcoma-leukemia virus: Lack of detectable RNase H and low activity with viral RNA and natural DNA templates. Lu-Hai Wang and Peter H. Duesberg, *J. Virol.* 12, 1512–1521, 1973.

58. Ribonucleic acid components of murine sarcoma and leukemia viruses. J. Maisel, V. Klement, M. M-C. Lai, W. Ostertag, and P. Duesberg, *PNAS* 70, 3536–3540, 1973.

59. Tracking defective tumor virus RNA. Peter H. Duesberg, Peter K. Vogt, Jan Maisel, Mike M-C. Lai, and E. Canaani, *in* Virus Research: Proceedings of the 2nd ICN-UCLA Symposium on Molecular Biology, eds. C. Fred Fox and William S. Robinson; Academic Press, New York, 327–338, 1973.

60. On the assembly of 60–70S RNA of avian RNA tumor viruses. E. Canaani, K. v. d. Helm, and P. Duesberg, *in* Virus Research: Proceedings of the 2nd ICN-UCLA Symposium on Molecular Biology, eds. C. Fred Fox and William S. Robinson; Academic Press, New York, 339–344, 1973.

61. The RNA of nondefective avian sarcoma viruses and corresponding transformation-defective segregants: A comparison by oligonucleotide fingerprinting and RNA-DNA hybridization. Michael M. C. Lai, Jürgen Horst, and P. H. Duesberg, *in* Virus Research: Proceedings of the 2nd ICN-UCLA Symposium on Molecular Biology, eds. C. Fred Fox and William S. Robinson; Academic Press, New York, 345–352, 1973.

62. On the mechanism of recombination between avian RNA tumor viruses. Peter K. Vogt and Peter H. Duesberg, *in* Virus Research: Proceedings of the 2nd ICN-UCLA Symposium on Molecular Biology, eds. C. Fred Fox and William S. Robinson; Academic Press, New York, 505–511, 1973.

63. The preferred role of 60–70S avian tumor virus RNA among natural RNAs as template for DNA polymerase of Rous sarcoma virus (RSV). E. Canaani and P. H. Duesberg, *in* Molecular Studies in Viral Neoplasia: 25th Symposium on Fundamental Cancer Research; The Williams and Wilkins Co., Baltimore, 97–114, 1974.

64. Tumor virus RNAs and tumor virus genes. Peter H. Duesberg, Mike M.-C. Lai, and Jan Maisel, *in* Modern Trends in Human Leukemia— Biological, Biochemical and Virological Aspects, *Hämatologie und Bluttransfusion* 14, eds. Rolf Neth, Robert C. Gallo, S. Spiegelman, and F. Stohlman, Jr.; J. F. Lehmanns Verlag, München, Germany, 133–147, 1974.

65. Evidence for crossing-over between avian tumor viruses based on analysis of viral RNAs. Karen Beemon, Peter Duesberg, and Peter Vogt, *PNAS* 71, 4254–4258, 1974.

66. Structure and molecular weight of the 60–70S RNA and the 30–40S RNA of the Rous sarcoma virus. Walter F. Mangel, Hajo Delius, and Peter H. Duesberg, *PNAS* 71, 4541–4545, 1974.

67. Properties and location of poly(A) in Rous sarcoma virus RNA. Lu-Hai Wang and Peter Duesberg, *J. Virol.* 14, 1515–1529, 1974.

68. Recombinants of avian tumor viruses: An analysis of their RNA. Peter Duesberg, Karen Beemon, Michael Lai, and Peter K. Vogt, *in* Mechanisms of Virus Disease, *ICN-UCLA Symposia on Molecular and Cellular Biology* 1, eds. William S. Robinson and C. Fred Fox; W. A. Benjamin, Inc., Menlo Park, CA, 287–302, 1974.

69. Recombinants of avian RNA tumor viruses: Characteristics of the virion RNA. Peter Duesberg, Karen Beemon, Michael Lai, and Peter K. Vogt, *in* Viral Transformation and Endogenous Viruses, eds. Albert S. Kaplan; Academic Press, New York, 137–153, 1974.

70. Electron microscope measurements of Rous sarcoma virus RNA. H. Delius, P. H. Duesberg, and W. F. Mangel, *Cold Spring Harbor Symp. Quant. Biol.* 39, 835–843, 1974.

71. Avian RNA tumor viruses: Mechanism of recombination and complexity of the genome. P. H. Duesberg, P. K. Vogt, K. Beemon, and M. Lai, *Cold Spring Harbor Symp. Quant. Biol.* 39, 847–857, 1974.

72. Translation of Rous sarcoma virus RNA in a cell-free system from ascites Krebs II cells. Klaus von der Helm and Peter H. Duesberg, *Proc. Natl. Acad. Sci. USA* 72, 614–618, 1975.

73. RNA of replication-defective strains of Rous sarcoma virus. Peter H. Duesberg, Sadaaki Kawai, Lu-Hai Wang, Peter K. Vogt, Helen M. Murphy, and Hidesaburo Hanafusa, *PNAS* 72, 1569–1573, 1975.

74. Base sequence differences between the RNA components of Harvey sarcoma virus. Jan Maisel, Edward M. Scolnick, and Peter Duesberg, *J. Virol.* 16, 749–753, 1975.

75. Elementary aspects of RNA tumor virus genetics. Peter K. Vogt and Peter H. Duesberg, *in* Chemical and Viral Oncogenesis, *Proceedings XI International Cancer Congress* 2, eds. Pietro Bucalossi, Umberto Veronesi, and Natale Cascinelli; Excerpta Medica, Amsterdam, 220–225, 1975.

76. Mapping RNase T[1]-resistant oligonucleotides of avian tumor virus RNAs: Sarcoma-specific oligonucleotides are near the poly(A) end and oligonucleotides common to sarcoma and transformation-defective viruses are at the poly(A) end. Lu-Hai Wang, Peter Duesberg, Karen Beemon, and Peter K. Vogt, *J. Virol.* 16, 1051–1070, 1975.

77. *In vitro* synthesis of full-length DNA transcripts of Rous sarcoma virus RNA by viral DNA polymerase. R. P. Junghans, P. H. Duesberg, and C. A. Knight, *PNAS* 72, 4895–4899, 1975.

78. Genomic complexities of murine leukemia and sarcoma, reticu-loendotheliosis, and visna viruses. Karen L. Beemon, Anthony J. Faras, Ashley T. Haase, Peter H. Duesberg, and Jan E. Maisel, *J. Virol.* 17, 525–537, 1976.

79. Location of envelope-specific and sarcoma-specific oligonucleotides on RNA of Schmidt-Ruppin Rous sarcoma virus. Lu-Hai Wang, Peter H. Duesberg, Sadaaki Kawai, and Hidesaburo Hanafusa, *PNAS* 73, 447–451, 1976.

80. RNA and proteins of the Kirsten sarcoma-xenotropic leukemia virus complex propagated in rat and duck cells. Donna M. Galehouse and Peter H. Duesberg, *Virology* 70, 97–104, 1976.

81. Distribution of envelope-specific and sarcoma-specific nucleotide sequences from different parents in the RNAs of avian tumor virus recom-binants. Lu-Hai Wang, Peter Duesberg, Pamela Mellon, and Peter K. Vogt, *PNAS* 73, 1073–1077, 1976.

82. Location of envelope-specific and other sequences on the RNA of Schmidt-Ruppin Rous sarcoma virus. Lu-Hai Wang, Peter H. Duesberg, Sadaaki Kawai, and Hidesaburo Hanafusa, *in* Comparative Leukemia Research 1975: 7th International Symposium on Comparative Leukemia Research, *Bibl. Haemat.* 43, eds. Johannes Clemmesen and David S. Yohn; S. Karger, Basel, Switzerland, 542–548, 1976.

83. Towards a complete genetic map of Rous sarcoma virus. Peter H. Duesberg, Lu-Hai Wang, Pamela Mellon, William S. Mason, and Peter K. Vogt, *in* Animal Virology, *ICN-UCLA Symposia on Molecular and Cellular Biology* 4, eds. David Baltimore, Alice S. Huang, and C. Fred Fox; Academic Press, New York, 107–125, 1976.

84. Differences in the glycoproteins of avian tumor virus recombi-nants: evidence for intragenic crossing over. D. M. Galehouse and P. H. Duesberg, *in* Animal Virology, *ICN-UCLA Symposia on Molecular and Cellular Biology* 4, eds. David Baltimore, Alice S. Huang, and C. Fred Fox; Academic Press, New York, 227–236, 1976.

85. The 30S Moloney sarcoma virus RNA contains leukemia virus nucleotide sequences. Dino Dina, Karen Beemon, and Peter Duesberg, *Cell* 9, 299–309, 1976.

86. Mapping oligonucleotides of Rous sarcoma virus RNA that seg-regate with polymerase and group-specific antigen markers in recom-binants. Lu-Hai Wang, Donna Galehouse, Pamela Mellon, Peter Duesberg, William S. Mason, and Peter K. Vogt, *PNAS* 73, 3952–3956, 1976.

288   Oncogenes, Aneuploidy, and AIDS

87. Sequences and functions of Rous sarcoma virus RNA. Peter H. Duesberg, Lu-Hai Wang, Karen Beemon, Sadaaki Kawai, and Hidesaburo Hanafusa, in Modern Trends in Human Leukemia II: Biological, Immunological,
Therapeutic and Virological Aspects, Hämatologie und Bluttransfusion 19,
eds. Ralph Neth, Robert C. Gallo, Klaus Mannweiler, and William C.
Moloney; J. F. Lehmanns Verlag, München, Germany, 327–340, 1976.

88. Cleavage map of linear mouse sarcoma virus DNA. Eli Canaani,
Peter Duesberg, and Dino Dina, PNAS 74, 29–33, 1977.

89. Murine sarcoma viruses: The helper-independence reported for a
Moloney variant is unconfirmed; distinct strains differ in the size of their
RNAs. Jan Maisel, Dino Dina, and Peter Duesberg, Virology 76, 295–312,
1977.

90. The genetic map of Rous sarcoma virus. Peter H. Duesberg, Lu-
Hai Wang, Pamela Mellon, William S. Mason, and Peter K. Vogt, in
Genetic Manipulation as it Affects the Cancer Problem: Proceedings of
the Miami Winter Symposia, January 10–14, 1977, Miami Winter Symposia 14, eds. J. Schultz and Z. Brada; Academic Press, New York,
161–179, 1977.

91. Murine leukemia viruses containing an ·-30 S RNA subunit of
unknown biological activity, in addition to the 38 S subunit of the viral
genome. Peter H. Duesberg and Edward M. Scolnick, Virology 83,
211–216, 1977.

92. The RNA of avian acute leukemia virus MC29. Peter H. Duesberg,
Klaus Bister, and Peter K. Vogt, PNAS 74, 4320–4324, 1977.

93. The terminal oligonucleotides of avian tumor virus RNAs are
genetically linked. Lu-Hai Wang, Peter H. Duesberg, Terry Robins, Hisao
Yokota, and Peter K. Vogt, Virology 82, 472–492, 1977.

94. Subgenomic, cellular Rous sarcoma virus RNAs contain oligonucleotides from the 3' half and the 5' terminus of virion RNA. Pamela
Mellon and Peter H. Duesberg, Nature (London) 270, 631–634, 1977.

95. Transformation-defective mutants of Rous sarcoma virus with src
gene deletions of varying length. Sadaaki Kawai, Peter H. Duesberg,
and Hidesaburo Hanafusa, J. Virol. 24, 910–914, 1977.

96. Glycoproteins of avian tumor virus recombinants: Evidence for
intragenic crossing-over. Donna M. Galehouse and Peter H. Duesberg,
J. Virol. 25, 86–96, 1978.

97. Identification of a 30S RNA with properties of a defective type C
virus in murine cells. Richard S. Howk, David H. Troxler, Douglas Lowy,
Peter H. Duesberg, and Edward M. Scolnick, J. Virol. 25, 115–123, 1978.

98. Structure of 50 to 70S RNA from Moloney sarcoma viruses. Jan Maisel, Welcome Bender, Sylvia Hu, P. H. Duesberg, and Norman Davidson, *J. Virol.* 25, 384–394, 1978.

99. Intracellular Rous sarcoma virus RNA: Subgenomic, poly(A)-tagged RNA species contain 5'-terminal oligonucleotides linked to sequences from the 3'-half of virion RNA. Pamela Mellon and Peter Duesberg, *in* Avian RNA Tumor Viruses: Proceedings of the ICREW-EMBO Workshop, Pavia, 9–12 September, 1977, eds. Sergio Barlati and Carlo de Giuli-Morghen; Piccin Medical Books, Padua, Italy, 88–94, 1978.

100. Oncogenic (*onc*) genes of sarcoma, leukemia and carcinoma viruses. Peter H. Duesberg, Peter K. Vogt, Klaus Bister, David Troxler, and Edward M. Scolnick, *in* Avian RNA Tumor Viruses: Proceedings of the ICREW-EMBO Workshop, Pavia, 9–12 September 1977, eds. Segio Barlati and Carlo de Giuli-Morghen; Piccin Medical Books, Padua, Italy, 95–111, 1978.

101. Specific RNA sequences and gene products of MC29 avian acute leukemia virus. Pamela Mellon, Anthony Pawson, Klaus Bister, G. Steven Martin, and Peter H. Duesberg, *PNAS* 75, 5874–5878, 1978.

102. Defining transforming (*onc*) genes and gene products of avian acute leukemia and carcinoma viruses. Peter Duesberg, Pamela Mellon, Tony Pawson, G. S. Martin, Klaus Bister, and Peter Vogt, *in* Persistent Viruses: Proceedings of the 1978 ICN-UCLA Symposia on Molecular and Cellular Biology held in Keystone, Colorado, February, 1978, *ICN-UCLA Symposia on Molecular and Cellular Biology* 5, eds. Jack G. Stevens, George J. Todaro, and C. Fred Fox; Academic Press, New York, 245–266, 1978.

103. Defective retrovirus-like 30S RNA species of rat and mouse cells are infectious if packaged by type C helper virus. Edward M. Scolnick, William C. Vass, Richard S. Howk, and Peter H. Duesberg, *J. Virol.* 29, 964–972, 1979.

104. A nonconditional replication-defective mutant of the Schmidt-Ruppin strain of Rous sarcoma virus. Peter K. Vogt, Michael Hayman, Eric Hunte, and Peter H. Duesberg, *Virology* 92, 285–290, 1979.

105. Specific RNA sequences of Rous sarcoma virus (RSV) recovered from tumors induced by transformation-defective RSV deletion mutant. Terry Robins and Peter Duesberg, *Virology* 93, 427–434, 1979.

106. Avian acute leukemia viruses MC29 and MH2 share specific RNA sequences: Evidence for a second class of transforming genes. Peter H. Duesberg and Peter K. Vogt, *PNAS* 76, 1633–1637, 1979.

107. Oncogenic (*onc*) genes of sarcoma, leukemia and carcinoma viruses. Peter H. Duesberg, Peter K. Vogt, Klaus Bister, David Troxler, and Edward M. Scolnick, *in* Oncogenic Viruses and Host Cell Genes: Proceedings of the 5th Oji International Seminar on Genetic Aspects of Friend Viruses and Friend Cells, Yamanaka-ko-mura, Japan, 1977, eds. Yoji Ikawa and Takeski Odaka; Academic Press, New York, 95–115, 1979.

108. Spleen focus-forming Friend virus: Identification of genomic RNA and its relationship to helper virus RNA. Leonard H. Evans, Peter H. Duesberg, David H. Troxler, and Edward M. Scolnick, *J. Virol.* 31, 133–146, 1979.

109. Avian oncovirus MH2: Preferential growth in macrophages and exact size of the genome. Sylvia S. F. Hu, Peter H. Duesberg, Michael M. C. Lai, and Peter K. Vogt, *Virology* 96, 302–306, 1979.

110. Anatomy of the RNA and gene products of MC29 and MH2, two defective avian tumor viruses causing acute leukemia and carcinoma: Evidence for a new class of transforming genes. P. Duesberg, P. Mellon, A. Pawson, K. Bister, and P. K. Vogt, *in* Modern Trends in Human Leukemia III: Newest Results in Clinical and Biological Research, *Haematology and Blood Transfusion* 23, eds. R. Neth, R. C. Gall, P.-H. Hofschneider, and K. Mannweiler; Springer-Verlag, New York, 241–260, 1979.

111. Oligoribonucleotide map and protein of CMII: Detection of conserved and nonconserved genetic elements in avian acute leukemia viruses CMII, MC29, and MH2. Klaus Bister, Hans-Christoph Löliger, and Peter H. Duesberg, *J. Virol.* 32, 208–219, 1979.

112. Structure and specific sequences of avian erythroblastosis virus RNA: Evidence for multiple classes of transforming genes among avian tumor viruses. Klaus Bister and Peter H. Duesberg, *PNAS* 76, 5023–5027, 1979.

113. Avian acute leukemia virus MC29: Conserved and variable RNA sequences and recombination with helper virus. Peter H. Duesberg, Klaus Bister, and Carlo Moscovici, *Virology* 99, 121–134, 1979.

114. Heteroduplex analysis of the RNA of clone 3 Moloney murine sarcoma virus. Yueh-Hsiu Chien, Inder M. Verma, P. H. Duesberg, and Norman Davidson, *J. Virol.* 32, 1028–1032, 1979.

115. Replication of spleen focus-forming Friend virus in fibroblasts from C57BL mice that are genetically resistant to spleen focus formation. Leonard H. Evans, Peter H. Duesberg, and Edward M. Scolnick, *Virology* 101, 534–539, 1980.

116. *env* gene of Rous sarcoma virus: Identification of the gene product by cell-free translation. Tony Pawson, Pamela Mellon, Peter H. Duesberg, and G. Steven Martin, *J. Virol.* 33, 993–1003, 1980.

117. Fujinami sarcoma virus: An avian RNA tumor virus with a unique transforming gene. Wen-Hwa Lee, Klaus Bister, Anthony Pawson, Terry Robins, Carlo Moscovici, and Peter H. Duesberg, *PNAS* 77, 2018–2022, 1980.

118. The RNAs of the defective and nondefective components of Friend anemia and polycythemia virus strains identified and compared, prototypes of a new class of retroviral transforming genes. Peter Duesberg, Leonard Evans, Michael Nunn, David Linemeyer, David Troxler, and Edward Scolnick, *in In vivo* and *in vitro* Erythropoiesis: The Friend System: Proceedings of the EMBO Workshop on Erythropoiesis and Differentiation in Friend Leukemia Cells, held in Urbino, Italy, 10–14 October 1979, *Symposia of the Giovanni Lorenzini Foundation* 5, eds. G. B. Rossi; Elsevier/North-Holland Biomedical Press, Amsterdam, 353–371, 1980.

119. Avian erythroblastosis virus RNA: Identification and comparison to nondefective helper and defective acute leukemia viral RNAs. Klaus Bister and Peter H. Duesberg, *in In vivo* and *in vitro* Erythropoiesis: The Friend System: Proceedings of the EMBO Workshop on Erythropoiesis and Differentiation in Friend Leukemia Cells, held in Urbino, Italy, 10–14 October 1979, *Symposia of the Giovanni Lorenzini Foundation* 5, eds. G. B. Rossi; Elsevier/North-Holland Biomedical Press, Amsterdam, 515–526, 1980.

120. Transforming genes of retroviruses. P. H. Duesberg, *Cold Spring Harbor Symp. Quant. Biol.* 44, 13–29, 1980.

121. Genetic structure of avian acute leukemia viruses. K. Bister and P. H. Duesberg, *Cold Spring Harbor Symp. Quant. Biol.* 44, 801–822, 1980.

122. RNAs of defective and nondefective components of Friend anemia and polycythemia virus strains identified and compared. L. Evans, M. Nunn, P. H. Duesberg, D. Troxler, and E. Scolnick, *Cold Spring Harbor Symp. Quant. Biol.* 44, 823–835, 1980.

123. Genetic structure of avian myeloblastosis virus, released from transformed myeloblasts as a defective virus particle. Peter H. Duesberg, Klaus Bister, and Carlo Moscovici, *PNAS* 77, 5120–5124, 1980.

124. Generation of nondefective Rous sarcoma virus by asymmetric recombination between deletion mutants. G. S. Martin, W.-H. Lee, and P. H. Duesberg, *J. Virol.* 36, 591–594, 1980.

125. Phosphorylation of the nonstructural proteins encoded by three avian acute leukemia viruses and by avian Fujinami sarcoma virus. Klaus Bister, Wen-Hwa Lee, and Peter H. Duesberg, *J. Virol.* 36, 617–621, 1980.

126. Fujinami sarcoma virus and sarcomagenic, avian acute leukemia viruses have similar genetic structures. Klaus Bister, Wen-Hwa Lee, Terry Robins, and Peter H. Duesberg, *in* Animal Virus Genetics: Proceedings of the 1980 ICN-UCLA Symposia on Animal Virus Genetics held in Keystone, Colo., March 9–14, 1980, *ICN-UCLA Symposia on Molecular and Cellular Biology* 5, eds. Bernard N. Fields, Rudolf Jaenisch, and C. Fred Fox; Academic Press, New York, 527–539, 1980.

127. OK10, an avian acute leukemia virus of the MC29 subgroup with a unique genetic structure. Klaus Bister, Gary Ramsay, Michael J. Hayman, and Peter H. Duesberg, *PNAS* 77, 7142–7146, 1980.

128. Transforming genes of retroviruses: Definition, specificity and relation to cellular DNA. Peter H. Duesberg and Klaus Bister, *in* Feline Leukemia Virus: Proceedings of the Third International Feline Leukemia Virus Meeting, St. Thomas, United States Virgin Islands, May 5–9, 1980, eds. William D. Hardy, Jr., Myron Essex, and Alexander J. McClelland; Elsevier North-Holland, New York, 273–292, 1980.

129. Transforming genes of retroviruses: Definition, specificity and relation to cellular DNA. Peter H. Duesberg and Klaus Bister, *in* Cancer Achievements, Challenges and Prospects for the 1980's: Proceedings of the 1980 International Symposium on Cancer, eds. J. Burchenal and H. Oettge; Grune & Stratton, New York, 111–136, 1981.

130. Biological activity of the spleen focus-forming virus is encoded by a molecularly cloned subgenomic fragment of spleen focus-forming virus DNA. David L. Linemeyer, Sandra K. Ruscetti, Edward M. Scolnick, Leonard H. Evans, and Peter H. Duesberg, *PNAS* 78, 1401–1405, 1981.

131. Temperature-sensitive mutants of Fujinami sarcoma virus: Tumorigenicity and reversible phosphorylation of the transforming p140 protein. Wen-Hwa Lee, Klaus Bister, Carlo Moscovici, and Peter H. Duesberg, *J. Virol.* 38, 1064–1076, 1981.

132. Transforming genes of retroviruses: Definition, specificity, and relation to cellular DNA. P. H. Duesberg and K. Bister, *in* Modern Trends in Human Leukemia IV: Latest Results in Clinical and Biological Research including Pediatric Oncology, *Haematology and Blood Transfusion* 26, eds. R. Neth, R. C. Gallo, T. Graf, K. Mannweiler, and K. Winkler; Springer-Verlag, Berlin, 383–396, 1981.

133. Structural and functional studies of the Friend spleen focus-

forming virus: Structural relationship of SFFV to dualtropic viruses and molecular cloning of a biologically active subgenomic fragment of SFFV DNA. L. H. Evans, P. H. Duesberg, D. L. Linemeyer, S. K. Ruscetti, and E. M. Scolnick, *in* Modern Trends in Human Leukemia IV: Latest Results in Clinical and Biological Research including Pediatric Oncology, *Haematology and Blood Transfusion* 26, eds. R. Neth, R. C. Gallo, T. Graf, K. Mannweiler, and K. Winkler; Springer-Verlag, Berlin, 472–478, 1981.

134. *src* genes of ten Rous sarcoma virus strains, including two reportedly transduced from the cell, are completely allelic; putative markers of transduction are not detected. Wen-Hwa Lee, Michael Nunn, and Peter H. Duesberg, *J. Virol.* 39, 758–776, 1981.

135. Two different designs of transforming genes in retroviruses. Klaus Bister and Peter H. Duesberg, *in* Antiviral Chemotherapy: Design of Inhibitors of Viral Functions: Proceedings of a Symposium on Antiviral Chemotherapy, held in Hamburg, Germany, August 27–29, 1980, eds. K. K. Gauri; Academic Press, New York, 1–10, 1981.

136. Structural relationship between a normal chicken DNA locus and the transforming gene of the avian acute leukemia virus MC29. Terry Robins, Klaus Bister, Claude Garon, Takis Papas, and Peter Duesberg, *J. Virol.* 41, 635–642, 1982.

137. Isolation of a transformation-defective deletion mutant of Moloney murine sarcoma virus. Leonard H. Evans and Peter H. Duesberg, *J. Virol.* 41, 735–743, 1982.

138. On the relationship between the transforming *onc* genes of avian Rous sarcoma and MC29 viruses and homologous loci of the chicken cell. P. Duesberg, T. Robins, W.-H. Lee, K. Bister, C. Garon, and T. Papas, *in* Expression of Differentiated Functions in Cancer Cells: Proceedings of the First Workshop on Cell Differentiation and Neoplastic Transformation held in Venice, Italy, April 6–10, 1981, eds. Roberto P. Revoltella; Raven Press, New York, 471–484, 1982.

139. Transforming genes of avian retroviruses and their relation to cellular prototypes. P. Duesberg, T. Robins, W.-H. Lee, C. Garon, T. Papas, and K. Bister, *in* Advances in Comparative Leukemia Research, 1981: Proceedings of the Xth International Symposium for Comparative Research on Leukemia and Related Diseases, held at the University of California, Los Angeles, August 31–September 4, 1981, eds. David S. Yohn and James R. Blakeslee; Elsevier Biomedical, New York, 279–296, 1982.

140. Acute leukemia viruses E26 and avian myeloblastosis virus have

related transformation-specific RNA sequences but different genetic structures, gene products, and oncogenic properties. Klaus Bister, Michael Nunn, Carlo Moscovici, Bernard Perbal, Marcel A. Baluda, and Peter H. Duesberg, *PNAS* 79, 3677–3681, 1982.

141. Genetic structure and transforming genes of avian retroviruses. Klaus Bister and Peter Duesberg, *in* Advances in Viral Oncology, *Oncogene Studies* 1, eds. George Klein; Raven Press, New York, 3–42, 1982.

142. DNA clone of avian Fujinami sarcoma virus with temperature-sensitive transforming function in mammalian cells. Wen-Hwa Lee, Chih-Ping Liu, and Peter Duesberg, *J. Virol.* 44, 401–412, 1982.

143. Nucleotide sequence analysis of the chicken c-*myc* gene reveals homologous and unique coding regions by comparison with transforming gene of avian myelocytomatosis virus MC29, Δ*gag-myc*. Dennis K. Watson, E. Premkumar Reddy, Peter H. Duesberg, and Takis S. Papas, *PNAS* 80, 2146–2150, 1983.

144. Transforming genes of avian retroviruses and their relation to cellular prototypes. P. Duesberg, T. Robins, W-H. Lee, C. Garon, T. Papas, and K. Bister, *in* Biochemical and Biological Markers of Neoplastic Transformation: Proceedings of the NATO Advanced Study Institute Meeting, Corfu, Greece, Sept. 28–Oct. 8, 1981, *NATO Advanced Science Institute Series: Series A, Life Sciences* 57, eds. Prakash P. Chandra; Plenum Press, New York, 409–431, 1983.

145. Viral oncogenes and cellular prototypes. P. Duesberg, M. Nunn, T. Biehl, W. Phares, and W.-H. Lee, *in* Modern Trends in Human Leukemia V: New Results in Clinical and Biological Research including Pediatric Oncology, *Haematology and Blood Transfusion* 28, eds. R. Neth, R. C. Gallo, T. Graf, K. Mannweiler, and K. Winkler; Springer-Verlag, Berlin, 163–172, 1983.

146. Structural relationship between the chicken DNA locus, proto-*fps*, and the transforming gene of Fujinami sarcoma virus (Δ*gag-fps*). Wen-Hwa Lee, William Phares, and Peter H. Duesberg, *Virology* 129, 79–93, 1983.

147. Retroviral transforming genes in normal cells? Peter H. Duesberg, *Nature (London)* 304, 219–225, 1983.

148. Genetic structure and gene products of erythroblastosis virus E26 and myeloblastosis virus AMV. Klaus Bister, Michael Nunn, Peter Duesberg, and Carlo Moscovici, *in* Tumor Viruses and Differentiation: Proceedings of the CETUS-UCLA Symposium held at Squaw Valley, California, March 21–27, 1982, *UCLA Symposia on Molecular and Cel-*

lular Biology: New Series 5, eds. Edward M. Scolnick and Arnold J. Levine; Alan R. Liss, Inc., New York, 289–297, 1983.

149. The low tumorigenic potential of PRCII, among viruses of the Fujinami sarcoma virus subgroup, corresponds to an internal (*fps*) deletion of the transforming gene. Peter H. Duesberg, William Phares, and Wen-Hwa Lee, *Virology* 131, 144–158, 1983.

150. Tripartite structure of the avian erythroblastosis virus E26 transforming gene. Michael F. Nunn, Peter H. Seeburg, Carlo Moscovici, and Peter H. Duesberg, *Nature (London)* 306, 391–395, 1983.

151. Avian carcinoma virus MH2 contains a unique transformation-specific sequence, *mht,* and shares the *myc* sequence with MC29, CMII, and OK10 viruses. Nancy C. Kan, Christos S. Flordellis, Claude F. Garon, Peter H. Duesberg, and Takis S. Papas, *PNAS* 80, 6566–6570, 1983.

152. A common *onc* gene sequence transduced by avian carcinoma virus MH2 and by murine sarcoma virus 3611. Nancy C. Kan, Christos S. Flordellis, George E. Mark, Peter H. Duesberg, and Takis S. Papas, *Science* 223, 813–816, 1984.

153. The 5' ends of the transforming gene of Fujinami sarcoma virus and of the cellular proto-*fps* gene are not colinear. Peter H. Seeburg, Wen-Hwa Lee, Michael F. Nunn, and Peter H. Duesberg, *Virology* 133, 460–463, 1984.

154. Nucleotide sequence of avian carcinoma virus MH2: Two potential *onc* genes, one related to avian virus MC29 and the other to murine sarcoma virus 3611. N. C. Kan, C. S. Flordellis, G. E. Mark, P. H. Duesberg, and T. S. Papas, *PNAS* 81, 3000–3004, 1984.

155. A relationship between the yeast cell cycle genes *CDC4* and *CDC36* and the *ets* sequence of oncogenic virus E26. Thomas A. Peterson, John Yochem, Breck Byers, Michael F. Nunn, Peter H. Duesberg, and Steven I. Reed, *Nature (London)* 309, 556–558, 1984.

156. Complete *env* gene deletions of three replication-defective strains of Rous Sarcoma Virus and a model for the origin of their genetic structures. Michael Nunn, Susan Chan, and Peter H. Duesberg, *Virology* 134, 466–471, 1984.

157. *myc*-related genes in viruses and cells. T. S. Papas, N. K. Kan, D. K. Watson, C. S. Flordellis, M. C. Psallidopoulos, J. Lautenberger, K. P. Samuel, and P. Duesberg, *in* Oncogenes and Viral Genes: Proceedings of a Cold Spring Harbor Meeting, September 1983, *Cancer Cells* 2, eds. George F. Vande Woude, A. J. Levine, W. C. Topp, and J. D. Watson; Cold Spring Harbor Laboratory, Cold Spring Harbor, NY, 153–163, 1984.

158. Are cellular proto-*onc* genes structural or functional equivalents of retroviral transforming genes? Peter Duesberg, Michael Nunn, Dennis Watson, Nancy Kan, Peter Seeburg, and Takis Papas, *in* Proceedings of the 75th Annual Meeting of the American Association for Cancer Research, Toronto, Canada, May 9–12, 1984, *Proceedings of the American Association for Cancer Research* 25, eds. P. N. Magee and M. Foti; Waverly Press, Baltimore, 402–404, 1984.

159. Avian erythroblastosis virus E26: nucleotide sequence of the tripartite *onc* gene and of the LTR, and analysis of the cellular prototype of the viral *ets* sequence. M. Nunn, H. Weiher, P. Bullock, and P. Duesberg, *Virology* 139, 330–339, 1984.

160. *Myc,* a genetic element that is shared by a cellular gene (proto-*myc*) and by viruses with one (MC29) or two (MH2) *onc* genes. T. S. Papas, N. C. Kan, D. K. Watson, J. A. Lautenberger, C. Flordellis, K. P. Samuel, U. G. Rovigatti, M. C. Psallidopoulos, J. Ascione, and P. H. Duesberg, *in* RNA Tumor Viruses, Oncogenes, Human Cancer and AIDS: On the Frontiers of Understanding: Proceedings of the International Conference on RNA Tumor Viruses in Human Cancer, Denver, Colorado, June 10–14, 1984, *Developments in Oncology* 28, eds. Philip Furmanski, Jean-Carol Hager, and Marvin A. Rich; Martinus Nijhoff Pub., Boston, 1–13, 1985.

161. Which cancers are caused by activated proto-*onc* genes? Peter H. Duesberg, Michael Nunn, Nancy Kan, Dennis Watson, Peter H. Seeburg, and Takis Papas, *in* RNA Tumor Viruses, Oncogenes, Human Cancer and AIDS: On the Frontiers of Understanding: Proceedings of the International Conference on RNA Tumor Viruses in Human Cancer, Denver, Colorado, June 10–14, 1984, *Developments in Oncology* 28, eds. Philip Furmanski, Jean-Carol Hager, and Marvin A. Rich; Martinus Nijhoff Pub., Boston, 168–190, 1985.

162. Two oncogenes in avian carcinoma virus MH2: *myc* and *mht.* T. S. Papas, N. C. Kan, D. K. Watson, C. Flordellis, J. A. Lautenberger, M. C. Psallidopoulos, U. G. Rovigatti, K. P. Samuel, R. Ascione, and P. H. Duesberg, *Anticancer Res.* 5, 73–80, 1985.

163. Activated proto-*onc* genes: Sufficient or necessary for cancer? Peter H. Duesberg, *Science* 228, 669–677, 1985.

164. Nucleotide sequence of two overlapping *myc*-related genes in avian carcinoma virus OK10 and their relation to the *myc* genes of other viruses and the cell. J. Hayflick, P. H. Seeburg, R. Ohlsson, S. Pfeifer-Ohlsson, D. Watson, T. Papas, and P. H. Duesberg, *PNAS* 82, 2718–2722, 1985.

165. Are activated proto-*onc* genes cancer genes? P. H. Duesberg, M. Nunn, Nancy Kan, D. Watson, P. H. Seeburg, and T. Papas, *in* Modern Trends in Human Leukemia VI: New Results in Clinical and Biological Research, including Pediatric Oncology, *Haematology and Blood Transfusion* 29, eds. Neth, Gallo, Greaves, and Janka; Springer-Verlag, Berlin, 9–27, 1985.

166. Oncogenes of avian acute leukemia viruses are subsets of normal cellular genes. T. S. Papas, N. C. Kan, D. K. Watson, J. A. Lautenberger, C. Flordellis, K. P. Samuel, U. G. Rovigatti, M. Psallidopoulos, R. Ascione, and P. H. Duesberg, *in* Modern Trends in Human Leukemia VI: New Results in Clinical and Biological Research, including Pediatric Oncology, *Haematology and Blood Transfusion* 29, eds. Neth, Gallo, Greaves, and Janka; Springer-Verlag, Berlin, 269–272, 1985.

167. Are activated proto-*onc* genes cancer genes? Peter H. Duesberg, Michael Nunn, Nancy Kan, Dennis Watson, Peter H. Seeburg, and Takis Papas, *in* Cell Transformation: Proceedings of the NATO Advanced Study Institute/FEBS/Gulbenkian Foundation Summer School on Cell Transformation, held September 2–12, 1984, Sintra-Estoril, Portugal, *NATO AIS Series: Series A, Life Sciences* 94, eds. J. Celis and A. Graessmann; Plenum Press, New York, 21–63, 1985.

168. Mutagenesis of avian carcinoma virus MH2: Only one of two potential transforming genes (Δgag-*myc*) transforms fibroblasts. Ren-Ping Zhou, Nancy Kan, Takis Papas, and Peter Duesberg, *PNAS* 82, 6389–6393, 1985.

169. Defining the borders of the chicken proto-*fps* gene, a precursor of Fujinami Sarcoma Virus. Samuel L. Pfaff, Ren-Ping Zhou, Judy C. Young, Joel Hayflick, and Peter H. Duesberg, *Virology* 146, 307–314, 1985.

170. The *ets* sequence from the transforming gene of avian erythroblastosis virus, E26, has unique domains on human chromosomes 11 and 21: Both loci are transcriptionally active. D. K. Watson, M. J. McWilliams-Smith, M. F. Nunn, P. H. Duesberg, S. J. O'Brien, and T. S. Papas, *PNAS* 82, 7294–7298, 1985.

171. Conserved chromosomal positions of dual domains of the *ets* protooncogene in cats, mice, and humans. Dennis K. Watson, Mary J. McWilliams-Smith, Christine Kozak, Roger Reeves, John Gearhart, Michael F. Nunn, William Nash, John R. Fowle, III, Peter Duesberg, Takis S. Papas, and Stephen J. O'Brien, *PNAS* 83, 1792–1796, 1986.

172. Harvey *ras* genes transform without mutant codons, apparently activated by truncation of a 5' exon (exon-1). Klaus Cichutek and Peter

H. Duesberg, *PNAS* 83, 2340–2344, 1986.

173. Viral *myc* genes and their cellular homologs. Takis S. Papas, James A. Lautenberger, Nancy C. Kan, Dennis K. Watson, Rebecca Van Beneden, Miltos Psallidopoulos, Robert J. Fisher, Shigeyoshi Fujiwara, Kenneth Samuel, Christos Flordellis, Ren-Ping Zhou, Peter Duesberg, Arun Seth, and Richard Ascione, *in* Oncogenes, *Gene Amplification and Analysis* 4, eds. Takis S. Papas and George F. Vande Woude; Elsevier, New York, 109–142, 1986.

174. Retroviruses as carcinogens and pathogens: Expectations and reality. Peter H. Duesberg, *Cancer Res.* 47, 1199–1220, 1987.

175. Cancer genes: Rare recombinants instead of activated oncogenes (A review). Peter H. Duesberg, *PNAS* 84, 2117–2124, 1987.

176. *ras* genes transform without mutant codons and are possibly activated by truncation of a newly defined *ras* exon. Peter H. Duesberg and Klaus Cichutek, *in* A Perspective on Biology and Medicine in the 21st Century: Proceedings of a Dedicatory Symposium sponsored by Eli Lilly & Co., held in Indianapolis on 27–30 October, 1985, *International Congress and Symposium Series* 121, eds. Irving S. Johnson; Royal Society of Medicine Services, London, 75–88, 1987.

177. A challenge to the AIDS establishment. Peter H. Duesberg, *Bio/Technology* 5, 1244, 1987.

178. Cancer genes generated by rare chromosomal rearrangements rather than activation of oncogenes. Peter H. Duesberg, *Med. Oncol. Tumor Pharmacother.* 4, 163–175, 1987.

179. Latent cellular oncogenes: The paradox dissolves. Peter H. Duesberg, *J. Cell. Sci. Suppl.* 7, 169–187, 1987.

180. Conversion of *ras* genes to cancer genes. K. Cichutek and P. H. Duesberg, *in* Modern Trends in Human Leukemia VII: New Results in Clinical and Biological Research including Pediatric Oncology, *Haematology and Blood Transfusion* 31, eds. Neth, Gallo, Greaves, and Kabisch; Springer-Verlag, Berlin, 477–481, 1987.

181. Cancer genes generated by rare chromosomal rearrangements rather than activation of oncogenes. P. H. Duesberg, *in* Modern Trends in Human Leukemia VII: New Results in Clinical and Biological Research including Pediatric Oncology, *Haematology and Blood Transfusion* 31, eds. Neth, Gallo, Greaves, and Kabisch; Springer-Verlag, Berlin, 493–507, 1987.

182. *myc* protooncogene linked to retroviral promoter, but not to enhancer, transforms embryo cells. R.-P. Zhou and P. H. Duesberg, *PNAS* 85, 2924–2928, 1988.

183. AIDS and the 'innocent' virus. Peter Duesberg, *New Scientist* 118 (1610), pp. 34–35, Apr. 28, 1988.

184. Retroviral transduction of oncogenic sequences involves viral DNA instead of RNA. David W. Goodrich and Peter H. Duesberg, *PNAS* 85, 3733–3737, 1988.

185. Die Onkogene machen es den Krebsforschern schwer. Peter H. Duesberg, *Selecta* 30, 182–183, 1988.

186. HIV is not the cause of AIDS. Peter Duesberg, *Science* 241, 514–516, 1988.

187. Two autonomous *myc* oncogenes in avian carcinoma virus OK10. Samuel L. Pfaff and Peter H. Duesberg, *J. Virol.* 62, 3703–3709, 1988.

188. The cause of AIDS (letter). Peter Duesberg, *Science* 242, 997–998, 1988.

189. Recombinant BALB and Harvey sarcoma viruses with normal proto-*ras*-coding regions transform embryo cells in culture and cause tumors in mice. Klaus Cichutek and Peter H. Duesberg, *J. Virol.* 63, 1377–1383, 1989.

190. Human immunodeficiency virus and acquired immunodeficiency syndrome: Correlation but not causation. Peter H. Duesberg, *PNAS* 86, 755–764, 1989.

191. Duesberg's *PNAS* paper (letter). Peter Duesberg, *Science* 243, 1125, 1989.

192. HIV und AIDS: Korrelation, aber nicht Ursache. Peter H. Duesberg, *AIDS-Forschung* 4, 115–130, 1989.

193. Cancer genes by illegitimate recombination. Peter H. Duesberg, Ren-Ping Zhou, and David Goodrich, *Annals of the New York Academy of Sciences* 567, 259–273, 1989.

194. Defective viruses and AIDS (letter). Peter Duesberg, *Nature (London)* 340, 515, 1989.

195. Questioning AIDS findings (letter). Peter Duesberg, *Sci. News* 136, 131, 1989.

196. Avian proto-*myc* genes promoted by defective or nondefective retroviruses are single-hit transforming genes in primary cells. Ren-Ping Zhou and Peter H. Duesberg, *PNAS* 86, 7721–7725, 1989.

197. Response of Prof. Dr. P. Duesberg to: Is HIV the cause of AIDS? An up-to-date reply to the theories of Duesberg, by Reinhard Kurth. Peter H. Duesberg, *AIDS-Forschung* 4, 515–516, 1989.

198. Response of Prof. Dr. P. Duesberg to: What actually are the postulates of causation? Some remarks on Duesberg's article "HIV and AIDS,

correlation but not causation," by Boris Velimirovic. Peter H. Duesberg, *AIDS-Forschung* 4, 521–522, 1989.

199. Does HIV Cause AIDS? (letter). Peter Duesberg, *JAIDS* 2, 514–515, 1989.

200. Duesberg Appeals (letter). Peter Duesberg, *The Scientist (Philadelphia)*, pp. 14, Oct. 16, 1989.

201. Noch einmal, HIV und AIDS (letter of response to Maelicke and Linz). P. H. Duesberg, *Nachr. Chem. Tech. Lab.* 37, 1302–1303, 1989.

202. Duesberg responds (letter). Peter H. Duesberg, *The AAAS Observer, Supplement to Science* (s8), pp. 2, Nov. 3, 1989.

203. Antecedents of a Nobel prize (letter). Peter H. Duesberg, *Nature* 343, 302–303, 1990.

204. Responding to the AIDS debate (letter). Peter H. Duesberg, *Naturwissenschaften* 77, 97–102, 1990.

205. Retroviral recombination during reverse transcription. David W. Goodrich and Peter H. Duesberg, *PNAS* 87, 2052–2056, 1990.

206. Quantitation of human immunodeficiency virus in the blood (letter). Peter H. Duesberg, *N. Engl. J. Med.* 322, 1466, 1990.

207. Evidence that retroviral transduction is mediated by DNA, not by RNA. David W. Goodrich and Peter Duesberg, *PNAS* 87, 3604–3608, 1990.

208. In Pursuit of Harmless Viruses: The Last Stand of the Microbe Hunters. Peter H. Duesberg, *raum & zeit (English edition)* 1 (5), pp. 4–8, 1990.

209. AIDS: Non-infectious deficiencies acquired by drug consumption and other risk factors. P. H. Duesberg, *Res. Immunol.* 141, 5–11, 1990.

210. Kümmerliche Resultate der Virus-AIDS-Hypothese. Peter H. Duesberg, *Diagonal (Switzerland)*, pp. 6–7, Apr., 1990.

211. Television as a forum for debate on HIV as the cause of Aids (letter to Lord Kilmarnock *et al.*). Peter Duesberg, Joan Shenton, and Michael Verny-Elliott, *The Independent (London)*, Jun. 20, 1990.

212. The link between HIV and Aids: dispatches from the research front (letter to Dr. F. M. Perutz). Peter Duesberg, *The Guardian (Manchester)*, Jun. 29, 1990.

213. Figuring out the Aids catch (letter to Dr. F. M. Perutz). Peter Duesberg, *The Guardian (Manchester)*, Jul. 31, 1990.

214. Is the AIDS Virus a Science Fiction? Peter H. Duesberg and Bryan J. Ellison, *Policy Review,* pp. 40–51, Summer, 1990.

215. Duesberg replies (letter). Peter H. Duesberg, *Nature (London)* 346, 788, 1990.

216. Is HIV the Cause of AIDS? Peter H. Duesberg and Bryan J. Ellison Respond to Their Critics. Peter H. Duesberg and Brian J. Ellison, *Policy Review,* pp. 781–83, Fall, 1990.

217. A retroviral promoter is sufficient to convert proto-*src* to a transforming gene that is distinct from the *src* gene of Rous sarcoma virus. Hong Zhou and Peter H. Duesberg, *PNAS* 87, 9128–9132, 1990.

218. Virus hunting and the scientific method (letter). Peter Duesberg, *Science* 251, 724, 1991.

219. AIDS epidemiology: Inconsistencies with human immunodeficiency virus and with infectious disease. Peter H. Duesberg, *PNAS* 88, 1575–1579, 1991.

220. Transforming function of proto-*ras* genes depends on heterologous promoters and is enhanced by specific point mutations. Asit K. Chakraborty, Klaus Cichutek, and Peter H. Duesberg, *PNAS* 88, 2217–2221, 1991.

221. Duesberg on AIDS and HIV (letter). Peter H. Duesberg, *Nature* 350, 10, 1991.

222. On *Virus Hunting* (book review). Peter Duesberg, *New York Native,* pp. 12, 14, Apr. 29, 1991.

223. A misleading AIDS rebuttal? Peter Duesberg and Bryan J. Ellison, *Los Angeles Times,* pp. E2, Jun. 9, 1991.

224. Biological warfare (letter of response to Randy Schekman). Peter Duesberg, *California Monthly* 101 (6), pp. 5, Jun., 1991.

225. AIDS-Epidemiologie: Widersprüchlichkeiten zur Annahme einer HIV-Ätiologie und Infektionskrankeit. Peter H. Duesberg, *AIDS-Forschung* 6, 299–306, 1991.

226. Can Alternative Hypotheses Survive in this Era of Megaprojects? Peter H. Duesberg, *The Scientist (Philadelphia),* pp. 12, Jul. 8, 1991.

227. Ist das Aids-Virus Science-fiction? Peter H. Duesberg, *in* Was macht den Menschen krank? 18 Kritische Analysen, eds. Klaus Jork, Bernd Kauffmann, Rocque Lobo, and Erika Schuchardt; Birkhäuser Verlag, Berlin, 199–224, 1991.

228. Professor, attorney clear up points on legal defense (letter to the Editor). Peter H. Duesberg and Harold Perry, *Oakland Tribune,* pp. A-10, Sep. 9, 1991.

229. Defense says only AIDS not infectious (letter to the Editor). Peter Duesberg, *San Francisco Examiner,* pp. A16, Aug. 30, 1991.

230. Tuberculosis meningitis in patients with and without human immunodeficiency virus infection. Michael. P. Dubé, Paul. D. Holtom, and Robert. A. Larsen, *Am. J. Med.* 93, 520–524, 1992.

231. Cancer genes by non-homologous recombination. Peter H. Duesberg, David Goodrich, and Ren-Ping Zhou, *Basic Life Sciences* 57, 197–211, 1992.

232. 'Encouragement' of a scientist's appeal (letter to the Editor). Peter Duesberg, *The Chronicle of Higher Education (Philadelphia)*, pp. B3, Jan. 15, 1992.

233. Dr. Gallos wilde Jagd nach dem Retrovirus. Peter Duesberg, *raum & zeit (Germany)* 55, 68–70, 72, 74, 1992.

234. Duesberg, pros & con: Professor Duesberg responds (letter). Peter H. Duesberg, *CalReport* 8 (2), pp. 2, Fall, 1992.

235. The role of drugs in the origin of AIDS. P. H. Duesberg, *Biomed. Pharmacother.* 46, 3–15, 1992.

236. HIV as target for zidovudine (letter to the Editor). Peter H. Duesberg, *Lancet* 339, 551, 1992.

237. "Psychologisches Gift" (letter). Peter H. Duesberg, *Der schweizerische Beobachter (Switzerland)*, pp. 7, Feb. 7, 1992.

238. HIV, AIDS, and zidovudine (letter to the Editor). Peter H. Duesberg, *Lancet* 339, 805–806, 1992.

239. A giant hole in the HIV-Aids hypothesis. Peter Duesberg, *Sunday Times (London)*, pp. 2.6, May 31, 1992.

240. Die Rolle rekreativer Drogen und Medikamenten bei "AIDS." Peter Duesberg, *raum & zeit (Germany)* 58, 30–41, 1992.

241. AIDS: the alternative view (letter to the Editor). Peter Duesberg, *Lancet* 339, 1547, 1992.

242. Questions about AIDS (letter to the Editor). Peter Duesberg, *Nature* 358, 10, 1992.

243. ¿Es el Virus del SIDA la Causa del SIDA? Peter Duesberg, *Medicina Holística: Revista de Medicinas Complementarias* 5 (29), pp. 36–47, 1992.

244. Unmutated proto-*src* coding region is tumorigenic if expressed from the promoter of Rous sarcoma virus: Implications for the gene-mutation hypothesis of cancer. Yue Wu, Hong Zhou, and Peter Duesberg, *PNAS* 89, 6393–6397, 1992.

245. Dispute on AIDS cause (letter). Peter H. Duesberg, *San Francisco Examiner*, Jul. 31, 1992.

246. The Debate Over AIDS (letter). Peter H. Duesberg and Bryan J.

Ellison, *Los Angeles Times,* Aug. 7, 1992.

247. Duesberg Replies (letter). Peter H. Duesberg, *San Francisco Chronicle,* pp. A26, September 17, 1992.

248. HIV-free AIDS reports (letter). Peter Duesberg, *Science* 257, 1848, 1992.

249. Doubts on Viral Theory (letter). Peter H. Duesberg, *New York Times,* pp. A16, September 29, 1992.

250. Latent viruses and mutated oncogenes: No evidence for pathogenicity. Peter H. Duesberg and Jody R. Schwartz, *Progress in Nucleic Acid Research and Molecular Biology* 43, 135–204, 1992.

251. Die Rolle von psychoaktiven Drogen und Medikamenten bei AIDS. Peter Duesberg, *AIDS-Forschung (AIFO)* 7, 631–641, 1992.

252. AIDS Acquired by Drug Consumption and Other Noncontagious Risk Factors. Peter H. Duesberg, *Pharmacology & Therapeutics* 55, 201–277, 1992.

253. HIV theory. Peter Duesberg, *The Daily Californian (Berkeley),* pp. 4, February 2, 1993.

254. HIV latency. Peter Duesberg, H., *Biotechnology* 11, 247, 1993.

255. HIV and the aetiology of AIDS. Peter Duesberg, *The Lancet* 341, 957–958, 1993.

256. AIDS theories. Peter Duesberg, *The Daily Californian (Berkeley),* pp. 5, April 20, 1993.

257. HIV history. Peter Duesberg, *Biotechnology* 11, 421, 1993.

258. Aetiology of AIDS. Peter Duesberg, *The Lancet* 341, 1544, 1993.

259. HIV and AIDS. Peter Duesberg, *Science* 260, 1705, 1993.

260. Peter Duesberg and the right of reply. Peter Duesberg, *Rethinking AIDS* 1, 1,4, 1993.

261. The HIV Gap in National AIDS Statistics. Peter Duesberg, *Bio/Technology* 11, 955–56, 1993.

262. The enigma of slow viruses. Peter Duesberg, *The Lancet* 342, 729, 1993.

263. HIV and AIDS. Peter Duesberg, *Commentary,* pp. 20–22, October, 1993.

264. AIDS—Causes and Consequences. Peter H. Duesberg, *Journal of Tumor Marker Oncology* 8, 47–58, 1993.

265. Can epidemiology determine whether drugs or HIV cause AIDS? Peter H. Duesberg, *AIDS-Forschung* 12, 627–635, 1993.

266. AIDS, guerra tra scienziati sulla vera causa della malattia. Peter Duesberg, *Corriere Della Sera/Salute* 5, 21–23, 1993.

267. Development of transforming function during transduction of proto-ras into Harvey sarcoma virus. M. Lang, I. Treines, P. H. Duesberg, R. Kurth, and K. Cichutek, *Proc. Natl. Acad. Sci. USA* 91, 654–658, 1994.

268. Results fall short for HIV theory. Peter H. Duesberg, *Insight* 10, pp. 27–29, February, 14, 1994.

269. Infectious AIDS—stretching the germ theory beyond its limits. Peter H. Duesberg, *Int. Arch. Allergy Immunol.* 103, 118–127, 1994.

270. Avian erythroblastosis virus E26: Only one (myb) of tow cell-derived coding regions is necessary for oncogenicity. Y. Wu and Duesberg P., *Proc. Natl. Acad. Sci. USA* 91, 4039–4043, 1994.

271. "The Duesberg-Phenomenon": Duesberg and Other Voices (letter). P. Duesberg, *Science* 267, 313, 1995.

272. AIDS: virus or drug induced? Peter Duesberg, *Am. J. Continuing Education Nursing* 7, 31–44, 1995.

273. AIDS Proposal. E. Baumann and et al., *Science* 267, 945–946, 1995.

274. Oncogenes and Cancer (letter). P. Duesberg, *Science* 267, 1407–1408, 1995.

275. The culprit is non-contagious risk factors. Peter Duesberg, *The Scientist* 9 (6), pp. 12, March 20, 1995.

276. Foreign-protein-mediated immunodeficiency in hemophiliacs with and without HIV. Peter Duesberg, *Genetica* 95, 51–70, 1995.

277. The Toxicity of Azidothymidine (AZT) on Human and Animal Cells in Culture at Concentrations Used for Antiviral Therapy. D. Chiu and P. Duesberg, *Genetica* 95, 103–109, 1995.

278. HIV as a surrogate marker for drug-use: a re-analysis of the San Francisco Men's Health Study. B.J. Ellison, A.B. Downey, and P.H. Duesberg, *Genetica* 95, 165–171, 1995.

279. DNA recombination is sufficienct for retroviral transduction. J.R. Schwartz, S. Duesberg, and P. Duesberg, *Proc. Natl. Acad. Sci. USA* 92, 2460–2464, 1995.

280. Preface. P. Duesberg, *Genetica* 95, 3, 1995.

281. AIDS Data (letter). P. Duesberg, *Science* 268, 350–351, 1995.

282. *AIDS: The good news is Hiv doesn't cause it. The bad news is "recreational drugs" and medical treatments like AZT do.* P. Duesberg and J. Yiamouyiannis. Health Action Press, Delaware, 1995.

283. HIV an illusion (letter). P. Duesberg and H. Bialy, *Nature* 375, 197, 1995.

284. Duesberg Responds (letter). P. Duesberg, *The Scientist* 9, 13, 1995.

285. Is HIV the cause of AIDS? (letter). P. Duesberg, *Lancet* 346, 1371–1372, 1995.

286. *Infectious AIDS: Have We Been Misled?* P.H. Duesberg. North Atlantic Books, Berkeley, 1995.

287. Commentary: non-HIV hypotheses must be studied more carefully. Peter Duesberg, *BMJ* 312, 210–211, 1996.

288. Duesberg and the right of reply according to Maddox-*Nature*. Peter H. Duesberg and Harvey Bialy, *in* AIDS: virus- or drug induced?, *Contemporary Issues in Genetics and Evolution* 5, eds. P. H. Duesberg; Kluwer Academic Publishers, Dordrecht/Boston/London, 111–125, 1996.

289. How much longer can we afford the AIDS virus monopoly? Peter H. Duesberg, *in* AIDS: virus- or drug induced? 5, eds. P. H. Duesberg; Kluwer Academic Publishers, Dordrecht, the Netherlands/Boston/London, 241–270, 1996.

290. *Inventing the AIDS VIrus*. Peter Duesberg. Regnery Publishing, Inc., Washington, DC, 1996.

291. Duesberg's questions. Peter Duesberg, *C&EN* 4, 40, 1996.

292. A debate over the causes of AIDS. Peter Duesberg, *San Francisco Chronicle (San Francisco)*, pp. A27, May 10, 1996.

293. AIDS and drugs. Peter Duesberg, *The New York Times (New York)*, pp. Book Review, p4, May 19, 1996.

294. "The AIDS Heresy": an exchange. Peter Duesberg and Richard Horton, *The New York Review* 43 (13), pp. 51, August 8, 1996.

295. Host range restrictions of oncogenes: myc genes transform avian but not mammalian cells and mht/raf genes transform mammalian but not avian cells. R. Li, R. P. Zhou, and P. H. Duesberg, *Proc. Natl. Acad. Sci. USA* 93, 7522–7527, 1996.

296. Duesberg's HIV. P. H. Duesberg, *Continuum* 4, 8–9, 1996.

297. The AIDS heresy: another exchange. P. H. Duesberg, *The New York Review*, September 19, 1996, 1996.

298. The drug-AIDS hypothesis. Peter H. Duesberg and David Rasnick, *International Journal of Medicine* 1, 26–64, 1997.

299. The drug-AIDS hypothesis. Peter Duesberg and David Rasnick, *Continuum (London)* 4, Supplement, 1–24, 1997.

300. Near enough is good enough? P. H. Duesberg, *Continuum* 4, 26, 1997.

301. The aneuploidy-cancer hypothesis (Abstract). Peter H. Duesberg, Ruhong Li, Alwin Kraemer, and Ruediger Hehlmann, *J Mol. Medicine*

(*JMM*) 75, B248, 1997.

302. AIDS - Inventing a Virus? P. H. Duesberg, *Medical Sentinel* 2, 107–108, 1997.

303. Dominant transformation by mutated human ras genes in vitro requires more than 100 times higher expression than is observed in cancers. Vivian Y. Hua, Wai Wang, K., and Peter H. Duesberg, *Proc. Natl. Acad. Sci. USA* 94, 9614–9619, 1997.

304. Aneuploidy correlated 100% with chemical transformation of Chinese hamster cells. R. Li, G. Yerganian, P. Duesberg, A. Kraemer, A. Willer, C. Rausch, and R. Hehlmann, *Proc Natl Acad Sci (USA)* 94, 14506–14511, 1997.

305. Genetic instability of cancer cells is proportional to their degree of aneuploidy. P. Duesberg, C. Rausch, D. Rasnick, and R. Hehlmann, *Proc Natl Acad Sci USA* 95, 13692–13697, 1998.

306. Bayesian projection of the acquired immune deficiency syndrome epidemic. P. H. Duesberg, *Applied Statistics (Royal Statistical Society)* 47, 488, 497–98, 1998.

307. The AIDS dilemma: drug diseases blamed on a passenger virus. P. H. Duesberg and D. Rasnick, *Genetica* 104, 85–132, 1998.

308. How aneuploidy affects metabolic control and causes cancer. David Rasnick and Peter Duesberg, *Biochem. J.* 340, 621–630, 1999.

Are centrosomes or aneuploidy the key to cancer? Peter Duesberg, *Science* 284, 2091–2092, 1999.

310. How aneuploidy may cause cancer and genetic instability. Duesberg, P., Rasnick, D., Li, R., Winters, L., Rausch, C., and Hehlmann, R. *Anticancer Research* 19, 4887–4906, 1999.

311. Aneuploidy vs. gene mutation hypothesis of cancer: recent study claims mutation but is found to support aneuploidy..., Li, R Sonik, A., Stindl, R., Rasnick, D., and Duesberg, P. *Proc Natl Acad Sci* 97, 3236–3241, 2000.

312. Aneuploidy precedes and segregates with chemical carcinogenesis. Duesberg, P., Li, R., Rasnick, D., Rausch, C., Willer, A., Kraemer, A., Yerganian, G., and Hehlmann, R. *Cancer Genet Cytogenet* 119, 83–93, 2000.

313. Duesberg, P., Li, R., Rausch, C., Willer, A., Kraemer, A., Yerganian, G., Hehlmann, R., and Rasnick, D. In: *Technological and Medical Implications of Metabolic Control Analysis,* Cornish-Bowden, A. J., and Cardenas, M. L., (Kluwer Academic Publishers,Dordrecht, Holland), pp. 83–89, 2000.

314. Rasnick, D., and Duesberg, P. H. In: *Technological and Medical Implications of Metabolic Control Analysis,* Cornish-Bowden, A. J., and Cardenas, M. L., (Kluwer Academic Publishers,Dordrecht, Holland), pp. 99–107, 2000.

315. Aneuploidy, the somatic mutation that makes cancer a species of its own. Duesberg, P., and Rasnick, D. *Cell Motil Cytoskeleton* 47, 81–107, 2000.

316. The Durban Declaration is not accepted by all. Stewart, G. T., Mhlongo, S., de Harven, E., Fiala, C., Koehnlein, C., Herxheimer, A., Duesberg, P., Rasnick, D., Giraldo, R., Kothari, M., et al. *Nature* 407, 286, 2000.

317. Explaining the high mutation rates of cancer cells to drug and multidrug resistance by chromosome reassortments that are catalyzed by aneuploidy. Duesberg, P., Stindl, R., and Hehlmann, R. *Proc. Natl. Acad. Sci. USA* 97, 14295–14300, 2000.

318. Origin of multidrug resistance in cells with and without multidrug resistance genes: Chromosome reassortments catalyzed by aneuploidy. Duesberg, P., Stindl, R., and Hehlmann, R. *Proc. Natl. Acad. Sci.USA* 98, 11283–11288, 2001.

319. Aneuploidy versus gene mutation as cause of cancer. Duesberg, P., Stindl, R., Li, R. H., Hehlmann, R., and Rasnick, D. Current Science 81, 490–500, 2001.

320. Specific aneusomies in Chinese hamster cells at different stages of neoplastic transformation, initiated by nitrosomethylurea. Fabarius, A., Willer, A., Yergenian, G., Hehlmann, R., and Duesberg, P. *Proc. Natl. Acad. Sci. USA* 99, 6778–6783, 2002.

321. Correspondence re: D. Zimonjic et al., Derivation of human tumor cells *in vitro* without widespread genomic instability. Li, R., Rasnick, D., and Duesberg, P. *Cancer Res.,* 61, 8838–8844, 2001. Cancer Res 62, 6345–6348; discussion 6348–6349, 2002.

322. Multistep carcinogenesis, a chain reaction of aneuploidizations. Duesberg, P., and Li, R. *Cell Cycle* 2, 202–210, 2003.

323. Are cancers dependent on oncogenes or aneuploidy? Duesberg, P. *Cancer Genet Cytogenet* 143, 89–91, 2003.

324. Instability of chromosome structure increases exponentially with degrees of aneuploidy. Fabarius, A., Hehlmann, R., and Duesberg, P. *Cancer Genet. Cytogenet.* 143, 59–72, 2003.

325. The chemical bases of the various AIDS epidemics: recreational drugs, anti-viral chemotherapy and malnutrition. Duesberg, P., Koehn-

lein, C., and Rasnick, D. *J. Biosci.* 28, 383–412, 2003.

326. Aneuploidy, the primary cause of the multilateral genomic instabilty of neoplastic and preneoplastic cells. Duesberg, P. H., Fabarius, A., and Hehlmann, R. *IUBMB Life* 56, 5–81, 2004.

Index